Anophthalmia

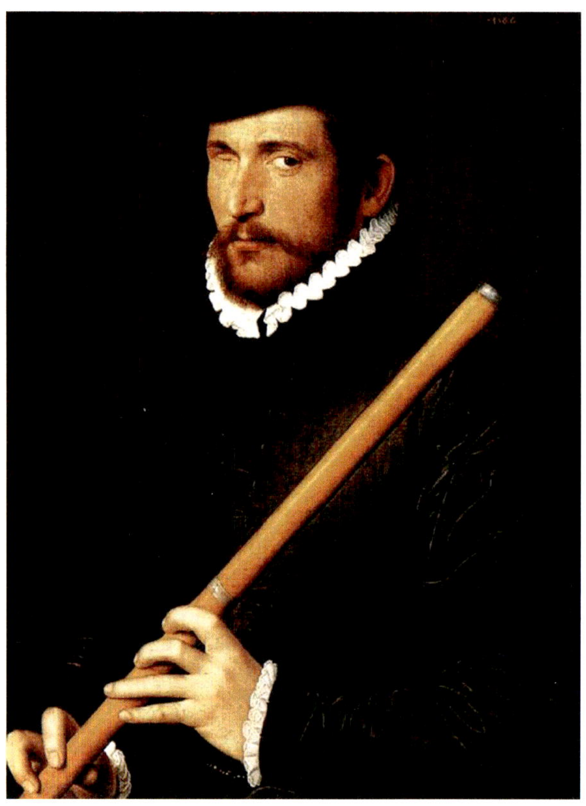

Portrait of a Flautist with One Eye, 1566, Anonymous Artist, Louvre Museum, Paris

Thomas E. Johnson
Editor

Anophthalmia

The Expert's Guide to Medical and Surgical Management

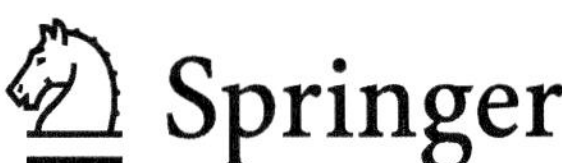

Editor
Thomas E. Johnson
Bascom Palmer Eye Institute
University of Miami
Miller School of Medicine
Miami, FL
USA

ISBN 978-3-030-29755-8 ISBN 978-3-030-29753-4 (eBook)
https://doi.org/10.1007/978-3-030-29753-4

This Springer imprint is published by the registered company Springer Nature Switzerland AG
The registered company address is: Gewerbestrasse 11, 6330 Cham, Switzerland

Dedicated to my daughter Olivia whose intellectual curiosity, passion for life, and empathy for others inspires me every day. Also dedicated to the rest of my wonderful family including my mom Anna, sister Janan, brother Lant, Maria, Dayra, and to the memory of my dad Arthur.

Foreword

End-stage ophthalmology: That is the title slide for the lecture I have presented for many years on the topics of evisceration, enucleation, and exenteration – operations of last resort when ocular disease has overwhelmed our abilities to salvage an eye. Unfortunately, unlike end-stage renal disease or end-stage cardiac disease, ophthalmologists do not have a biological alternative, such as a kidney or heart transplant, to restore useful function when vision has been lost or a sick eye has become a liability or even a threat to life.

In *Anophthalmia: The Expert's Guide to Medical and Surgical Management*, Dr. Thomas Johnson and his collaborators present a comprehensive approach to managing these always discouraging scenarios. The scope of the book goes considerably beyond the wherefores and standard techniques for removing a diseased eye, including detailed coverage of tertiary care such as congenital anophthalmia, socket expansion, osseointegration, implant exchange, and corneal tattooing. The authors also emphasize the critical partnership between the surgeon and the ocularist, whose skill and artistry are fundamental to a satisfactory functional and aesthetic outcome. Readers should be interested to learn how the expertise of ocularists can be traced to doll-making and dentistry.

As with any area of medicine, ambiguities and controversies remain, such as whether to perform an evisceration or an enucleation in certain circumstances to minimize the risk of sympathetic ophthalmia. After a detailed, balanced review in Chapters 1 and 3 of publications dating back more than two centuries, the authors of Chapter 3 "generally favor enucleation." Personally, I *generally* favor evisceration, which has served my patients well for the past 35 years, but perhaps I have simply been lucky. Another minor quibble is the preference in Chapter 8 for lining an exenterated socket with split-thickness skin grafts over allowing the cavity to heal by second intention. In the Upper Midwest, granulated sockets tend to be less sensitive to winter temperatures than skin grafts on bone. My hardy heartland patients seem not to be troubled by postoperative orbital wound care, and long-term tumor surveillance is rarely problematic with the availability of sophisticated imaging. However, in the absence of unimpeachable level 1 evidence for much of what we do, *vive la différence*!

I particularly appreciate the book's historical perspectives, which emphasize the physical and emotional insults of losing an eye along with the creative approaches that our predecessors have devised and attempted, over many centuries and often unsuccessfully, to improve on wearing a black patch. The wisdom of Carl Becker, quoted in Chapter 1, warrants highlighting: "History prepares us to live more humanely in the present and to meet rather than foretell the future." One hopes, however, that the future will include new technologies and treatments that will render anophthalmia a much less assaultive and distressing condition for both patients and physicians than it is today.

George B. Bartley, MD
The Louis and Evelyn Krueger Professor
of Ophthalmology, Mayo Clinic
Rochester, MN, USA

Chief Executive Officer,
American Board of Ophthalmology
Bala Cynwyd, PA, USA

Preface

The loss of an eye is tragic. Not only do patients suffer a significant functional disability, but also live the rest of their lives with a cosmetic deformity with the real probability of discomfort and inflammation. In the not-so-distant past, ophthalmologists might admit defeat, remove the eye, and then forget about the patient, directing their efforts toward treating eyes that still have vision. Eye removal surgery was often delegated to beginning ophthalmology residents as a way for them to learn surgery with minimal risk. Bad functional and cosmetic outcomes were common, with inflamed sockets, volume loss, implant shifting, eyelid abnormalities, and resultant difficulties in wearing an ocular prosthesis.

But times have changed. We now realize that the loss of an eye is not the final stage of the patients' ophthalmology care. It is a new beginning, a new phase. Improved orbital implants, more refined surgical techniques, recognition of problems causing anophthalmic socket problems, and superior ocular prosthesis fabrication have tremendously improved the quality of life for anophthalmic patients. True, the gift of sight has been lost. But the gifts of comfort, freedom from infection and inflammation, and good cosmesis are now possible, boosting patients' comfort and self-esteem and allowing them to live more fulfilling lives.

The authors of this book have attempted to create a resource that comprehensively covers the field of anophthalmia: Historical perspectives, indications for eye removal along with surgical techniques, prosthesis making, anophthalmic socket care and maintenance, and surgical procedures to correct anophthalmic socket defects are described. Congenital anophthalmia is reviewed. Newer techniques such as osseointegration are illustrated. It provides a quick reference for medical students, ophthalmology residents and fellows, ophthalmologists, psychologists, and everyone else taking care of these patients. In this changing field, we hope newer advancements will allow us to update this book every few years!

I am greatly indebted to my authors for their hard work in contributing to this book. Also thank you to the editors and staff at Springer, including Tracy Marton,

Caitlin Prim, Melanie Zerah, Rekha Udaiyar, Jeffrey Taub, and staff at SPi Technologies India Private Ltd, including Srijanani Balagopal. Also special thanks to our medical illustrator Alison Bozung.

Miami, FL, USA Thomas E. Johnson, MD

Contents

Contributors

Chrisfouad R. Alabiad, MD University of Miami Miller School of Medicine, Bascom Palmer Eye Institute, Miami, FL, USA

Zakeya Mohammed Al-Sadah, MD Ophthalmic Plastic and Reconstructive Surgery, Department of Ophthalmology, Bascom Palmer Eye Institute, University of Miami Miller School of Medicine, Miami, FL, USA

Mohammed Salman AlShakhas, BDS Department of Oral and Maxillofacial Surgery, University of Alabama at Birmingham, Birmingham, AL, USA

Apostolos G. Anagnostopoulos, MD University of Miami, Bascom Palmer Eye Institute, Ophthalmic Plastic and Reconstructive Surgery, Miami, FL, USA

Yasser Bataineh, BCO, BCCA International Ocular Center, Miami, FL, USA

Nathan W. Blessing, MD Dean McGee Eye Institute, University of Oklahoma College of Medicine, Department of Ophthalmology, Oklahoma City, OK, USA

Elin Bohman, MD St. Erik Eye Hospital, Oculoplastic and Orbital Services, Stockholm, Sweden

Catherine J. Choi, MD, MS Ophthalmic Plastic and Reconstructive Surgery, Department of Ophthalmology, Bascom Palmer Eye Institute, University of Miami Miller School of Medicine, Miami, FL, USA

Janet L. Davis, MD University of Miami Miller School of Medicine, Bascom Palmer Eye Institute, Miami, FL, USA

Benjamin Erickson, MD Stanford Byers Eye Institute, Department of Ophthalmology, Palo Alto, CA, USA

Virginia A. Jacko, MS Miami Lighthouse for the Blind and Visually Impaired, Miami, FL, USA

Thomas E. Johnson, MD Bascom Palmer Eye Institute, University of Miami Miller School of Medicine, Miami, FL, USA

Audrey C. Ko, MD University of Iowa Hospitals and Clinics, Department of Ophthalmology and Visual Sciences, Iowa City, IA, USA

Andrea Lora Kossler, MD Oculofacial Plastic Surgery & Orbital Oncology, Byers Eye Institute, Stanford University, Stanford, CA, USA

Michelle W. Latting, MD Bascom Palmer Eye Institute, University of Miami Miller School of Medicine, Miami, FL, USA

Bradford W. Lee, MD, MSc Bascom Palmer Eye Institute, University of Miami, Miami, FL, USA

Wendy W. Lee, MD, MS Bascom Palmer Eye Institute, University of Miami Miller School of Medicine, Miami, FL, USA

Alexandra E. Levitt, MD Bascom Palmer Eye Institute, University of Miami, Miami, FL, USA

Ji Kwan Park, MD, MPH Loma Linda University Eye Institute, Department of Ophthalmology, Loma Linda, CA, USA

Keith Pine, BSc, MBA, PhD University of Auckland, School of Optometry and Vision Science, Grafton, Auckland, New Zealand

Andrew J. Rong, MD Oculoplastic Surgery, Bascom Palmer Eye Institute, Miami, FL, USA

Erin M. Shriver, MD, FACS University of Iowa, Department of Ophthalmology and Visual Sciences, Iowa City, IA, USA

Ann Q. Tran, MD Bascom Palmer Eye Institute, University of Miami Miller School of Medicine, Miami, FL, USA

Brian C. Tse, MD Bascom Palmer Eye Institute, University of Miami Miller School of Medicine, Miami, FL, USA

Sara Tullis Wester, MD Bascom Palmer Eye Institute, Department of Oculoplastics, Miami, FL, USA

Kelly H. Yom, BA University of Iowa Hospitals and Clinics, Department of Ophthalmology and Visual Sciences, Iowa City, IA, USA

Chad Zatezalo, MD The Zatezalo Group, Oculoplastics Private Practice, North Bethesda, MD, USA

Lily Zhang, BS University of Miami Miller School of Medicine, Bascom Palmer Eye Institute, Miami, FL, USA

Part I
Clinical Foundations

Chapter 1
Introduction and Historical Perspectives

Ji Kwan Park and Thomas E. Johnson

Introduction

The art of successfully removing a diseased eye has long been underappreciated. In years past, enucleation was a type of surgery given to first-year ophthalmology residents. What could ever go wrong? The eye was removed, a spherical implant was inserted deep into the muscle cone, and the tissues were closed. The risk was minimal, and the rest of the patients' functional and cosmetic rehabilitation was left in the hands of the ocularist.

Over time, however, almost all of these patients developed significant functional and cosmetic problems. Invariably, the implant would migrate, the inferior fornix would shorten, the lower lid would sag, and the superior fornix would deepen. There would be no way to hide the fact that the patient had an "artificial eye." However, that was the standard of care, and we just accepted that those problems were just part of losing an eye.

The psychological effects of eye loss can be quite serious. Loss of self-esteem is common. The cosmetic deformities of the anophthalmic socket syndrome affect patients' employability, their ability to find a romantic partner successfully, and their ability to make new friends. Feelings of inferiority based on the cosmetic appearance of their eyes may prevent them from achieving their full potential and meeting their goals.

Ophthalmologists recognized these problems and began working on ways to improve the outcomes of eye removal surgery. Implants were improved in an attempt

J. K. Park (✉)
Loma Linda University Eye Institute, Department of Ophthalmology, Loma Linda, CA, USA
e-mail: jkpark@llu.edu

T. E. Johnson
Bascom Palmer Eye Institute, University of Miami Miller School of Medicine, Miami, FL, USA
e-mail: tjohnson@med.miami.edu

T. E. Johnson (ed.), *Anophthalmia*,
https://doi.org/10.1007/978-3-030-29753-4_1

to increase prosthesis motility and to replace volume lost due to fat atrophy in the anophthalmic socket. Wrapping materials were employed so that extraocular muscles could be attached, improving socket motility and helping to prevent implant migration. Integrated implants were invented to impart more movement to the overlying prosthesis. Porous integrated implants were developed to allow tissue and vascular ingrowth into the implants, making them a living part of the body and more resistant to extrusion and migration.

Ocularists also improved the fabrication of their prostheses. Better curing of the acrylic material decreased inflammatory responses, resulting in healthier and less inflamed sockets. Impressions were made to allow the custom-fitting of the artificial eye. Patient education improved, and regular prosthesis polishing and cleaning also resulted in healthier sockets.

Early Historical Perspectives

The earliest manuscripts on ocular surgery come from a collection of laws in old Babylonian and Sumerian codes between 3000 BCE and 2250 BCE. One law stated that "if a man destroys the eye of another man, they shall destroy his eye." The law also punished the surgeon, who also served as a temple priest, by cutting off his fingers if he "fails to open an abscess with a bronze lancet and destroys the eye." As early as 2600 BCE, the Chinese devoted a god in the interest of oculists [1, 2]. The oldest known prosthetic eye is dated between 2900 and 2800 BCE (Fig. 1.1) [3, 4]. In 1650 BCE, Egyptians removed the eye from the dead and filled the orbit with wax and precious stones (to simulate the iris) during the process of mummification. Around 500 BCE, Egyptian and Roman priests employed ocular decorations made of clay and held in place by adhesives or thongs to cover phthisical globes [5–7]. Eye removal surgery and cosmetic prostheses were not described until the late sixteenth century in Europe [6, 7].

The *ekblepharon* was the first external prosthesis described by Frenchman Ambroise Paré (1510–1590). The painted leather patch was worn over the disfigured eye and held in place by a metal wire that wrapped around the head (Fig. 1.2a) [8]. In 1749, Burchard Mauchart of Tübingen, Germany, described a prosthesis that would fit in the eye socket. The *hypoblepharae* was a gold shell with the iris painted in colored enamel (Fig. 1.2b). In the seventeenth century, skilled Venetian and German glassblowers made more realistic prosthetic eyes [7]. Lorenz Heister of Nuremberg in 1752 recorded that he preferred the glass eyes over metal prostheses that repelled tear fluids and lost their brightness over time. In 1880, Herman Snellen invented the "Reform" eye, a hollow glass eye with round edges, to improve comfort and facilitate restoration of the socket volume (Fig. 1.2c). Duponcet of Paris also published one of the earliest books on the fabrication of glass prosthetic eyes in 1818. Ludwig Müller-Ur (1811–1888) developed the cryolite glass eye, which was made of arsenic oxide and sodium aluminum fluoride. These glass eyes were exported across the world from the late nineteenth century until the beginning of

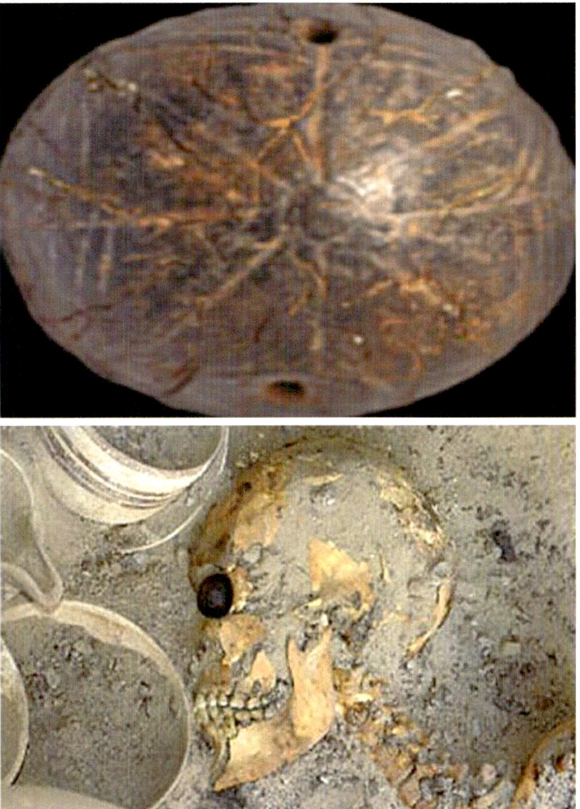

Fig. 1.1 The world's earliest known prosthetic eye was made of a mixture of natural tar and animal fat overlaid with a thin layer of gold. The central corneal circle had radial lines fanning out like the rays of the sun and represented light emanating from the eye. Fine lines were drawn to simulate conjunctival vessels. A small hole on each side of the half sphere allowed golden threads to pass through and hold it in place. The prosthesis also had imprints from chronic skin contact and marks suggestive of an abscess of the eyelids. Archeologists believe it was worn by a young ancient Persian priestess who lived between 2900 and 2800 BCE. (Images reproduced with permission)

World War II, when all trade with Germany ceased (Fig. 1.2d). British dental technicians discovered polymethylmethacrylate (PMMA) as an alternative material to make eye prostheses in the 1930s. PMMA was not only well tolerated by the orbital tissues but also allowed for molding and curing of the prosthesis. For the first time, a custom-fit prosthesis was made from an impression of the patient's socket. Fritz Jardon, who immigrated to the United States from Germany, also developed PMMA prosthetic eyes and improved impression techniques [7, 9]. By the early 1940s, scleral cosmetic lenses were introduced as these plastic shells eliminated the risk of breakage and injury to the eyes [10]. Advances in orbital implants also led to the development of a combined ocular prosthesis by Ruedemann in 1946 (Fig. 1.2e) [12, 13].

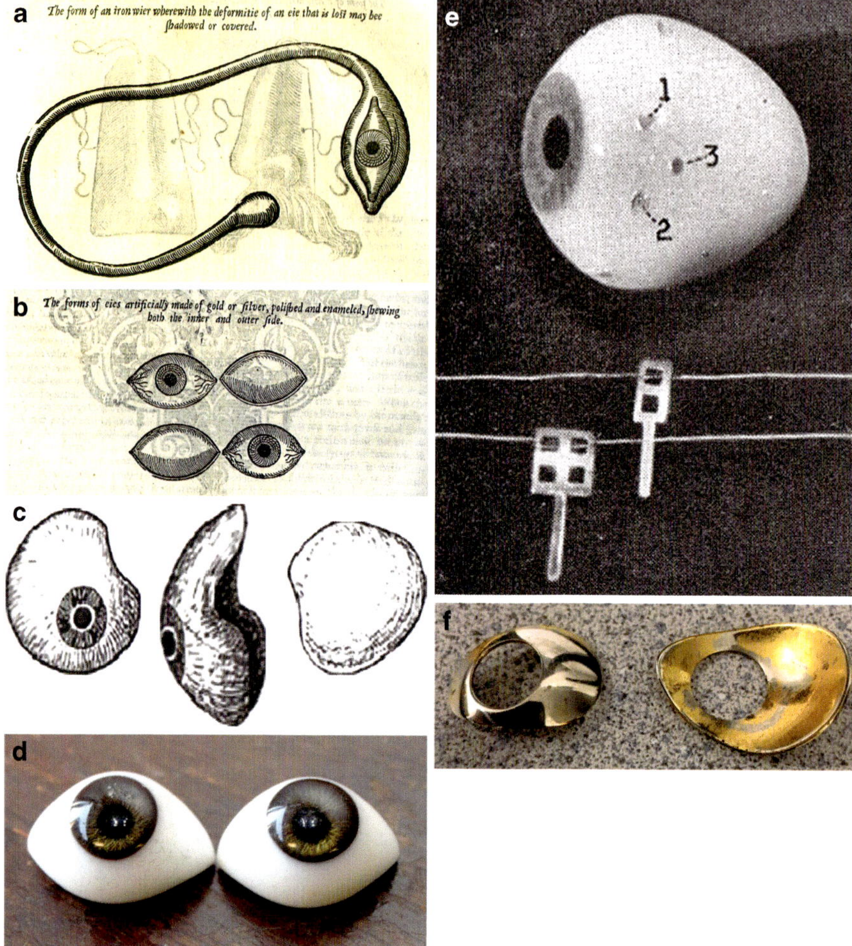

Fig. 1.2 (**a**) The *ekblepharon*. This painted leather patch was worn over the disfigured eye and held in place by a metal wire that wrapped around the head. (**b**) The *hypoblepharae* was a gold shell with the iris painted in colored enamel. It was the first prosthesis that would fit in the eye socket. (**c**) Snellen's *Reform* glass eyes had round edges to improve comfort and facilitate the restoration of the socket volume [11]. (Image courtesy of Arbaz Sajjad, MD). (**d**) A glass eye made in the early twentieth century from Germany. (**e**) A combined motility implant and ocular prosthesis was introduced by Ruedemann in 1946. Numbers 1 and 2 indicate the holes used to pass the needle and secure the metal muscle paddle, which is anchored at the hole labeled as number 3. A high rate of infection, difficulty with alignment, and inability to remove the prosthesis limited its use [12, 13]. Image reproduced with permission. (**f**) A gold-plated ocular conformer was used in 1929. In 1902, Fox believed that the conformer aided in tissue healing following his gold sphere placement [14, 15]. (Image courtesy of Michael O. Hughes, BCO)

Extirpation

Extirpation was a subtotal exenteration traditionally performed without anesthesia. In 1583, Georg Bartisch, of Dresden, Germany, first described the surgical technique in his book, the *Augendienst*. The operation was reiterated by Johannes Lange (1485–1565), of Lowenberg, Silesia (Germany) [1, 16]. The surgery was so excruciatingly painful that the patient had to be tied down and bled to a state of delirium before the operation. A thick suture was passed through the globe to exert forward traction, while a curved knife was passed into the orbit. Hemostasis was achieved with ice water. The operation not only removed the globe but also sacrificed the conjunctiva, orbital fascia, and portions of the extraocular muscles (Fig. 1.3a–c). The socket was then allowed to spontaneously granulate, and the surgery left the conjunctival fornices unsuitable for ocular prosthesis wear [1, 5]. Instead, an external prosthesis complete with eyelids, lashes, and a painted globe was held in position with an external strap [7]. This surgical procedure was rejected by many physicians and declared as "inhuman except under the greatest and most urgent necessity." The last recorded extirpation was performed by John Whitaker Hulke of Moorfields Eye Hospital, London, in 1848 [5, 6], suggesting that extirpation had been a common surgical practice for over two and a half centuries!

Enucleation

Enucleation refers to the removal of the globe and its contents with the preservation of the surrounding periorbital and orbital structures. In the first known description of enucleation recorded in 1826, Cleoburey (Saxon) stated that the conjunctiva should be divided with a thin, sharp-pointed knife followed by the detachment of all the muscles that are inserted into the globe. Further dissection was carried out toward the posterior part of the orbit to divide the optic nerve. He stated, "The nerve will be easily divided by directing the knife back into the orbit on the nasal side of the globe, as the optic nerve is situated nearer on this side [1, 17]." However, his technique was later dismissed owing to the final result being a deep-set, immobile prosthesis [6].

Enucleation surgery in this era resulted in a large amount of blood loss and a high complication rate. Complications included postoperative infection, meningitis, and sometimes mortality. The sockets were often left without an implant, and this caused the ocular prosthesis to sink back and with a resultant deep superior sulcus deformity. Nonetheless, enucleation was deemed necessary to prevent the contralateral eye from developing sympathetic ophthalmia following trauma [15, 18, 19]. In 1841, O'Ferral (Dublin) and Bonnet (Paris) introduced a more anatomic approach that laid the foundation for modern enucleation. O'Ferral reported that by separating a new fascial tissue called "tunica vaginalis oculi" from the sclera, and then severing the muscles at their insertion to the globe, the surgeon could remove the

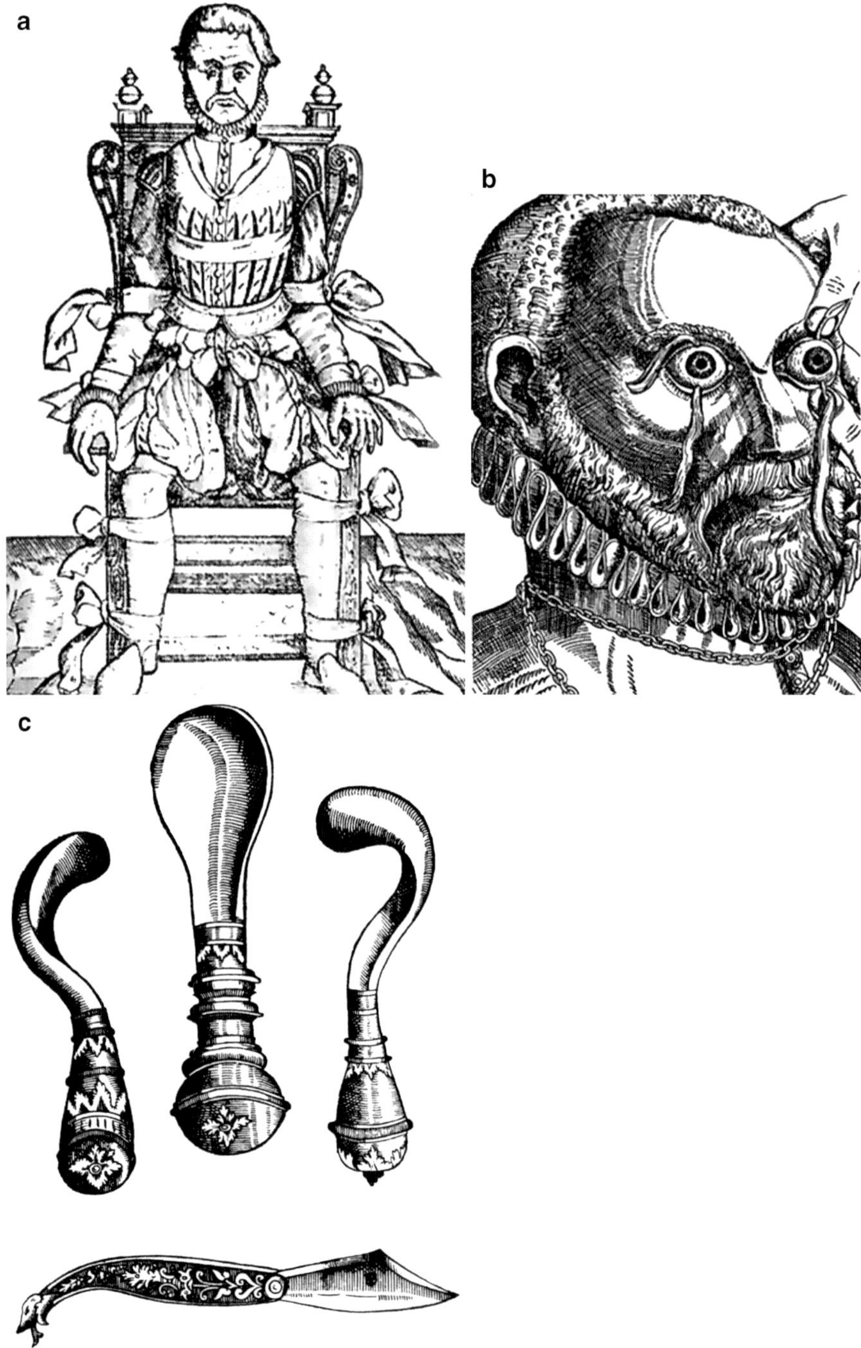

Fig. 1.3 (**a**) Preparing for extirpation, as described by Georg Bartisch in his book the *Augendienst* in 1583. (**b**) Passing a suture through the globe followed by forwarding traction and severing the optic nerve and surrounding tissues with a curved knife to remove the eye. (**c**) Surgical instruments used to perform the extirpation

globe with minimal blood loss. This "new" fascia was described by Rene Tenon in 1806 and is now known as Tenon's capsule [5]. In 1842, Stoeber also described his technique of "shelling the eyeball" within the Tenon's capsule. In 1855, Critchett reported several successful enucleations for nonmalignant ocular conditions [1].

In 1906, Gallemaerts introduced an interim prosthesis that was placed between the closed bulbar conjunctiva and the palpebral conjunctiva. Holes were drilled through the center of this temporary prosthesis, which allowed the drainage of secretions. This device was initially criticized as a source of infection that caused severe sepsis and the eventual death of a patient [7]. However, most surgeons soon understood that the insertion of a conformer between the lids helps to tamponade postoperative conjunctival edema and it prevents socket contracture (Fig. 1.2f) [1, 14]. In 1847, the introduction of general anesthesia with ether and chloroform changed the field of surgery drastically, including advances in eye removal surgery [6].

Evisceration

Evisceration involves the removal of the intraocular content while leaving the sclera, the attached extraocular muscles, and the optic nerve intact. The cornea may or may not be removed. The first evisceration was accredited to James Beer in 1817. While performing an iridectomy for acute angle glaucoma, his case was complicated by an expulsive hemorrhage that necessitated the removal of the contents of the globe [1, 8]. In 1874, Noyes routinely performed evisceration on patients with severe ocular infections. He reported excellent cosmetic outcomes, with no cases of sympathetic ophthalmia [1, 20]. In 1884, Philip Henry Mules placed a hollow glass sphere into the scleral cavity after the removal of the cornea and the intraocular contents [21]. His technique not only replaced the lost orbital volume, it also reduced the incidence of socket contraction [7]. Various orbital implants were developed after his revolutionary discovery and are discussed in Chap. 10. Further advances in the surgical techniques led to the modern approach in evisceration without keratectomy as described by Burch in 1939 [22]. In 1956, Berens published a large case series of successful eviscerations with keratectomy and reported no cases of sympathetic ophthalmia and a low rate of implant extrusion [23].

The perpetual controversy over evisceration versus enucleation has been ongoing for more than a century. In 1887, Frost reported a series of patients who developed sympathetic ophthalmia after evisceration. Although he considered evisceration to be inferior to the enucleation, he complimented on the excellent outcomes of using Mules' glass sphere following evisceration. He proposed that a good cosmetic prognosis may convince patients to choose surgery after eye trauma rather than to keep the injured eye and take the risk of losing the fellow eye from sympathetic ophthalmia [24]. However, surgeons in this era objected to the use of evisceration due to concerns for the development of sympathetic ophthalmia, the spread of a previously undetected intraocular tumor, and the loss of ocular tissues for pathologic studies. In 1898, the Ophthalmological Society of the United Kingdom assigned a committee to compare a simple excision of the eyeball, evisceration with or without the insertion of an implant, enucleation with the insertion of an implant in Tenon's capsule, and other procedures. The committee decided that the simple enucleation of the globe within Tenon's capsule with or without implant placement was the most appropriate procedure. George Edmund de Schweinitz presented similar conclusions at the International Congress in 1900. However, some members felt that evisceration was not sufficiently recognized. They filed a minority report stating that the excision should be limited to cases of intraocular and orbital malignancies, extensive lacerated or contused wounds of the sclera, markedly shrunken globes, and sympathetic ophthalmia [1]. Nonetheless, most surgeons in Great Britain, Europe, and the United States were in favor of enucleation due to the fear of sympathetic ophthalmia that was prevalent in the literature between 1887 and 1908 [25, 26]. This resulted in a near abandonment of evisceration for more than half a century, and it was considered a substandard procedure by World War I. Only a few ophthalmologists stood firm and advocated for evisceration [22, 26]. Some authors continued to report isolated cases of sympathetic ophthalmia following evisceration until the 1970s [26].

In 1963, Ruedemann questioned the validity of previous case reports in an attempt to reignite interest in evisceration. He found that 17 out of 47 reported cases since 1887 did not meet his diagnostic criteria for sympathetic ophthalmia. These cases not only lacked sufficient clinical details to support the diagnosis but rarely reported exam findings of the uninjured eye. The histopathological results were routinely missed in the case reports. For example, one contributor sent a biopsy of the anterior chamber for analysis but discarded the posterior segment contents. While most patients had eviscerations following severe eye trauma, Ruedemann speculated that some of the patients instead received incomplete enucleations [26]. Other authors believe that early ophthalmologists often confused sympathetic ophthalmia with a variety of other types of uveitis [27]. In Ruedemann's report of 506 cases of evisceration, not a single case of sympathetic ophthalmia was found. In 1972, Green also admitted that his reported cases of sympathetic ophthalmia might have been initiated by the original trauma rather than the evisceration itself [26].

Between the late 1970s and early 2000s, more surgeons were performing eviscerations, although the total number of eye removal surgeries decreased [28–30]. Hansen et al. attributed such a shift in practice to the general acceptance by surgeons who favored enhanced cosmetic and motility outcomes following eviscerations [28]. In 1985, a questionnaire sent out by the American Society of Ophthalmic Plastic and Reconstructive Surgery (ASOPRS) found that none of the 140 respondents had seen a case of sympathetic ophthalmia after evisceration [31]. A similar but larger survey in the late 1990s revealed 5 recalled cases of sympathetic ophthalmia out of 841 eviscerations, 3 of which were post-trauma-related. Despite the increasing number of eviscerations performed across the United States, no cases of sympathetic ophthalmia were reported between 1972 and 1997. In 1999, Levine et al. did not find any cases of sympathetic ophthalmia in his review of 90 evisceration surgeries over a 35-year period. He concluded that evisceration is a safe procedure with a low risk for sympathetic ophthalmia [32]. Although retinal surgery is now suggested as the leading cause of sympathetic ophthalmia [33–35], reports of sympathetic ophthalmia after evisceration are not unheard of in the twenty-first century [36–41]. A number of unsuspected malignant melanomas following eviscerations have been reported since the early 1900s [42–48]. Historically, the incidence of this finding was about 0.5% [49]. Some authors believe that this condition is underreported, and the risk of accidentally eviscerating an eye with an intraocular tumor may be higher than the risk of sympathetic ophthalmia [45].

Exenteration

Orbital exenteration refers to complete removal of the globe, eyelids, muscles, fat, and nerves of the orbit. The first reported exenteration was described by Gooch in 1767 [50]. Langenbeck in 1821 and Dupuytren in 1833 further advanced this surgical technique [51]. Collis in 1864 and von Arlt in 1874 described detailed surgical steps of exenteration, most of which are still used today. In 1888, Jacobson reported an exenteration of an orbital "rodent ulcer" using the Arlt method. After cutting the outer commissure to the margin of the orbit, the lids were folded back upon the cheek and the forehead. The orbital tissues were dissected beyond the conjunctival fornices and away from the globe. The tumor or the orbital contents were seized and drawn forward using a pair of forceps with hooks at the tip of each blade, also known as a vulsellum. A blunt elevator was used to separate the mass from each outer wall. The optic nerve and the muscles were then severed with a sharp pair of curved scissors. When the tumor was adherent to the periosteum, it was incised at its margin with a scalpel [52]. His technique had been influenced by the "lid-sparing technique" introduced by Streatfeild in 1872, where the upper and the lower eyelids were sutured together to cover the exenterated socket. At about the same time, Noyes included the eyelids during exenterations. He made the initial incisions vertically through the middle of the upper and lower eyelids. A knife was used to deeply dissect the orbit along the roof and the floor. Horizontal cuts were made through the inner and outer angles. The orbital contents were then separated from the medial and lateral walls without any tissue collapse. The cuts were made diagonally to reach the apex of the orbit [53]. In 1909, Golovine reported an extended orbital exenteration, which included the removal of the adjacent maxillary sinuses [54].

Most surgeons in the early 1800s reserved orbital exenteration for malignant tumors involving the orbit and the periorbital tissue. The empty socket was allowed to epithelialize spontaneously by the granulation tissues [55]. By the early 1900s, many surgeons found that the cicatricial healing of the surrounding soft tissues caused postoperative discomfort and resulted in poor cosmesis. Some patients and family members were appalled at the hollow appearance of the desquamating orbital cavity and found the routine care of the exenterated socket distasteful [56, 57]. The Ollier-Thiersch split-thickness graft, which was first introduced in 1872, was used to line the orbital cavity, but the technique was not well-accepted [56, 58]. The

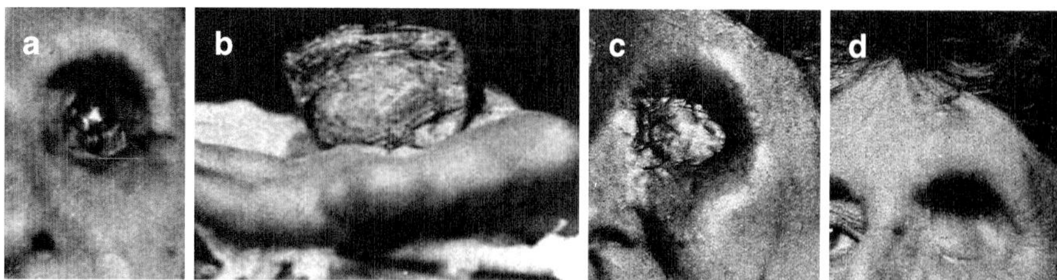

Fig. 1.4 (**a**) Cicatrization of the surrounding tissues drew the facial skin and soft parts into the orbit and caused pain. (**b**) In 1919, Davis harvested a pedunculated flap of thick fat and skin from the abdominal wall and implanted it to an incision on the palm. (**c**) Once the circulation was established, the flap was transferred and shaped to fit the defect in the orbital cavity. The sutures were then removed after 10–14 days. (**d**) Twelve months later, the skin remained soft and covered the cavity without puckering the surrounding tissues [56]

Schirmer method filled the cavity with a free fat graft and then covered the orbital opening with a pedunculated flap from the forehead or cheek. This technique, however, left extensive facial scars [56, 59]. In 1919, Davis introduced a double transfer method using a pedunculated flap from the abdominal wall to cover the orbital cavity (Fig. 1.4) [56]. Numerous primary reconstructive methods, including primary skin grafts, temporalis muscle flaps, pectoralis major muscle flaps, and single flap repairs, were introduced throughout the twentieth century [57, 59–61]. Exenteration and reconstruction techniques are further discussed in Chap. 9.

Conclusion

As historian Carl L. Becker would say, "the value of history is not scientific but moral … it prepares us to live more humanely in the present and to meet rather than to foretell the future." Surgeons from every era strived to meet a moral standard to find the best approach to remove a patient's eye while maintaining the pristine condition of the anophthalmic socket to preserve the patient's comfort, aesthetic appearance, vision in the contralateral eye, and overall health. As technology advanced, new techniques were developed, and existing methods were modified, resulting in a variety of surgical options to achieve better outcomes. Ocularists also searched for new methods and materials to create natural-appearing, comfortable eye prostheses. Some surgical techniques and certain prostheses surpassed the test of time and remained unchanged over a century. By understanding the history of anophthalmia, we are ready to utilize present techniques and also face the future.

References

1. Luce CM. A short history of enucleation. Int Ophthalmol Clin. 1970;10(4):681–7.
2. Wheeler JR. History of ophthalmology through the ages. Br J Ophthalmol. 1946;30(5):264.

3. Moghadasi AN. Artificial eye in Burnt City and theoretical understanding of how vision works. Iran J Public Health. 2014;43(11):1595. Copyrighted image reproduced with permission.
4. Farrokh K. The world's oldest known artificial eye [Internet]. Kaveh Farrokh. 2006 [cited 2018 Aug 28]. Available from: http://kavehfarrokh.com/iranica/maps-of-iran-5000-bc-651-ad/the-worlds-oldest-known-artificial-eye/.
5. Sami D, Young S, Petersen R. Perspective on orbital enucleation implants. Surv Ophthalmol. 2007;52(3):244–65.
6. Calvano CJ. Smith and Nesi's ophthalmic plastic and reconstructive surgery. New York: Springer Science & Business Media; 2012.
7. Kelley JJ. History of ocular prostheses. Int Ophthalmol Clin. 1970;10(4):713–9.
8. Beer GJ. Geschichte der Augenkunde überhaupt und der Augenheilkunde insbesondere: Eine Einladungs-Schrift zur Eröffnung d. Clinic für d. Augenkrankheiten. V. Haykul; 1813.
9. Pine KR, Sloan BH, Jacobs RJ. Clinical ocular prosthetics. New York: Springer; 2015.
10. Espy JW. Cosmetic scleral contact lenses and shells. Am J Ophthalmol. 1968;66(1):95–100.
11. Sajjad A. Ocular prosthesis-a simulation of human anatomy: a literature review. Cureus. 2012;4(12):e74. Permission granted by the author and publisher.
12. Ruedemann AD. Plastic eye implant. Am J Ophthalmol. 1946;29(8):947–52. Copyrighted image reproduced with permission under license number 4425650517351.
13. Gougelmann HP. The evolution of the ocular motility implant. Int Ophthalmol Clin. 1976;10:689–711.
14. Sherman AE. The retracted eye socket. Am J Ophthalmol. 1952;35(1):89–101.
15. Hughes OH. Incorporating gold into ocular prosthetics. J Ophthalmic Prosthet. 2010;15:31–43. Author's personal collection. Permission granted by the author.
16. Shastid TH. History of ophthalmology. In: The American encyclopedia and dictionary of ophthalmology, vol. 11. Chicago: Cleveland Press; 1917. p. 8524–904.
17. Snyder C. An operation designated the extirpation of the eye. Arch Ophthalmol. 1965;74(3):429–32.
18. Hughes MO. Eye injuries and prosthetic restoration in the American Civil War years. J Ophthalmic Prosthet. 2008;13:17–28.
19. Harlan GC. Article IV. Am J Med Sci (1827–1924). 1879;(154):383.
20. King JH Jr, Wadsworth JAC. An atlas of ophthalmic surgery. 3rd ed. Philadelphia: JB Lippincott; 1981.
21. Mules P. Evisceration of the globe with artificial vitreous. Ophthalmol Soc UK. 1885;5:200–8.
22. Burch FE. Evisceration of the globe with scleral implant and preservation of the cornea. Trans Am Ophthalmol Soc. 1939;37:272.
23. Berens C, Carter GZ, Breakey AS. Evisceration: experience with a steel-mesh capped hollow plastic implant. Trans Am Ophthalmol Soc. 1956;54:337.
24. Frost WA. What is the best method of dealing with a lost eye? BMJ. 1887;2013:1153–4.
25. Migliori ME. Enucleation versus evisceration. Curr Opin Ophthalmol. 2002;13(5):298–302.
26. Ruedemann AD Jr. Sympathetic ophthalmia after evisceration. Trans Am Ophthalmol Soc. 1963;61:274.
27. Du Toit N. Evisceration and sympathetic ophthalmia: is there a risk? University of Cape Town [dissertation]. [Riga, Lavita]: Lambert Academy Publishing; 2009. [cited 2018 Oct 13]. Available from: https://pdfs.semanticscholar.org/1096/7415a8d87123d07l6494d53d681c7eca969b.pdf.
28. Hansen AB, Petersen C, Heegaard S, Prause JU. Review of 1028 bulbar eviscerations and enucleations, changes in aetiology and frequency over a 20-year period. Acta Ophthalmol Scand. 1999;77(3):331–5.
29. Saeed MU, Chang BY, Khandwala M, Shivane AG, Chakrabarty A. Twenty year review of histopathological findings in enucleated/eviscerated eyes. J Clin Pathol. 2006;59(2):153–5.
30. Rasmussen ML, Prause JU, Johnson M, Kamper-Jørgensen F, Toft PB. Review of 345 eye amputations carried out in the period 1996–2003, at Rigshospitalet, Denmark. Acta Ophthalmol. 2010;88(2):218–21.
31. Walter WI. Update on enucleation and evisceration surgery. Ophthal Plast Reconstr Surg. 1985;1:243–52.

32. Levine MR, Pou CR, Lash RH. The 1998 Wendell Hughes Lecture. Evisceration: is sympathetic ophthalmia a concern in the new millennium? Ophthal Plast Reconstr Surg. 1999;15(1):4–8.
33. Kilmartin DJ, D DICK AN, Forrester JV. Sympathetic ophthalmia risk following vitrectomy: should we counsel patients? Br J Ophthalmol. 2000;84(5):448–9.
34. Kilmartin DJ, Dick AD, Forrester JV. Prospective surveillance of sympathetic ophthalmia in the UK and Republic of Ireland. Br J Ophthalmol. 2000;84(3):259–63.
35. Ozbek Z, Arikan G, Yaman A, Oner H, Bajin MS, Saatci AO. Sympathetic ophthalmia following vitreoretinal surgery. Int Ophthalmol. 2010;30(2):221–7.
36. Du Toit N, Motala MI, Richards J, Murray AD, Maitra S. The risk of sympathetic ophthalmia following evisceration for penetrating eye injuries at Groote Schuur Hospital. Br J Ophthalmol. 2008;92:61–3.
37. Freidlin J, Pak J, Tessler HH, Putterman AM, Goldstein DA. Sympathetic ophthalmia after injury in the Iraq War. Ophthal Plast Reconstr Surg. 2006;22(2):133–4.
38. Griepentrog GJ, Lucarelli MJ, Albert DM, Nork TM. Sympathetic ophthalmia following evisceration: a rare case. Ophthalmic Plast Reconstr Surg. 2005;21(4):316–8.
39. Androudi S, Theodoridou A, Praidou A, Brazitikos PD. Sympathetic ophthalmia following postoperative endophthalmitis and evisceration. Hippokratia. 2010;14(2):131–2.
40. Zhang Y, Zhang MN, Jiang CH, Yao Y. Development of sympathetic ophthalmia following globe injury. Chin Med J. 2009;122(24):2961–6.
41. Buller AJ, Doris JP, Bonshek R, Brahma AK, Jones NP. Sympathetic ophthalmia following severe fungal keratitis. Eye. 2006;20(11):1306.
42. Kita Y, Yabe H, Shikishima K, Takahashi K. A case of malignant melanoma occurring 63 years after evisceration. Nippon Ganka Gakkai Zasshi. 2001;105(1):52–7.
43. Schwartz GP, Schwartz LW. Acute angle closure glaucoma secondary to a choroidal melanoma. Eye Contact Lens. 2002;28(2):77–9.
44. Akaishi PM, Kitagawa VM, Chahud F, Cruz AA. Malignant melanoma in anophthalmic socket post-evisceration: case reports and literature review. Arq Bras Oftalmol. 2004;67(6):969–72.
45. Eagle RC, Grossniklaus HE, Syed N, Hogan RN, Lloyd WC, Folberg R. Inadvertent evisceration of eyes containing uveal melanoma. Arch Ophthalmol. 2009;127(2):141–5.
46. Bembridge BA, McMillan J. Malignant melanoma occurring after evisceration. Br J Ophthalmol. 1953;37(2):109.
47. Moro F, Ruffato C. Malignant melanoma of the choroid of long duration; orbital evisceration 19 years after diagnosis. Boll Ocul. 1952;31(11):661.
48. Smith B, Soll DB. Malignant melanoma of choroid: report of a case discovered after evisceration. Am J Ophthalmol. 1960;50(2):330–3.
49. Makley TA, Teed RW. Unsuspected intraocular malignant melanomas. AMA Arch Ophthalmol. 1958;60(3):475–8.
50. Frezzotti R, Bonanni R, Nuti A, Polito E. Radical orbital resections. Adv Ophthalmic Plast Reconstr Surg. 1992;9:175–92.
51. Kademani D, Tiwana P. Atlas of oral and maxillofacial surgery. St. Louis: Elsevier Health Sciences; 2015.
52. Jacobson WH. Some points of practical importance in the operative treatment of rodent ulcer. Ann Surg. 1888;8(2):101.
53. Noyes HD. A text-book on diseases of the eye. New York: William Wood & Company; 1890. p. 502.
54. Golovine SS. Orbito-sinus exenteration. Ann Ocul. 1909;141:413–31.
55. Mouriaux F, Barraco P, Patenôtre P, Pellerin P. L'exentération orbitaire. 2001.
56. Davis JS. Plastic surgery: its principles and practice. Philadelphia: Blakiston; 1919. p. 381–3. Public domain.
57. Beare R. Surgery of the orbital region: flap repair following exenteration of the orbit. Proc R Soc Med. 1969;62:1087–90.
58. Ameer F, Singh AK, Kumar S. Evolution of instruments for harvest of the skin grafts. Indian J Plast Surg. 2013;46(1):28.

59. McLaren LR. Primary skin grafting after exenteration of the orbit. Br J Plast Surg. 1958;11:57–61.
60. Ariyan S. The pectoralis major myocutaneous flap. Plast Reconstr Surg. 1979;63(1):73–81.
61. Reese AB. Exenteration of the orbit: with transplantation of the temporalis muscle. Am J Ophthalmol. 1958;45(3):386–90.

Chapter 2
Clinical Decision-Making

Nathan W. Blessing

Introduction

The decision to remove a patient's eye or orbit can be challenging clinically for the physician and emotionally for the patient. For these reasons, careful consideration must be given to the specific indications for eye removal, the surgical methods employed, and the expected rehabilitative process for the patient. Goals of eye removal surgery may include the elimination of chronic pain and suffering, complete removal of a malignancy to prevent disease progression, reduction of the risk of sympathetic ophthalmia, or prevention of the spread of a potentially life-threatening infection. A careful discussion of the risks, benefits, and alternatives to eye removal should be extensively reviewed with every patient with particular attention paid to the postsurgical rehabilitative course. Wherever possible, patients should be included in the clinical decision-making process with appropriate preoperative illustration of orbital implants and prostheses. This is especially important in cases where the eye or orbit being removed is still functioning at a reasonable level. This chapter addresses the indications for eye removal with consideration given to an appropriate surgical approach to achieve clinical goals while mitigating unnecessary patient rehabilitation.

Indications for Eye Removal

The clinical scenarios which might dictate the removal of a patient's eye may be broadly grouped into four categories: infectious, neoplastic, traumatic, and palliative. Although the utilized surgical approach always results in the removal of a

---

N. W. Blessing (✉)
Dean McGee Eye Institute, University of Oklahoma College of Medicine, Department of Ophthalmology, Oklahoma City, OK, USA
e-mail: nathan-blessing@dmei.org

T. E. Johnson (ed.), *Anophthalmia*,
https://doi.org/10.1007/978-3-030-29753-4_2

patient's eye, the clinical goals dictating the approach may differ considerably between patients. Blindness in the absence of persistent pain or ongoing infection unresponsive to local antibiotic therapy is not an indication for eye removal, and phthisical patients with cosmetic concerns can often be addressed using a cosmetic scleral shell as long as corneal sensation is absent or significantly diminished.

Infectious

A number of infectious organisms may affect the eye and surrounding orbit and can arise from invasive surgical procedures (e.g., cataract surgery, glaucoma surgery, intravitreal injections), chronic contact lens wear with poor hygiene, traumatic imbrication with organism-laden foreign material, endogenous spread from a remote infection (endocarditis, fungemia), or local spread from an adjacent sinus (*Mucor*, *Aspergillus*). Atypical infections that may result in eye removal also include parasites (*Toxocara canis*, *Baylisascaris procyonis*) and protozoa (*Acanthamoeba*).

Surgical removal of the eye is indicated in three scenarios. First, if an infection causes the eye to perforate and the visual potential of the eye is poor due to either chronic long-standing disease or irreparable intraocular damage, then removal of the eye is indicated to reduce the risk of sympathetic ophthalmia with subsequent loss of vision in the contralateral eye. Second, if an infected eye or orbit with low visual potential has failed to respond to more conservative medical or surgical therapy and there is risk for intracranial progression, then the eye may be removed to prevent further infectious morbidity or mortality. In cases of intraocular infection, the visual potential is often poor, and the patient may have significant pain. Additionally, the presence of a glaucoma shunt or other foreign bodies may predispose the development of orbital cellulitis and possible extensive orbital scarring which may impede the patient's anophthalmic rehabilitation. In these cases, early intervention is considered to prevent additional orbital morbidity. In cases of rhino-orbital fungal disease, a patient's orbit may be involved to the extent that medical therapy is ineffective, but the orbit and eye are functioning normally. In these cases, eye removal is indicated to prevent intracranial spread and is often difficult for the patient from an emotional standpoint. Similarly, patients with periorbital necrotizing fasciitis may develop orbital involvement (Fig. 2.1). The third scenario whereby eye removal may be considered is chronic indolent infection causing significant pain. In these cases, although there may be some visual potential, a patient may elect for eye removal for palliative reasons (covered later in this chapter).

Neoplastic

Neoplasms may arise in the eye or orbit either primarily, via adjacent spread, or via hematogenous metastasis. When a primary intraocular neoplasm such as uveal melanoma or retinoblastoma cannot be treated with more conservative therapy, eye removal is indicated to prevent regional or distant metastasis. In other instances, an

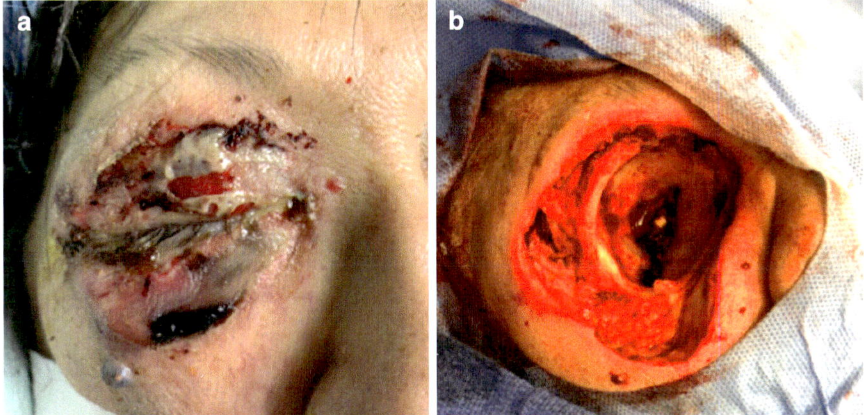

Fig. 2.1 Right periorbital necrotizing fasciitis with both orbital and ocular involvement (**a**) and the same patient immediately following extensive periorbital debridement with concurrent orbital exenteration (**b**)

extraocular malignancy arising from the ocular surface may progress to the point of failure of local medical control such as topical chemotherapy. Additionally, disease from the adjacent facial structures such as the paranasal sinuses and facial skin may have invaded the orbit to such an extent that both the eye and the orbit may be removed to achieve local disease control.

Occasionally, appropriate treatment of an intraocular or orbital malignancy may result in the removal of a comfortable eye that sees perfectly well. In these instances, it is important to counsel the patient appropriately regarding the benefits of early elimination of a potentially fatal malignancy versus the risk of inaction with subsequent morbidity and mortality.

Traumatic

Globe trauma with secondary rupture is a significant cause of ocular morbidity resulting in eye removal. Although the degree of trauma may vary, the typical underlying concern is the development of sympathetic ophthalmia in the contralateral eye. This may result from irreparable posterior ruptures or globe trauma so severe that the sclera is shredded resulting in diffuse uveal exposure. In either instance, the surgical goal is to remove the eye and especially the uvea while identifying and utilizing the extraocular muscles for future implant motility wherever possible. Additionally, blunt anterior trauma can result in dehiscence of a previously placed full-thickness corneal transplant with expulsive suprachoroidal hemorrhage. These cases are often amenable to primary evisceration and should be performed expediently to prevent secondary infection (Fig. 2.2).

Primary enucleation should be avoided except in cases where delaying surgery will result in an increased risk of sympathetic ophthalmia or infection (e.g., diffuse ante-

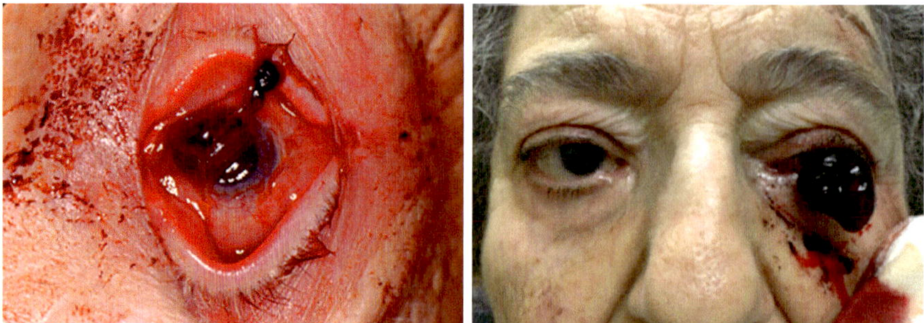

Fig. 2.2 Two patients with a history of prior penetrating keratoplasty who sustained blunt trauma to the globe with subsequent graft dehiscence and expulsion of intraocular contents; both were successfully treated via evisceration

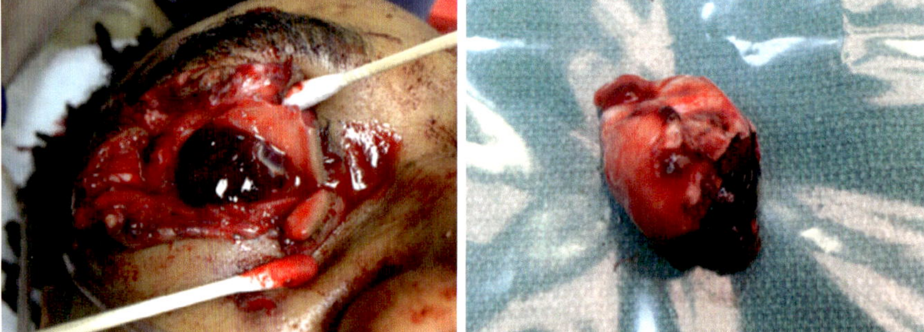

Fig. 2.3 External photo showing a gunshot injury to the right side of the face and orbit (left). The eyelids are extensively damaged as is the anterior aspect of the globe. Gross photo showing the same globe immediately following enucleation surgery (right). The anterior portion of the globe was irreparably damaged, and there were few identifiable structures remaining

rior rupture in a persistently intubated patient with other medical comorbidities). Patient decision-making is critical in proposing primary enucleation in an unsalvageable eye. In situations where patients cannot personally consent due to capacity, such as following a severe trauma with traumatic brain injury, the decision to primarily remove a patient's eye should be undertaken only after several independent physicians have deemed and documented that the eye is unsalvageable and poses a significant risk to the patient (Fig. 2.3). Large irreparable posterior ruptures can often be observed for 1 week while a patient deliberates the prospect of eye removal surgery.

Palliative

In some patients, an eye with either very poor vision or no vision may develop intractable pain or become cosmetically disfiguring. The patient's particular circumstances will dictate whether surgery is advisable and which technique should be employed. However, in cosmetically disfiguring cases, surgery is not always necessary. In cases where a globe is phthisical but painless, an assessment of corneal sensation should be performed, as diminished or absent corneal sensation may allow the patient to tolerate a cosmetic scleral shell without the need for invasive surgery (Fig. 2.4).

In other cases a long-standing painless but blind eye may develop intractable pain for which topical and medical therapy fail. Examples include patients with a history of neovascular glaucoma in which the intraocular pressure is significantly elevated, congenital glaucoma patients who develop profound buphthalmos with mechanical lagophthalmos (Fig. 2.5), or patients with blind phthisical eyes who develop suprachoroidal hemorrhage. B-scan ultrasound can help to elucidate anatomical changes consistent with the development of pain when the ocular media is

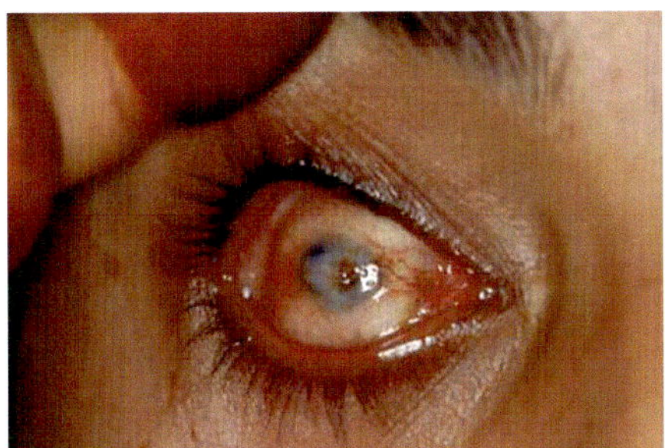
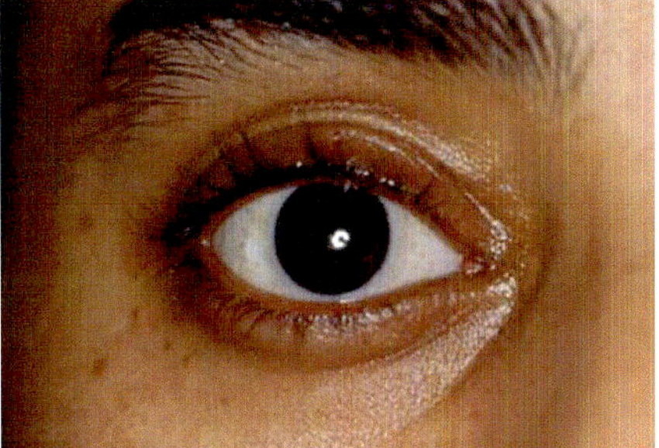

Fig. 2.4 External photo of the right eye demonstrating a phthisical globe with a shrunken and opacified cornea (left). The same patient after scleral shell fitting (right)

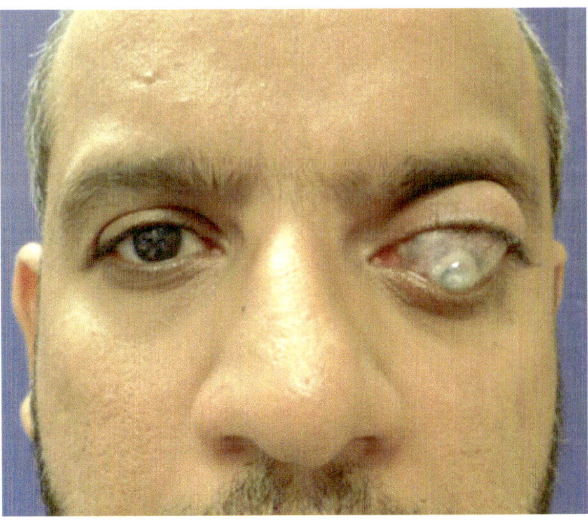

Fig. 2.5 External photo of a patient with a long-standing history of congenital glaucoma in the left eye which responded poorly to treatment. He subsequently developed buphthalmos with extensive scleral thinning and chronic irritation. He was successfully treated via enucleation

otherwise opacified and can be employed to detect new hemorrhage inside an eye. These patients may initially respond to medical therapy but ultimately develop chronic pain for which globe removal would be advantageous. Some patients may develop discomfort due to chronic corneal disease such as band keratopathy or bullous keratopathy and may be amenable to local treatment with EDTA chelation, superficial keratectomy, stromal keratotomy, or Gundersen flap placement. Such patients often experience significant pain relief with topical anesthetic placement. However, some patients may complain of chronic intractable pain but no anatomical explanation for the patient's pain is evident (Fig. 2.6). These patients often have vague complaints such as a headache which may originate in the region near the suspect eye. Caution should be taken in recommending eye removal surgery in such cases unless the patient and provider are reasonably convinced that the patient's chronic pain is a result of the eye in question. All efforts should be made to medically control suspected non-ocular pain prior to pursuing eye removal, as the surgery itself may result in significant postoperative discomfort. In patients with truly painful eyes, the postoperative discomfort is typically less than the pain they were experiencing pre-procedure, and eye removal results in the elimination of their chronic pain. Patients whose symptomatology is non-ocular in origin may continue to complain of persistent chronic pain despite having an anophthalmic socket.

Finally, some patients may have such significant ocular morbidity with poor visual potential that the ongoing pain necessary to achieve ocular stability outweighs the potential visual benefits of retaining the eye. An example might include an elderly patient with a history of penetrating keratoplasty who develops a corneal ulcer, endophthalmitis, and panophthalmitis with worsening pain despite maximal medical therapy (Fig. 2.7a). These patients may elect for expedient eye removal to ameliorate their pain, whereas a younger and healthier patient may elect to continue

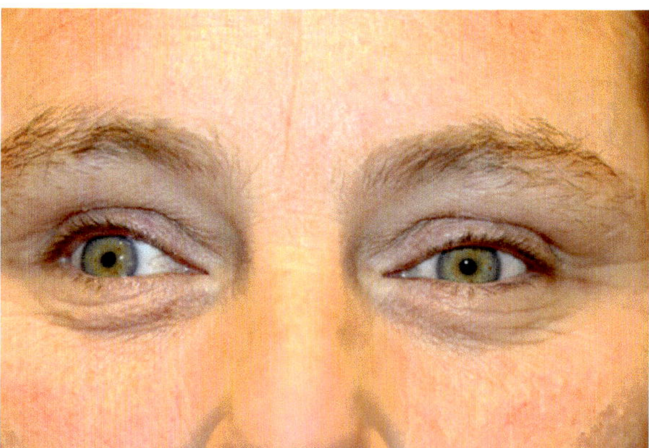

Fig. 2.6 External photo of a patient referred for headaches thought secondary to her blind and exotropic right eye which on examination was anatomically normal other than extensive retinal scarring from a prior traumatic injury. Subsequent investigation revealed symptomatology classic for cluster-type headaches which were successfully treated by a neurologist with expertise in headache treatment

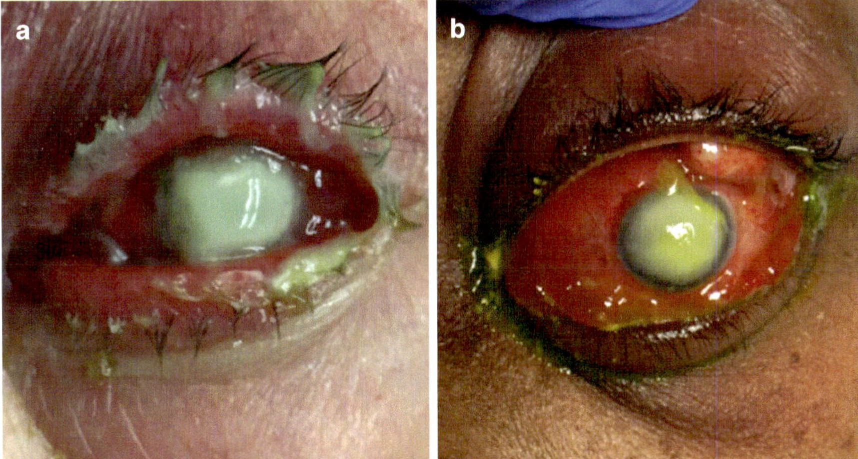

Fig. 2.7 Two patients with extensive panophthalmitis refractory to medical therapy referred for palliative eye removal

all efforts to save their vision (Fig. 2.7b). In these cases, it is most appropriate that the patient understands their visual potential and the necessary surgical steps and timeline required to potentially save the eye. It is the patient that must decide that the pain they are experiencing outweighs any residual visual potential.

Choice of Surgical Technique

Choosing a surgical technique to remove a particular patient's eye is dependent upon the condition of the patient's sclera and the degree of orbital involvement. The particulars of each individual surgical technique are addressed in their own respective chapters, but in general patients with diffuse orbital malignancies are best treated via exenteration in order to obtain adequate surgical margins. When choosing between evisceration and enucleation, consideration should be given to the condition of the patient's sclera, particularly the degree of phthisis, buphthalmos, or traumatic damage. Phthisical eyes with significant scleral contraction cannot retain a large enough implant via evisceration to permit adequate anophthalmic rehabilitation without using a very large prosthesis. Some drawbacks of a large prosthesis include poor motility and chronic elongation and relaxation of the supporting lower eyelid. As such, phthisical eyes are best addressed via enucleation. Additionally, buphthalmic eyes from longstanding congenital glaucoma often have significant scleral enlargement and thinning and are best treated via enucleation. Eyes with intraocular neoplasms are always treated via enucleation in order to obtain adequate surgical margins and prevent unnecessary exposure of the open orbit to a potentially invasive malignancy. Traumatic anterior globe ruptures can be treated via evisceration so long as there is adequate sclera to permit placement of a reasonably sized orbital implant (at least 14–16 mm in diameter). Evisceration is often considered in elderly patients with significant medical comorbidities and those on blood thinners who would benefit from a shorter, less invasive surgery and is the technique of choice in patients with dehisced penetrating keratoplasty grafts and expulsive choroidal hemorrhages.

With regard to infected eyes, a technique is chosen which will eliminate the offending infectious agent with the least risk for persistent infection and the best anophthalmic outcome. It is critical to identify the offending organism and their antibiotic sensitivities wherever possible. A pan-sensitive bacteria may be easily eliminated with placement of a donor sclera and a porous implant for optimal anophthalmic socket topography and motility. However, a resistant bacteria may easily colonize a porous implant resulting in subsequent anophthalmic socket infection and implant exposure. In these cases, it is best to either place a smooth implant that will extrude easily if infection persists or to stage the socket reconstruction with secondary implant placement. In patients who do not desire rehabilitation, implant placement can be deferred indefinitely.

Further Reading

1. Al-Farsi HA, Sabt BI, Al-Mujaini AS. Orbital implant exposure following enucleation or evisceration. Oman J Ophthalmol. 2017;10:87–90.
2. Brownstein S, Jastrzebski A, Saleh S, et al. Unsuspected and misdiagnosed posterior uveal melanoma following enucleation and evisceration in Ottawa-Gatineau. Can J Ophthalmol. 2018;53:155–61.
3. Chan SWS, Khattak S, Yucel N, Gupta N, Yucel YH. A decade of surgical eye removals in Ontario: a clinical-pathological study. Can J Ophthalmol. 2017;52:486–93.
4. Chaudhry IA, AlKuraya HS, Shamsi FA, Elzaridi E, Riley FC. Current indications and resultant complications of evisceration. Ophthalmic Epidemiol. 2007;14:93–7.
5. Custer PL. Enucleation: past, present, and future. Ophthalmic Plast Reconstr Surg. 2000;16:316–21.
6. Eagle RC Jr, Grossniklaus HE, Syed N, Hogan RN, Lloyd WC 3rd, Folberg R. Inadvertent evisceration of eyes containing uveal melanoma. Arch Ophthalmol. 2009;127:141–5.
7. Idowu OO, Ashraf DC, Kalin-Hajdu E, Ryan MC, Kersten RC, Vagefi MR. Efficacy of care for blind painful eyes. Ophthalmic Plast Reconstr Surg. 2019;35:182–6.
8. Kitzmann AS, Weaver AL, Lohse CM, Buettner H, Salomao DR. Clinicopathologic correlations in 646 consecutive surgical eye specimens, 1990–2000. Am J Clin Pathol. 2003;119:594–601.
9. Kord Valeshabad A, Naseripour M, Asghari R, et al. Enucleation and evisceration: indications, complications and clinicopathological correlations. Int J Ophthalmol. 2014;7:677–80.
10. Lemaitre S, Lecler A, Levy-Gabriel C, et al. Evisceration and ocular tumors: what are the consequences? J Fr Ophtalmol. 2017;40:93–101.
11. Lin CW, Liao SL. Long-term complications of different porous orbital implants: a 21-year review. Br J Ophthalmol. 2017;101:681–5.
12. Nunery WR, Cepela MA, Heinz GW, Zale D, Martin RT. Extrusion rate of silicone spherical anophthalmic socket implants. Ophthalmic Plast Reconstr Surg. 1993;9:90–5.
13. Schellini S, Jorge E, Sousa R, Burroughs J, El-Dib R. Porous and nonporous orbital implants for treating the anophthalmic socket: a meta-analysis of case series studies. Orbit. 2016;35:78–86.
14. Soares IP, Franca VP. Evisceration and enucleation. Semin Ophthalmol. 2010;25:94–7.
15. Yousuf SJ, Jones LS, Kidwell ED Jr. Enucleation and evisceration: 20 years of experience. Orbit. 2012;31:211–5.

Chapter 3
Sympathetic Ophthalmia

Chrisfouad R. Alabiad, Lily Zhang, and Janet L. Davis

Introduction

Definition Sympathetic ophthalmia [SO] is a bilateral, diffuse, granulomatous uveitis following trauma or surgery in one eye. The eye with a history of injury is referred to as the "exciting" or "inciting" eye, and the contralateral eye is known as the "sympathizing" eye. Descriptions of sympathetic ophthalmia have been linked back far in history to Hippocrates where reports of injury to one eye were said to put "the other eye in great danger" [1]. In 1840, William Mackenzie coined the term "sympathetic ophthalmitis," and by 1905, Fuchs described the classic histopathology of SO with inflammatory infiltration of the uvea and formation of nodular depigmented aggregations beneath the retinal pigment epithelium, now known as Dalen-Fuchs nodules.

Immunopathogenesis The etiology is not fully understood but is believed to be due to an acquired T-cell-mediated immune reaction to previously unexposed ocular antigens after penetrating trauma or injury. The precise antigen causing this reaction is unknown, but self-antigens found in the lens [2, 3], retina [4, 5], RPE [6], and uveal tract [7] have been implicated.

C. R. Alabiad · L. Zhang · J. L. Davis (✉)
University of Miami Miller School of Medicine, Bascom Palmer Eye Institute, Miami, FL, USA
e-mail: jdavis@med.miami.edu

T. E. Johnson (ed.), *Anophthalmia*,
https://doi.org/10.1007/978-3-030-29753-4_3

Background: Epidemiology and Risk Factors

Immune Privilege The eye is one of the few structures in the body heralded as an immune-privileged site. Sir Peter Medawar demonstrated this in 1948 after a homologous graft of skin transplanted to the anterior chamber of the eye failed to elicit signs of tissue rejection [8]. This results from (1) blood tissue barriers from tight junctions at the levels of the retinal vascular endothelium [9] and the retinal pigment epithelium (RPE); (2) the lack of intraocular lymphatic drainage [10]; and (3) an immunosuppressive ocular microenvironment [11–15]. When these antigens escape the intraocular environment via violation of globe integrity, the antigens are subject to exposure to the host's immune system as they drain through conjunctival lymphatic channels, abrogating the immune privilege. This is hypothesized to stimulate an autoimmune reaction against intraocular tissue, specifically, the uvea.

Etiology In the past, the leading cause of sympathetic ophthalmia was penetrating trauma. Recent studies have shown conflicting data on whether surgical or accidental trauma is now the most common risk factor. Kilmartin et al. reported vitreoretinal surgery as the main risk factor in the UK [16]. The change in the principal etiology has been attributed to increased prevalence of ocular surgery and better management and prevention of ocular injuries. Other studies have found trauma still to be the most prevalent cause [17]. Sympathetic ophthalmia has also been described in relation to non-penetrating injuries including intravitreal injections [18], non-penetrating procedures including irradiation for melanoma [19], plaque brachytherapy [20], and laser cyclodestructive procedures [21], as well as infectious and noninfectious keratitis [22, 23]. The mechanism for immune exposure in these cases is hypothesized to be due to ocular antigens entering the systemic circulation through the vortex veins after leaving the intraocular compartment through the trabecular meshwork.

Incidence and Prevalence Sympathetic ophthalmia is rare and its incidence is therefore difficult to confirm. Recent estimates are that the 1-year incidence is a minimum of 0.03 per 100,000 people [16]. Because SO may be a lifelong illness, the prevalence is higher, approximately 0.3% of uveitis in the general population [16]. Among patients with eye injuries, the incidence ranges from 0% to 3.1% [24]. It has no racial, gender, or age predilection other than differences in demographics related to the frequency of ocular trauma and surgeries.

HLA Association Certain patients may be more at risk for SO because of HLA Class II antigens. Moderately strong HLA associations with SO have been described for HLA-DRB1*04 and HLA-DQB1*03 [25, 26]. Similar HLA haplotypes in patients are associated with Vogt-Koyanagi-Harada disease (VKH), a panuveitis with many features resembling SO [25, 26]. Other than HLA restriction limiting the number of people at risk and the need for an inciting event, another factor assumed to contribute to the current low incidence of sympathetic ophthalmia is improvement in surgical techniques, including management of open globe injuries.

Reduction of Risk of SO

Risk-Benefit Considerations In the setting of ocular trauma, the Ocular Trauma Score [OTS] is often used to predict visual prognosis [27]. When OTS suggests poor long-term visual prognosis and the eye is severely damaged, surgical removal of the injured eye is often performed to reduce the risk of sympathetic ophthalmia. There is at least some evidence to suggest that HLA typing of patients could help clinicians assess individual risk of SO more precisely [see above]. Once a decision has been made to remove an injured eye to reduce the risk of sympathetic ophthalmia, the main surgical options are enucleation and evisceration.

Controversies in Surgical Technique and Timing It is controversial whether enucleation is preferable to evisceration in reducing the risk of SO. Optimal timing for the procedure after the initial insult is also a concern. Given the low incidence of disease, a prospective study to compare surgical techniques and timing is not feasible. Traditional teaching is that removal of the inciting eye by evisceration or enucleation within 2 weeks of injury is necessary to reduce the risk of SO. Advantages of each technique have been well described and are addressed in detail in another chapter. Evisceration is felt by many practitioners to be faster, simpler, and less invasive and to provide better cosmesis and prosthetic motility. Regarding risk of SO, there are two major concerns about evisceration: (1) scleral emissary channels may retain antigens that will continue to promote SO, and (2) previously sequestered intraocular antigens may be released during evisceration and actually cause SO or permit dissemination of an unsuspected intraocular tumor. Case reports of SO after evisceration have been reported as far back as the 1800s [28] with a handful of reports thereafter [29–32]. Because of the concerns about SO after evisceration, the authors of this manuscript generally favor enucleation. In a retrospective analysis, most patients at risk for SO did undergo enucleation; however, Zheng and Wu recommended evisceration over enucleation when patients were reliable for follow-up due to the low incidence of SO [33].

Modification of Evisceration Technique to Reduce Risk If evisceration is elected, modifications in technique may reduce the risk of antigenic exposure. Scraping the scleral bed free of pigment and applying absolute alcohol to the scleral bed after evisceration may denature residual retinal and uveal proteins adherent to sclera and decrease their antigenicity. The authors also suggest that surgeons treat previous surgical or traumatic sclerotomies either with application of absolute alcohol or with focal excision of sclera. In addition, preoperative preparation should include a dilated fundus examination to rule out intraocular tumor, or B-scan ultrasonography should be performed.

Limitations in Risk Reduction It must be emphasized that removal of the injured eye is only recommended when the eye has poor prognosis for visual function and reconstruction is impossible. If sympathetic ophthalmia occurs, the inciting eye may have better visual function than the sympathizing eye [34]; therefore, many patients and doctors will reasonably choose not to enucleate an injured eye. Additionally, enucleation may not always protect against SO [33] as a case of SO has been reported as early as 5 days after injury [35]. Prophylactic corticosteroids do not prevent the development of sympathetic ophthalmia [36].

Lifelong Risk of SO The risk for developing sympathetic ophthalmia after an ocular trauma is lifelong as demonstrated by a case of SO reported 66 years after traumatic injury. It remains to be determined if there will be an increase in the incidence of SO in years to come. Though techniques of intraocular surgery are improving as well as trauma prevention and surgical management, current ophthalmic practice includes an increasing number of intraocular surgeries that manipulate retinal/uveal tissues, such as pars plana vitrectomy, intravitreal injections, laser procedures, and plaque radiation therapy.

Elective Intraocular Surgery in Severely Damaged Eyes Providers managing monocular patients, regardless of etiology, should carefully consider the potential risk of SO when offering intraocular therapies such as repeated pars plana vitrectomy in eyes with very low visual potential, which might incite SO in a normal fellow eye. Minimizing the number of surgical entries into a severely damaged eye may be prudent. As above, HLA typing may help individualize risk.

Presentation and Diagnosis

Time to Onset Most patients (90%) who develop sympathetic ophthalmia will present within 1 year of the inciting injury. The majority of cases (65%) present between 2 and 8 weeks [37]. Documented cases have ranged in presentation from 5 days to 66 years [38]. Cases resulting from trauma have been found to present earlier than surgically induced cases, with a median of 6.5 months after the inciting trauma compared to a median of 14.3 months after surgery [17].

Clinical Diagnosis Diagnosis of sympathetic ophthalmia is usually made by history and clinical examination. History of trauma is significant in differentiating from other similar presentations including Vogt-Koyanagi-Harada syndrome and sarcoidosis. While extraocular manifestations are quite rare, there may be findings similar to VKH, including sensorineural hearing loss, alopecia, poliosis, and vitiligo.

Ocular Features Onset may be acute or insidious onset. Although this is a bilateral process, symptoms and signs of disease may be asymmetric. Severely damaged inciting eyes may be difficult to assess for inflammation. Symptoms vary in intensity between patients and include photophobia, blurry vision, and pain. In addition to a decrease in visual acuity, there may be changes in intraocular pressure, which may be elevated due to trabeculitis or decreased due to ciliary body dysfunction.

Examination of the anterior segment may disclose mutton fat keratic precipitates, anterior chamber cell and flare, posterior synechiae, and iris thickening. Examination of the posterior segment may demonstrate vitritis, cream-/yellow-colored subretinal infiltrates colloquially known as Dalen-Fuchs nodules but is a histopathologic term (Fig. 3.1), exudative/serous retinal detachments (Fig. 3.2), and optic nerve edema.

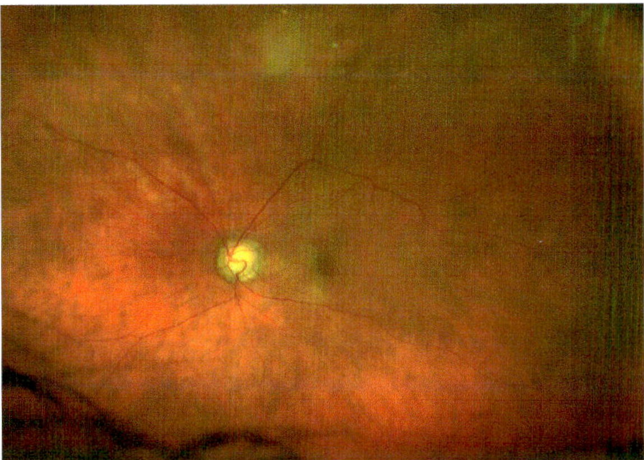

Fig. 3.1 Fundus photo, left eye. Sympathetic ophthalmia. Although there is only trace vitreous haze, the choroid appears thickened and infiltrated by focal yellow lesions despite the use of high doses of oral corticosteroids for 3 weeks. There is glaucomatous cupping of the optic nerve. Sympathetic ophthalmia developed in the aftermath of glaucoma surgery, endophthalmitis, and pars plana vitrectomy of the right eye

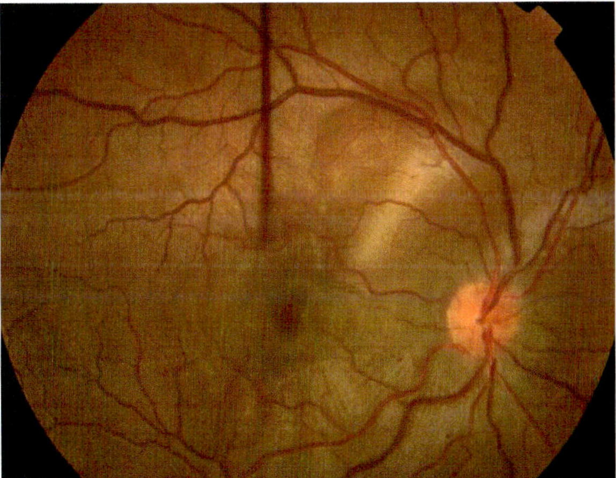

Fig. 3.2 Fundus photo, right eye. Sympathetic ophthalmia. There are collections of subretinal fluid surrounding the optic nerve. Vessels and nerves are healthy and the media is clear. This presentation resembles the acute phases of VKH. The diseases are differentiated by the history of ocular injury or surgery and by the greater frequency of neurologic and dermatologic manifestations in VKH

Because the principal site of inflammation is in the uvea and retina rather than in the vitreous cavity, the amount of cellular inflammation may be less than expected despite severe posterior disease, and the view into the fundus may be quite clear, confounding diagnosis.

Ancillary Testing Ophthalmic imaging provides supportive findings for SO. Fluorescein angiography (FA) shows hyperfluorescent leakage in the venous phase that continues to the late phase (Fig. 3.3a). Indocyanine green angiography (ICG) shows hypofluorescent areas that represent choroidal inflammatory cellular infiltration and edema [39] (Fig. 3.3b). Ocular coherence tomography (OCT) can demonstrate serous retinal detachments and choroidal infiltration that can be used to monitor progression and response to treatment [40]. Although the exudative changes usually resolve quickly and could be monitored clinically, it is important to monitor SO with simultaneous FA/ICG to confirm that uveal inflammation has subsided (Figs. 3.4 and 3.5).

Prognosis When poorly controlled or left untreated, this lifelong uveitic process carries significant ocular morbidity with poor visual prognosis. Sight-threatening consequences include cataract, secondary glaucoma, cystoid macular edema, optic nerve pallor, choroidal neovascular membrane and subretinal fibrosis in the macula or in the peripapillary region (Fig. 3.6), choroidal atrophy, and depigmentation of the RPE and choroid akin to the "sunset glow" fundus seen in VKH. Changes in pigmentation may be slow to develop and difficult to recognize but are a sign of inadequate control. Fundus photography can be used to document progressive choroidal depigmentation associated with suboptimally controlled disease (Fig. 3.7). Phthisis may occur solely from the uveitis [41].

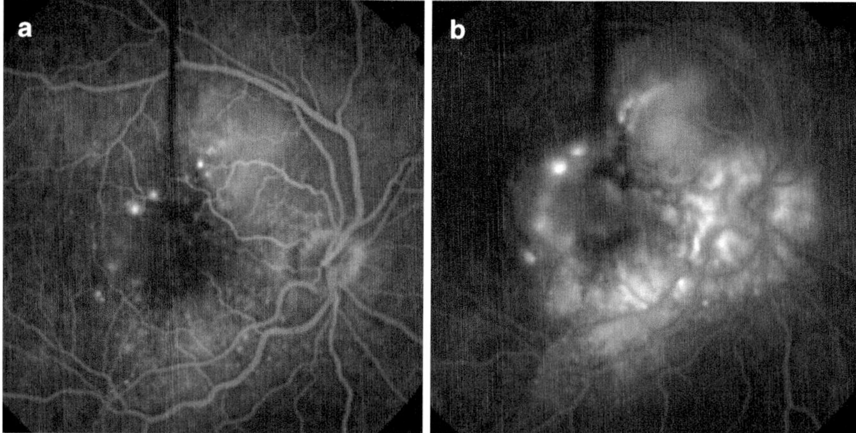

Fig. 3.3 Fluorescein angiogram of the eye in Fig. 3.2. (**a**) Early phase FA. Pinpoint choroidal leaks are present posteriorly and more diffuse leakage is starting. (**b**) Late phase FA. Pooling under the retina increases with retinal elevation. There is a vertical artifact from the fixation device

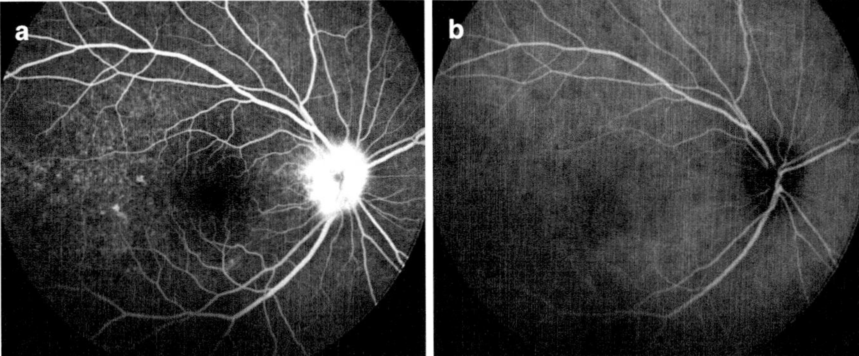

Fig. 3.4 FA and simultaneous indocyanine angiogram of right eye. Sympathetic ophthalmia in the initial stages of treatment with non-corticosteroid systemic immunomodulatory therapy. (**a**) There is speckled hyperfluorescence temporally related to choroidal leakage and RPE changes, but no pooling. The optic nerve leaks. (**b**) ICG reveals that the choroidal inflammation remains active with many small choroidal infiltrates

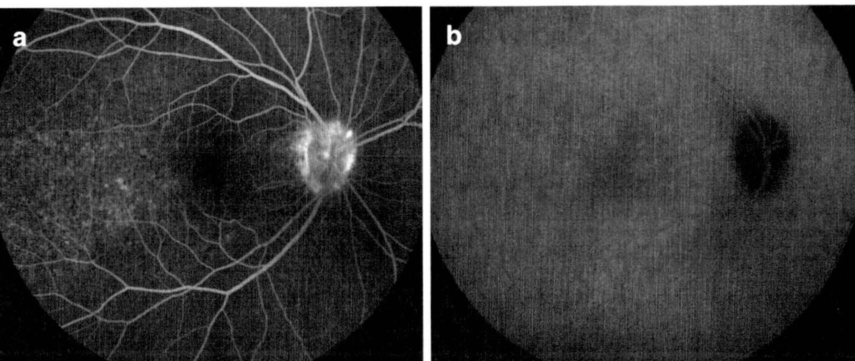

Fig. 3.5 FA and ICG. Same eye as Fig. 3.4 after additional treatment. These images are from later in the angiogram when pathologic leakage would normally be more visible. (**a**) The RPE is altered in the temporal macula, but there is less choroidal leakage, and the optic nerve no longer leaks. (**b**) ICG shows resolution of the choroidal infiltrates. There is satisfactory control of the acute inflammation

Management

Importance of Initial Therapy Sympathetic ophthalmia responds best to early, intense treatment with systemic corticosteroid and non-corticosteroid immunosuppression as demonstrated by controlled inflammation and retention of visual function in patients who receive early treatment. Most patients maintain functional visual acuity, with many patients achieving a final visual acuity of 20/60 or better [17, 36, 42]. Long-term remission off corticosteroids and immunomodulation is possible [43]; however, it must be emphasized that SO is usually a lifelong disease.

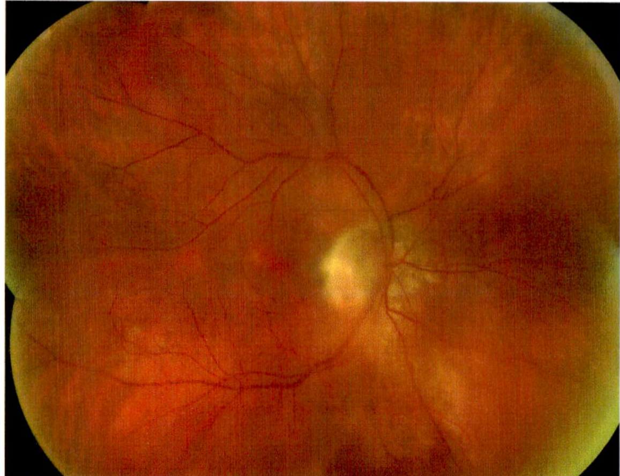

Fig. 3.6 Fundus photo, right eye. Sympathetic ophthalmia, acute stage. Yellow choroidal infiltrates are seen, but in addition, there is peripapillary fibrosis. These fibrotic rings usually have a neovascular component and typically progress to involve the center of the macula. Immunomodulatory therapy and anti-VEGF therapy may both be needed to control the process. Pigmentary changes are beginning inferonasal to the optic nerve

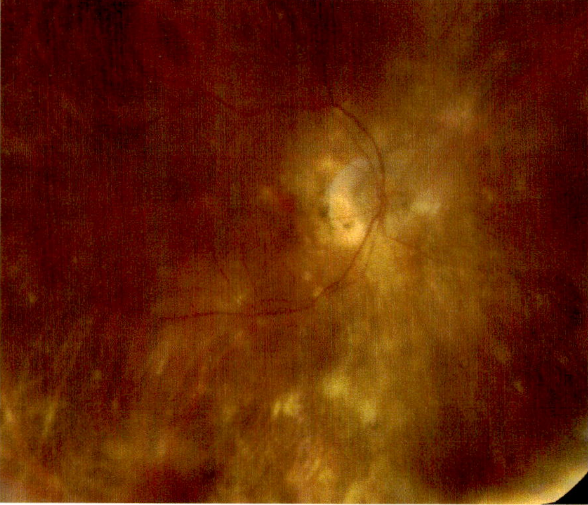

Fig. 3.7 Same eye as in Fig. 3.6. Sympathetic ophthalmia, convalescent phase. The patient had difficult tolerating any immunomodulatory therapy due to bone marrow suppression and was ultimately switched to adalimumab with improved control. The peripapillary neovascularization has been controlled by multiple anti-VEGF injections and is regularly monitored with OCT. There are extensive pigmentary changes related to the prolonged choroidal inflammation. The findings are concerning for progressive loss of retinal function

Serial follow-up is required to monitor for disease control and for side effects from treatment.

Choice of Initial Therapy Sympathetic ophthalmia treatment calls for systemic immunosuppression through the use of corticosteroids and immunomodulatory agents. Treatment for the acute phase of the disease includes high-dose oral prednisone up to 1 mg/kg/day [36]. Exudative detachment or vision loss from choroidal infiltrates may benefit from treatment with intravenous steroids 0.5–1 gram daily for 3 days [44]. Topical corticosteroids and cycloplegics help treat the anterior uveitis and prevent formation of posterior synechia. The speed of action of corticosteroids is unique among available agents, and it is very difficult to replace them with non-corticosteroid systemic immunomodulatory agents in the initial phases of treatment. Once corticosteroid treatment has been initiated, immunomodulatory therapy should be started as soon as possible, anticipating that long-term treatment will be needed and that the alternative drugs will require a longer time to become effective.

Preparatory to Medical Treatment Although corticosteroids must often be started urgently, it is important to obtain laboratory testing in all patients suspected of sympathetic ophthalmia to assess them for conditions that may be affected by treatment. Recommended tests include complete blood count, comprehensive metabolic panel, urinalysis, FTA with reflex RPR, hepatitis B surface antigen, hepatitis C antibody, HIV antibody, and urine pregnancy test. An interferon-gamma release assay test for tuberculosis is more practical than a PPD as the results will not be affected if the blood is drawn before corticosteroids are started, whereas the TB skin test might fail to show a reaction if large doses of corticosteroids are being given. A chest X-ray should be scheduled. There should be consideration of age-appropriate vaccinations with recombinant or killed vaccines before immunosuppression deepens; live vaccines are contraindicated while on therapy.

Non-corticosteroid Systemic Immunomodulatory Therapy Several immunomodulatory agents have been used as steroid-sparing long-term agents for sympathetic ophthalmia including mycophenolate mofetil [45], azathioprine [46], cyclosporine [47], tacrolimus [48], and chlorambucil [49]. These agents are introduced in an effort to fully taper the patient off corticosteroids and thus avoid devastating long-term complications of steroid use. Management of these agents is most appropriately reserved for an experienced uveitis or rheumatology practitioner as they require frequent monitoring to assess for compromise of the hematologic, renal, and hepatic systems. Dosing is adjusted according to the clinical activity of the uveitis, so communication between the ophthalmologist, usually a retina or uveitis specialist, and a managing rheumatologist is particularly important. Vote et al. published an algorithm in 2004 for the medical management of sympathetic ophthalmic using corticosteroids and non-corticosteroid drugs without consideration of biologic agents [50]. The current 2016 consensus guidelines for treatment of noninfectious intermediate, posterior, and panuveitis should be consulted for additional information regarding current therapies. [51]. There are case reports of the use of tumor necrosis factor-α (TNF-α) inhibitors in refractory SO in pediatric and adult patients [52–54]. Insight into the cytokine and chemokine milieu of SO [55] may help identify efficacious targeted therapies with fewer systemic side effects than conventional corticosteroid and non-corticosteroid drugs.

Intraocular Treatment of SO Corticosteroid drug delivery intravitreal implants have been used in SO to reduce or eliminate systemic corticosteroid treatment [56–58]. Intravitreal injections of triamcinolone acetonide may also decrease the dose of systemic steroid needed to treat SO [40, 59]. These agents are best used as adjuncts rather than primary therapy. In addition to the inadvisability of short-duration therapies for a long-duration disease, the risk of complications or infection with intravitreally delivered drugs in monocular patients may be unacceptable.

References

1. Albert DM, Diaz-Rohena R. A historical review of sympathetic ophthalmia and its epidemiology. Surv Ophthalmol. 1989;34(1):1–14.
2. Blodi FC. Sympathetic uveitis as an allergic phenomenon; with a study of its association with phacoanaphylactic uveitis and a report on the pathologic findings in sympathizing eyes. Trans Am Acad Ophthalmol Otolaryngol. 1959;63:642–9.
3. Little J, Ikeda A, Zwaan J, Langman J. The immunologic specificity of human lens proteins. Exp Eye Res. 1965;4(3):187–95.
4. von Sallmann L, Meyers RE, Stone SH, Lerner EM 2nd. Retinal and uveal inflammation in monkeys following inoculation with homologous retinal antigen. Arch Ophthalmol. 1969;81(3):374–82.
5. Rao NA, Robin J, Hartmann D, Sweeney JA, Marak GE Jr. The role of the penetrating wound in the development of sympathetic ophthalmia experimental observations. Arch Ophthalmol. 1983;101(1):102–4.
6. Marak GE Jr, Font RL, Johnson MC, Alepa FP. Lymphocyte-stimulating activity of ocular tissues in sympathetic ophthalmia. Investig Ophthalmol. 1971;10(10):770–4.
7. Mills PV, Shedden WI. Serological studies in sympathetic ophthalmitis. Br J Ophthalmol. 1965;49:29–33.
8. Medawar PB. Immunity to homologous grafted skin; the fate of skin homografts transplanted to the brain, to subcutaneous tissue, and to the anterior chamber of the eye. Br J Exp Pathol. 1948;29(1):58–69.
9. Campbell M, Humphries P. The blood-retina barrier: tight junctions and barrier modulation. Adv Exp Med Biol. 2012;763:70–84.
10. Streilein JW, Wilbanks GA, Cousins SW. Immunoregulatory mechanisms of the eye. J Neuroimmunol. 1992;39(3):185–200.
11. Taylor AW, Streilein JW, Cousins SW. Immunoreactive vasoactive intestinal peptide contributes to the immunosuppressive activity of normal aqueous humor. J Immunol. 1994;153(3):1080–6.
12. Taylor AW, Streilein JW, Cousins SW. Identification of alpha-melanocyte stimulating hormone as a potential immunosuppressive factor in aqueous humor. Curr Eye Res. 1992;11(12):1199–206.
13. Wenkel H, Streilein JW. Evidence that retinal pigment epithelium functions as an immune-privileged tissue. Invest Ophthalmol Vis Sci. 2000;41(11):3467–73.

14. Taylor AW, Streilein JW, Cousins SW. Alpha-melanocyte-stimulating hormone suppresses antigen-stimulated T cell production of gamma-interferon. Neuroimmunomodulation. 1994;1(3):188–94.
15. Kawanaka N, Taylor AW. Localized retinal neuropeptide regulation of macrophage and microglial cell functionality. J Neuroimmunol. 2011;232(1–2):17–25.
16. Kilmartin DJ, Dick AD, Forrester JV. Prospective surveillance of sympathetic ophthalmia in the UK and Republic of Ireland. Br J Ophthalmol. 2000;84(3):259–63.
17. Galor A, Davis JL, Flynn HW Jr, Feuer WJ, Dubovy SR, Setlur V, et al. Sympathetic ophthalmia: incidence of ocular complications and vision loss in the sympathizing eye. Am J Ophthalmol. 2009;148(5):704–10 e2.
18. Brouzas D, Koutsandrea C, Moschos M, Papadimitriou S, Ladas I, Apostolopoulos M. Massive choroidal hemorrhage after intravitreal administration of bevacizumab (Avastin) for AMD followed by contralateral sympathetic ophthalmia. Clin Ophthalmol. 2009;3:457–9.
19. Fries PD, Char DH, Crawford JB, Waterhouse W. Sympathetic ophthalmia complicating helium ion irradiation of a choroidal melanoma. Arch Ophthalmol. 1987;105(11):1561–4.
20. Ahmad N, Soong TK, Salvi S, Rudle PA, Rennie IG. Sympathetic ophthalmia after ruthenium plaque brachytherapy. Br J Ophthalmol. 2007;91(3):399–401.
21. Roberts MA, Rajkumar V, Morgan G, Laws D. Sympathetic ophthalmia secondary to cyclodiode laser in a 10-year-old boy. J AAPOS. 2009;13(3):299–300.
22. Guerriero S, Montepara A, Ciraci L, Monno R, Cinquepalmi V, Vetrugno M. A case of sympathetic ophthalmia after a severe acanthamoeba keratitis. Eye Contact Lens. 2011;37(6):374–6.
23. Shen J, Fang W, Jin XH, Yao YF, Li YM. Sympathetic ophthalmia caused by a severe ocular chemical burn: a case report and literature review. Int J Clin Exp Med. 2015;8(2):2974–8.
24. Chu XK, Chan CC. Sympathetic ophthalmia: to the twenty-first century and beyond. J Ophthalmic Inflamm Infect. 2013;3(1):49.
25. Kilmartin DJ, Wilson D, Liversidge J, Dick AD, Bruce J, Acheson RW, et al. Immunogenetics and clinical phenotype of sympathetic ophthalmia in British and Irish patients. Br J Ophthalmol. 2001;85(3):281–6.
26. Davis JL, Mittal KK, Freidlin V, Mellow SR, Optican DC, Palestine AG, et al. HLA associations and ancestry in Vogt-Koyanagi-Harada disease and sympathetic ophthalmia. Ophthalmology. 1990;97(9):1137–42.
27. Kuhn F, Maisiak R, Mann L, Mester V, Morris R, Witherspoon CD. The Ocular Trauma Score (OTS). Ophthalmol Clin N Am. 2002;15(2):163–5, vi.
28. Migliori ME. Enucleation versus evisceration. Curr Opin Ophthalmol. 2002;13(5):298–302.
29. Ruedemann AD. Sympathetic ophthalmia after evisceration. Trans Am Ophthalmol Soc. 1963;61:274–314.
30. Ikui H, Ueno K. Six cases of sympathetic ophthalmia developing after evisceration. Nihon Ganka Kiyo. 1965;16(8):458–67.
31. Green WR, Maumenee AE, Sanders TE, Smith ME. Sympathetic uveitis following evisceration. Trans Am Acad Ophthalmol Otolaryngol. 1972;76(3):625–44.
32. Griepentrog GJ, Lucarelli MJ, Albert DM, Nork TM. Sympathetic ophthalmia following evisceration: a rare case. Ophthalmic Plast Reconstr Surg. 2005;21(4):316–8.
33. Zheng C, Wu AY. Enucleation versus evisceration in ocular trauma: a retrospective review and study of current literature. Orbit. 2013;32(6):356–61.
34. Gasch AT, Foster CS, Grosskreutz CL, Pasquale LR. Postoperative sympathetic ophthalmia. Int Ophthalmol Clin. 2000;40(1):69–84.
35. Bilyk JR. Enucleation, evisceration, and sympathetic ophthalmia. Curr Opin Ophthalmol. 2000;11(5):372–86.
36. Chan CC, Roberge RG, Whitcup SM, Nussenblatt RB. 32 cases of sympathetic ophthalmia. A retrospective study at the National Eye Institute, Bethesda, Md., from 1982 to 1992. Arch Ophthalmol. 1995;113(5):597–600.
37. Marak GE Jr. Recent advances in sympathetic ophthalmia. Surv Ophthalmol. 1979;24(3):141–56.

38. Zaharia MA, Lamarche J, Laurin M. Sympathetic uveitis 66 years after injury. Can J Ophthalmol. 1984;19(5):240–3.
39. Bernasconi O, Auer C, Zografos L, Herbort CP. Indocyanine green angiographic findings in sympathetic ophthalmia. Graefes Arch Clin Exp Ophthalmol. 1998;236(8):635–8.
40. Chan RV, Seiff BD, Lincoff HA, Coleman DJ. Rapid recovery of sympathetic ophthalmia with treatment augmented by intravitreal steroids. Retina. 2006;26(2):243–7.
41. Chang GC, Young LH. Sympathetic ophthalmia. Semin Ophthalmol. 2011;26(4–5):316–20.
42. Makley TA Jr, Azar A. Sympathetic ophthalmia. A long-term follow-up. Arch Ophthalmol. 1978;96(2):257–62.
43. Payal AR, Foster CS. Long-term drug-free remission and visual outcomes in sympathetic ophthalmia. Ocul Immunol Inflamm. 2017;25(2):190–5.
44. Hebestreit H, Huppertz HI, Sold JE, Dammrich J. Steroid-pulse therapy may suppress inflammation in severe sympathetic ophthalmia. J Pediatr Ophthalmol Strabismus. 1997;34(2):124–6.
45. Lau CH, Comer M, Lightman S. Long-term efficacy of mycophenolate mofetil in the control of severe intraocular inflammation. Clin Exp Ophthalmol. 2003;31(6):487–91.
46. Hakin KN, Pearson RV, Lightman SL. Sympathetic ophthalmia: visual results with modern immunosuppressive therapy. Eye (Lond). 1992;6(Pt 5):453–5.
47. Nussenblatt RB, Palestine AG, Chan CC. Cyclosporin A therapy in the treatment of intraocular inflammatory disease resistant to systemic corticosteroids and cytotoxic agents. Am J Ophthalmol. 1983;96(3):275–82.
48. Ishioka M, Ohno S, Nakamura S, Isobe K, Watanabe N, Ishigatsubo Y, et al. FK506 treatment of noninfectious uveitis. Am J Ophthalmol. 1994;118(6):723–9.
49. Miserocchi E, Baltatzis S, Ekong A, Roque M, Foster CS. Efficacy and safety of chlorambucil in intractable noninfectious uveitis: the Massachusetts Eye and Ear Infirmary experience. Ophthalmology. 2002;109(1):137–42.
50. Vote BJ, Hall A, Cairns J, Buttery R. Changing trends in sympathetic ophthalmia. Clin Exp Ophthalmol. 2004;32(5):542–5.
51. Dick AD, Rosenbaum JT, Al-Dhibi HA, Belfort R Jr, Brezin AP, Chee SP, et al. Guidance on noncorticosteroid systemic immunomodulatory therapy in noninfectious uveitis: fundamentals of care for uveitis (FOCUS) initiative. Ophthalmology. 2018;125(5):757–73.
52. Kim JB, Jeroudi A, Angeles-Han ST, Grossniklaus HE, Yeh S. Adalimumab for pediatric sympathetic ophthalmia. JAMA Ophthalmol. 2014;132(8):1022–4.
53. Ramirez ED, Guijarro Gonzalez JJ, Vicuna RG. Postsurgical sympathetic ophthalmia refractory to treatment: the response to infliximab. Retin Cases Brief Rep. 2012;6(2):169–71.
54. Gupta SR, Phan IT, Suhler EB. Successful treatment of refractory sympathetic ophthalmia in a child with infliximab. Arch Ophthalmol. 2011;129(2):250–2.
55. Furusato E, Shen D, Cao X, Furusato B, Nussenblatt RB, Rushing EJ, et al. Inflammatory cytokine and chemokine expression in sympathetic ophthalmia: a pilot study. Histol Histopathol. 2011;26(9):1145–51.
56. Jonas JB, Rensch F. Intravitreal steroid slow-release device replacing repeated intravitreal triamcinolone injections for sympathetic ophthalmia. Eur J Ophthalmol. 2008;18(5):834–6.
57. Mahajan VB, Gehrs KM, Goldstein DA, Fischer DH, Lopez JS, Folk JC. Management of sympathetic ophthalmia with the fluocinolone acetonide implant. Ophthalmology. 2009;116(3):552–7 e1.
58. Mansour AM. Dexamethasone implant as sole therapy in sympathetic ophthalmia. Case Rep Ophthalmol. 2018;9(2):257–63.
59. Jonas JB. Intravitreal triamcinolone acetonide for treatment of sympathetic ophthalmia. Am J Ophthalmol. 2004;137(2):367–8.

Chapter 4
Psychological and Cognitive Adjustment to Vision Loss

Virginia A. Jacko

As a successful executive at one of our major institutions of higher education, toward the end of my 20-year career I learned I had a degenerative eye disease most likely resulting in total blindness. The first person I phoned was my mother. Looking back, I ask myself "How was I able to cope with this diagnosis?" I wonder sometimes if it was the reaction my mother had when she responded to my initial phone call telling her of the diagnosis. I said, "Mother, I just got my diagnosis, and I am going to go totally blind!" She responded in her very pragmatic style, "Well, I will just have to pray that you then do big things for the blind!" I know that at the time, quite frankly, she annoyed me because I expected some pity, some sadness, or maybe even some motherly love. Looking back, what she was saying was, "I have confidence in you, and you will learn about blindness and then help others." This was the best thing she could have said because it made me proactive, and I did not waste any time figuring out what I needed to do. I learned that the Miami Lighthouse for the Blind and Visually Impaired (Fig. 4.1) was a founder of the University of Miami Bascom Palmer Eye Institute where my ophthalmologist was on the faculty. I also learned that the Miami Lighthouse was the first private agency in the USA to rehabilitate blind adults for competitive mainstream employment, so it seemed reasonable that I enroll as a client.

As soon as I could wrap up crucial university business and identify my interim replacement, I began a four-month rehabilitation program at Miami Lighthouse for the Blind. During this period, I lost all of my vision except for light perception. At Miami Lighthouse, I learned personal management, which gave me the training I needed for my independent living skills such as grooming including putting on my makeup, cooking, writing checks, addressing envelopes, telephone skills, and shopping. I learned how to use all Microsoft Office applications with supplemental screen-reading software called JAWS. My physical adjustment to blindness required

V. A. Jacko (✉)
Miami Lighthouse for the Blind and Visually Impaired, Miami, FL, USA
e-mail: vjacko@miamilighthouse.org

T. E. Johnson (ed.), *Anophthalmia*,
https://doi.org/10.1007/978-3-030-29753-4_4

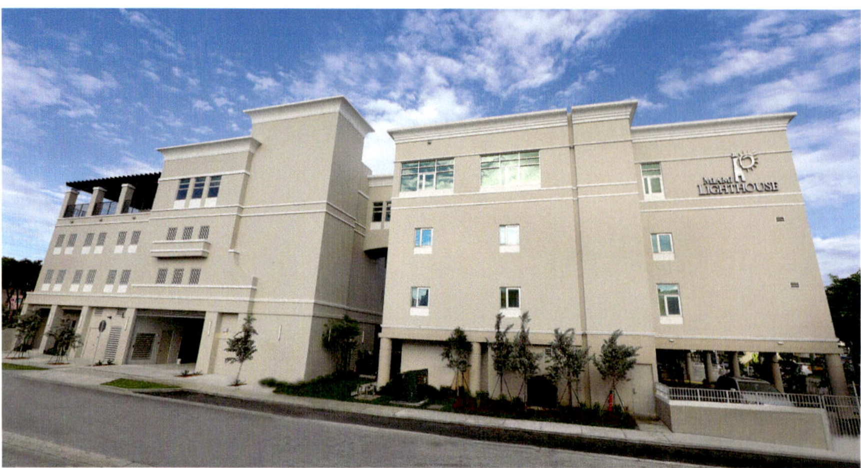

Fig. 4.1 Miami lighthouse for the blind in Miami, Florida

that I learn how to use the white cane. One-on-one Orientation and Mobility classes involved learning how to safely take the stairs and cross busy intersections, walk down the sidewalk to the park and take public transportation without the assistance of a sighted guide. Going to these classes, I met others who were successful despite having lost their eyesight, and this interaction motivated me to be the very best blind person I could be. At the end of my program, when I was told, "You would be a great guide dog user," I was shocked. That was not on my radar; however, I traveled to New York and went to an accredited guide dog school, Guiding Eyes for the Blind, lived there for nearly a month and returned to Miami with my first guide dog. I had no idea how the orientation and mobility instruction I received at Miami Lighthouse would enable me to travel safely with a guide dog, including traveling to France and throughout the USA.

Now as President and CEO of the Miami Lighthouse for the Blind, I use the executive skills I gained in my sighted career; this is not a change for me. However, access to information is quite different. I read through my computer or use other innovative technology like the OrCam. This is a pair of glasses with a tiny camera mounted on the front and a small CPU with a few buttons that enable me to have it read text on a page or identify faces. I have, in essence, trained the computer for face recognition of my colleagues and acquaintances. I use an iPhone, like everyone else, but the setting of "voice over" enables me to get auditory feedback instead of reading the phone screen. Recent technology innovations like these help the blind to be independent users; however, training on these devices is critical.

A few years ago, I received a phone call from a hospital administrator in ophthalmology. The call went like this "Virginia, we have a patient coming out of surgery, and we need to tell the patient's wife and mother that he is totally blind. Could you come over?" Looking back and thinking about the perspective of this family, I heard on the phone tremendous hope with these words: "Perhaps if they see you, they will have confidence that their loved one will be okay despite being blind."

While this relates to my personal response to blindness, I observed that for many that lose their eyesight, who are not born blind, my adjustment to blindness was a personal journey, and for each person the adjustment time and the social, emotional and cognitive process is different. For the patient I mentioned above, the family was not ready to hear about vision rehabilitation or engage with a person with a guide dog. Over time, the patient and family pursued our services and he became a beneficiary of our Miami Lighthouse rehabilitation programs. He physically adjusted to using a white cane and progressed to getting a guide dog. He became an outstanding computer user despite being blind. Of course, as an engineer, in his sighted career he used the computer, and at Miami Lighthouse he learned how to do it with screen-reading software. This means he memorized lots of keystroke commands to interface with the monitor and to ask the monitor, in essence, to give auditory information as to what was on the monitor. He had to go through an adjustment period; some call it "the grieving" process. Today, I can describe him as a highly confident, independent person who just happens to be blind.

Helen Keller used the phrase "House of Light." About 100 years ago the New York Lighthouse began and then the Chicago Lighthouse followed by Miami Lighthouse. Lighthouses in the U.S. are all autonomous. Initially, Miami Lighthouse was called the Florida Association of Workers for the Blind because during the early years the blind gathered, practiced their Braille, and made things like brooms and mops. With advances in technology, this sheltered workshop employment model diminished. Outside the USA, some cultures still have the blind making brooms. Recently, traveling to Israel, I visited the Muslim Institute for the Blind in Jerusalem where the blind make brooms for most cleaning applications. What is noteworthy for me is the importance of the blind having a purpose, a destination, and a community. Whether in Jerusalem or in the USA, the blind seek to be productive and independent. At this Institute, the blind were very productive.

In the USA with an emphasis on integrated, competitive employment and with the accommodations required under the Americans with Disabilities Act, the blind can have mainstream jobs if they received vision rehabilitation and vocational training, such as computer training.

With technology, the blind have access to information that enables them to read, to use an iPhone, to use a computer and with training to get mainstream, competitive employment. All of these skills require training. Center-based training on independent living skills, computer use, orientation and mobility and more enables the blind to meet others who have achieved excellent independent living skills.

New technology recently introduced such as the OrCam MyEye enables the blind to read documents, recognize faces, and identify previously entered consumer products such as money notes and credit cards to make shopping easier, and more. OrCam MyEye is a tiny smart camera with a small speaker that attaches to eyeglass frames attached by a cable to a mini-computer device that can fit in your pocket. Another innovation is a subscription service called AIRA that utilizes a tiny camera mounted to eyeglass frames enabling the blind subscriber to have access to a personal agent at a remote location who describes the environment through a camera on the glasses or using an iPhone camera, thus enabling the agent to describe to the subscriber of the service what the agent is seeing.

While every state has a school for the blind to train and educate schoolchildren, most large communities also have an agency serving the blind. The website of VisionServe Alliance (www.visionservealliance.org) provides a listing of agencies throughout the country that offer programs and services for the blind.

Programs offered by Miami Lighthouse are typical of the types of vision rehabilitation services available.

Children's Programs:

- Blind Babies Early Intervention Program provides home visitations and early intervention support to children from birth to 5 years of age, playgroups, family support groups, and consultative services with professionals. Our peer-reviewed article provides further information about our Babies Program [1].
- Pre-Kindergarten for three- and four-year-olds. Pre-Braille readiness and Braille instruction are part of the curriculum at Miami Lighthouse adapted for every age and ability.
- Summer Training and Recreation Program for children ages 5–13 is designed to enhance literacy skills, sharpen students' life skills, learn Braille and technology, and improve physical fitness through structured activities.
- Braille and Technology Literacy is a year-round program for children ages 5–13. Children learn computer technology and hone their Braille reading and writing skills. For a child who is blind and print impaired (cannot read large print), Braille reading and writing is literacy and talking books can supplement Braille books but are not a substitute for Braille.
- Family support and community outreach presentations.
- Pre-Employment Transition Services for students and youth enhance each individual's abilities to be successful in competitive employment, training, and academic settings.

Adult Programs:

- Orientation and Mobility instruction helps an individual gain better spatial awareness and travel independence to enable the blind or visually impaired maneuver in a sighted world.
- Personal Management and Communications teach individuals of all ages how to remain in their own home and establish an independent life.
- Job Readiness employment training helps analyze an individual's skills and interests in conjunction with today's business environment.
- Music program and state-of-the-art production studio allow teens and adults to learn performance, recording, sound engineering, and business skills. Our peer-reviewed article describes how people in our program who are visually impaired acquire marketable skills that lead to employment and independence [2].
- Computer and Technology training help a visually impaired individual to utilize technology to lead a more independent life.
- GED/Adult Basic Education, in partnership with Miami-Dade County Public Schools, provides blind and visually impaired adults the education needed to obtain their GED. English as a Second Language classes are offered for students whose first language is Spanish or Creole.

- Senior Group Health and Activities Program (SGA) offers leisure activities that also aid in improving one's life skills, including music, macramé, jewelry making, and other tactile arts, field trips, and counseling regarding disease management. Our peer-reviewed article demonstrates how participation in the arts provides positive outcomes for adults with visual impairments [3].

Our Senior Groups Health and Activities program addresses the issue that social opportunities for interaction among adults affected by sudden loss of useful vision or blindness throughout most of their life often results in greater independence and other outcomes related to adjustment to blindness. The positive outcomes shown in our journal article continue as demonstrated by recently collected data. Surveys from the past 4 years for over 400 Senior Group and Health Activities participants found that:

- 99% of clients felt that the program directly related to them remaining independent in their daily lives
- 99% of clients felt the program was beneficial to them and the time they spent here was valuable to their overall well-being
- 98% of clients felt they were making progress through the program in their skills[1]

It is generally accepted, and research confirms that people with disabilities, like the blind, tend to more frequently suffer from social isolation and loneliness that often lead to depression. Our Senior Group Health and Activities Program article cited above quoted one program participant, "When I lost my sight, I thought it was all over for me. I went into a deep depression." Another program participant was described as extremely depressed when she began the program. This client remained active in the program and subsequently encouraged others with their adjustment to vision loss. The article also stated that participants in our program demonstrated increased feelings of self-esteem, which reflected a more positive self-image, a greater acceptance of their blindness and a willingness to help their peers overcome similar obstacles. By attending a center-based program, feelings of social isolation can be mitigated, relationships can be created, and in some cases peer mentors become role models.

These outcomes related to seniors demonstrate the importance for visually impaired people of all age groups to seek vision rehabilitation programs and take advantage of available resources in order to obtain the skills to lead independent and productive lives.

Other resources for blind individuals include two consumer groups: the National Federation of the Blind (www.nfb.org) and the American Council of the Blind (www.acb.org). Both sites have links to other resources for the blind. The American Foundation for the Blind's (www.afb.org) goal is to ensure that individuals who are blind or visually impaired have access to the information, technology, education, and legal resources they need to lead independent and productive lives and to provide a national clearing house for information about vision loss.

---

[1] Blind Babies play program article.

Blind individuals in Miami-Dade County, Florida, can contact Miami Lighthouse for the Blind and Visually Impaired, 601 SW 8th Avenue, Miami, Florida 33130, 305-856-2288, www.miamilighthouse.org. We offer vision rehabilitation training for the blind and visually impaired of all ages in our community ranging from blind babies to seniors with age-related vision loss.

References

1. Jacko VA, Mayros R, Brady-Simmons C, Chica I, Moore JE. Blind babies play program: a model for affordable, sustainable early childhood literacy intervention through play and socialization. J Vis Impair Blind. 2013;107(3):238–42.
2. Jacko VA, Cobo H, Cobo A, Fleming R, Moore JE. Mainstream employment in music production for individuals who are visually impaired: development of a model training program. J Vis Impair Blind. 2010;104(9):519–22.
3. McKenzie AR, Palma T. Intervention through art for adults who are blind or visually impaired. J Assoc Educ Rehabil Blind Vis Impair. 2009;2(1):9–11.

Chapter 5
History of Ocular Implants

Kelly H. Yom and Audrey C. Ko

Prehistory/Before Ocular Implants

Throughout human history, the removal of an offending or disfigured eye has been well documented. In fact, it is thought that a rudimentary version of an enucleation was one of the earliest ocular surgeries performed by mankind. Of course, with the removal of an eye comes the natural desire to replace what was lost, whether for functional, cosmetic, or psychological reasons. Although the ocular implant as we know it was not conceived until 1885, any number of materials have been historically implanted in anophthalmic sockets in attempts to do so, including wool, clay, sponge, rubber, paraffin, ivory, cork, cartilage, fat, bone, and metals such as gold, silver, platinum, aluminum, or vitallium [1, 2].

The earliest documented cases of ocular implants come from ancient Egyptian civilizations. Mummies have been excavated with artificial eyes found in the sockets made of precious metals, gemstones, and obsidian (Fig. 5.1) [3]. These artificial eyes are thought to have been implanted after death as a decorative means to allow the soul of the owner to see and navigate its way into the afterlife; there was little indication that intraorbital implants were routinely inserted into the sockets of living people.

Prior to the nineteenth century, surgical eye removal was rarely performed due to a high risk of uncontrolled bleeding and poor pain control [5]. Even when the operation – called extirpation – was performed, it was a crude procedure that did not spare the conjunctiva or the extraocular muscles and resulted in the orbital cavity granulating in on itself. As such, eye removal techniques were not yet sophisticated enough to create an acceptable soft tissue space for the introduction of an ocular

K. H. Yom · A. C. Ko (✉)
University of Iowa Hospitals and Clinics, Department of Ophthalmology and Visual Sciences, Iowa City, IA, USA
e-mail: kelly-yom@uiowa.edu; audrey-ko@uiowa.edu

T. E. Johnson (ed.), *Anophthalmia*,
https://doi.org/10.1007/978-3-030-29753-4_5

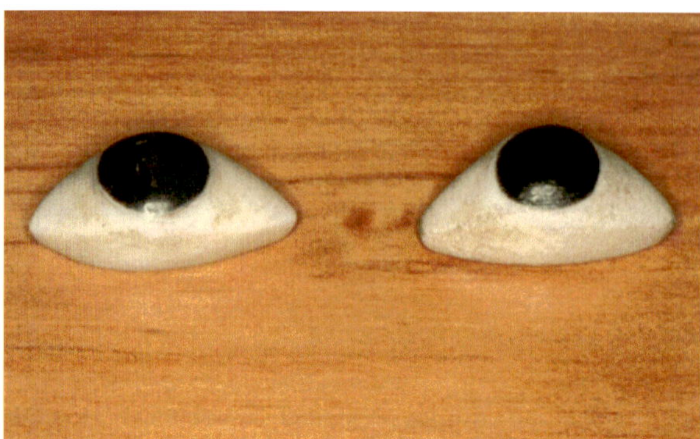

Fig. 5.1 Prosthetic eyes such as these – made from wax, glass, and onyx – are some of the oldest artificial eyes known to exist. (Image from Pine et al. [4] © Springer)

implant. Instead, the replacement of ocular contents took the form of thin, shell-shaped ocular prosthetics that were worn in the socket in front of either the disfigured eye or contracted orbital cavity after eye removal [3].

This type of indwelling ocular prosthetic first emerges in the medical literature of the sixteenth century. It is during this time that the French surgeon Ambroise Paré wrote about the many patients requiring anophthalmic care that he had encountered in his career as a military surgeon [1]. In 1575, he published a detailed account of ocular prostheses in use at the time, where he described the use of an "enblepharon" or "hypoblepharon" to be worn inside the socket over a phthisical shrunken globe [5]. These were shells made of gold or silver and colored with enamel and paint to mimic the color and texture of the remaining eye (Fig. 5.2) [6].

Simultaneously, elsewhere in Europe, Venetian glassblowers skilled in the making of doll eyes also had begun to make glass shells for use as human ocular prosthetics, although the glassmaking formulas and techniques were kept highly confidential and only passed down through the generations as family trade secrets [3]. These glass shells were brighter, more reflective, and more closely resembled natural eyes than the metal alternatives. However, they were quite brittle, had sharp edges, and were notoriously uncomfortable to wear, causing them to be irritating at best and dangerous at worst [5]. Moreover, because they were so thin, they did little to replace orbital volume, causing patients to have a significant enophthalmic appearance. Attempts to find alternative materials such as rubbers or celluloids were not fruitful, and glass remained the only viable option for ocular prostheses until the mid-1900s [3].

Italy remained the epicenter of artificial eye making for centuries until, in the 1820s, a generation of Parisian ocularists emerged with superior glassblowing techniques [7]. Glassmakers such as Hazard-Mirault, Desjardins, and Boissoneau in France came to rival those in Venice and eventually came to dominate the field [1]. Boissoneau in particular not only coined the term "ocularist" but was instrumental in shaping the theory and core tenets of the profession [8]. Then, in 1835, the epicenter shifted again when a German glassblower name Ludwig Muller Uri

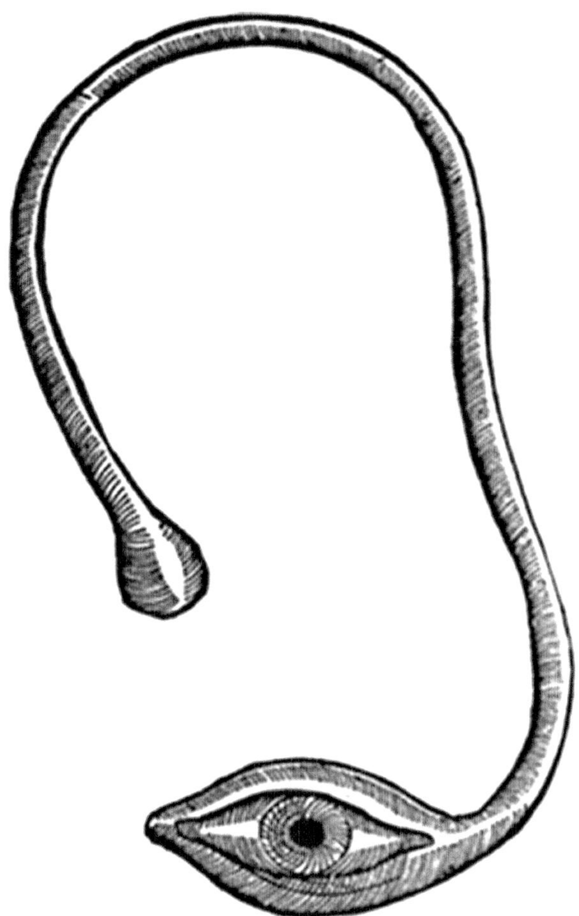

Fig. 5.2 One of Paré's designs for his ocular prostheses, meant to be worn in the eye socket with the metal arm wrapping around the head to secure it in place. This design was published in 1614 after his death. (Image from Pine et al. [4] © Springer)

developed a new cryolite glass, which not only mimicked the color of the sclera, but was lighter, sturdier, and less corrosive to the tissues of the eye socket than the previously used lead oxide glass [1, 4]. In addition to the invention of this superior glass material, Muller-Uri also redefined the way that the iris was painted onto the prosthetic, using colored glass instead of pigments. His techniques made the prosthetic more lifelike than any of its predecessors, and Muller-Uri's technique is still used to this day. Apprentices would flock to Germany to train under Muller-Uri, and Germany became the world's leader in glass manufacturing skills [1]. German craftsmen toured the world, making artificial eyes. They could be custom fit to individual patients' sockets, or doctors could order a stock of pre-made artificial eyes from which the best fit for a patient would be found.

The First Ocular Implant

It was not until the modern surgical techniques of enucleation and evisceration emerged in the mid-nineteenth century that the use of ocular implants did as well. The first-ever evisceration was reported in 1817 by James Bear for the management of expulsive hemorrhage, with J.F. Noyes describing the first planned, routine evisceration as a treatment for ocular infection in 1874; the enucleation, as we know it, was established in 1841 by the simultaneous but separate writings of O'Ferrall and Bonnet [9]. While these first decades of eviscerations and enucleations did not see the use of ocular implants, they were important in setting the stage for the spread and standardization of these eye removal techniques.

Subsequently, with the increase in popularity and availability of eye removal surgery, more and more patients were having intraocular contents or entire globes removed from the socket, only to find that the thin shells of the ocular prostheses at the time did little to restore the normal contours and protrusion of the eye socket. This left patients with a markedly sunken appearance to their removed eye. It quickly became clear that eye removal without implantation resulted in the retraction of Tenon's capsule, socket granulation, orbit disfiguration, and eyelid displacement. This only served to emphasize the inadequacy of the ocular prostheses alone, as they failed to replace the significant amounts of volume being lost from the orbit.

In response to this issue, spherical orbital implants were used for the first time in 1885 to replace volume in the orbit. P.H. Mules was the first to establish this milestone technique for evisceration in which a hollow, silicate glass sphere (which came to be known as the "Mules sphere") was inserted in the scleral cavity after removal of the cornea and intraocular contents [10]. The subsequent year, a similar hollow glass sphere was used as the orbital implant in an enucleation procedure, making the surgeon, William Adam Frost, the first to describe the placement of an implant into Tenon's capsule of an enucleated socket [11]. These orbital implants were novel in that they were able to minimize socket retraction and intraorbital fat redistribution, thus preventing a subsequent superior sulcus deformity and resulting enophthalmos. Additionally, because the orbital implant was positioned posteriorly behind the prosthesis, the implant provided enhanced foundational support for the prosthetic and allowed future prostheses to be thinner and lighter, reducing weight on the lower lid and any resulting ectropion [12].

Even though the postoperative volume-filling benefits of the Mules spheres were immediately evident, these pioneering implants were associated with a number of adverse events. For example, the first implants had an initial extrusion rate of up to 90%; this rate decreased to 21% by 1898 and further dropped to less than 10% by 1944 with improvements in aseptic surgical technique [7, 13, 14]. The Mules spheres would also occasionally break during trauma or implode with extreme temperature changes due to their fragile glass composition and hollow cavity. Finally, in the early 1900s, the newly adopted internal spherical glass orbital implants were paired for the first time with external ocular prostheses. However, because the Mules spheres were smooth glass surfaces without any connection to the remaining rectus muscles nor to the overlying prosthetic, there was virtually no motility of the prosthetic eye. The next major milestone in orbital implants would have to address these issues – extrusion, frailty, and poor motility.

One initially proposed surgical solution was to imbricate or overlap the rectus muscles and sew them to each over the anterior surface of the ocular implant, essentially "locking" the implant within the muscle cone [7, 15]. By adding another tissue layer between the external environment and the ocular implant, this technique was theorized to prevent extrusion by mechanically securing the implant in place. However, in practice, the imbricated muscles created a posteriorly directed pressure that caused migration of the implant superotemporally, between the superior and lateral recti muscles [15]. In an effort to further stabilize the implant in place and prevent both extrusion in the anterior direction and displacement in the superotemporal direction, the Wheeler implant was designed in 1938 [16]. This implant was designed with four grooves meant to receive the rectus muscles and prevent rotation or migration of the implant within the muscle cone. While the clover-like shape was revolutionary and would come to inspire future iterations of implants, the Wheeler implant itself was composed of a cork material which was inevitably rejected by the body, so never gained much popularity beyond its prototype phase.

The Emergence of Acrylics

With the beginning of WWII in 1939, the number of wartime causalities increased demand for artificial eyes. Unfortunately, German manufactured glass artificial eyes became harder and harder to find, as wartime shortages had limited the availability of German goods. German glassblowers stopped touring the United States, stockpiles of German glass eyes dwindled, and American ocularists were hard-pressed to find other solutions [3]. This led the United States to invest in the research and development of alternative materials to glass for the orbital implants. One effort, led largely by the US Naval Dental and Medical School, focused on making both orbital implants and prosthetics out of acrylic resin [4]. One type of resin, poly methyl methacrylate (PMMA), had already found popularity in the field of dentistry as a material for dentures [1]. The first orbital implant made of PMMA was a solid, lightweight sphere in 1976, and it was quickly discovered that ocular hardware made out of plastic afforded distinct advantages over those made of glass – they were easily and cheaply manufactured, virtually unbreakable, and were inert to etching by ocular fluids [7]. Silicone also quickly gained popularity for many of the same reasons (Fig. 5.3) [7]. In a matter of years, these plastics replaced glass as the preferred material for the ocular prosthesis in the US. The pliable nature of the acrylic allowed greater customization in the shape of the prosthetic eye, which allowed for the conceptualization of new designs of implants and prostheses to promote motility of the prosthetic eye.

These implants, like the ones made of glass before them, had no means of having the recti muscles attached to them – in other words, they were non-integrated.

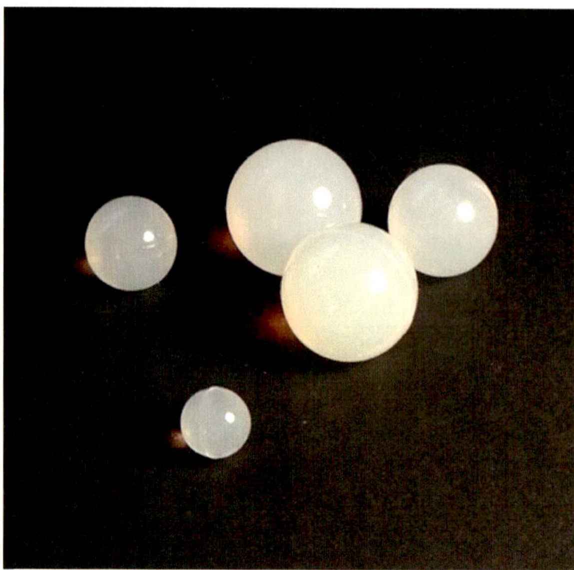

Fig. 5.3 Orbital implants made of silicone. (Image from Baino and Potestio [17]. © Elsevier)

Securing the recti muscles to the implant itself was the next proposed advancement. This would mean both diminish the risk of extrusion and enhance motility, as the recti muscles would be able to provide traction to the orbital implant, transmitting conjugate movements the prosthetic in sync with the contralateral eye. One way that this was achieved with these solid, nonporous materials was by wrapping the implant in mesh, autologous fascia, or donor sclera, providing a surgeon a surface directly on the implant to suture the muscles to.

In Search of Increased Motility

With the increased material pliability of PMMA came an explosion of different implant designs, each one highly focused on maximizing the mobility of the prosthetic. Each of these designs, whether successful or not, imparts a lesson on what the ideal orbital implant should and should not be able to do.

The first type of these were implants that had a direct mechanical connection to the prosthesis and were called exposed-integrated implants. In 1945, Ruedemann fabricated a combined ocular implant and ocular prosthesis [15]. The posterior portion of the device was made to be attached to the muscle cone, while the anterior portion consisted of the cosmetic portion of the prosthesis. This design was ultimately abandoned due to an inability to remove the prosthesis and issues with positional deviations. Two years later, in 1947 Cutler created the first peg-type implant (Cutler II), where the PMMA implant had an exposed face with a square receptacle, meant to receive a square peg protruding from the posterior side of the prosthesis [18]. This design, along with variations from Hughes, Whitney, Stone, and Rolf, made it clear that the direct coaptation of the prosthesis and the implant allowed for improved mobility. However, exposed-integrated implants, due to the chronically exposed conjunctival surface, were associated with high rates of infection, recurrent granulation, and excessive secretions, which caused subsequent dehiscence and extrusion [15, 16]. As a result, exposed-integrated implants were rather quickly dismissed as a safe and viable option for ocular implantation.

An alternative and concurrently evolved design was the quasi-integrated, or buried-integrated, orbital implant. The first buried-integrated implant reportedly used was in 1945 by Cutler (Cutler I) [7]. This PMMA implant had a central concavity over which the conjunctiva was closed. A prosthesis was then designed with a knob on its posterior aspect, made to fit into the concavity of the implant. This was the first predecessor to the Allen implant, which is one of the most common implants still used today. In 1946, the first prototype of the Allen implant was drafted (Fig. 5.4) [7]. What differentiated the Allen implant from its predecessor was that the protrusion originated from the implant and was received by a concavity in the prosthetic – the reverse of the Cutler I [7]. The Tenon's and conjunctiva were closed over the protrusion of the implant, making it a quasi-integrated orbital implant. The design of the Allen implant was also inspired by the Wheeler implant, with four grooves corresponding to the four recti muscles. Moreover, because the irregular anterior surface coaptated with the grooves in the prosthesis, any motion of the

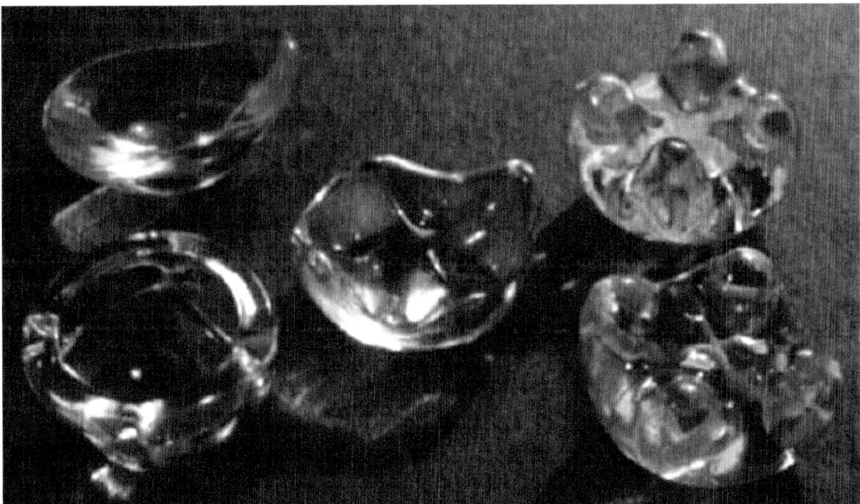

Fig. 5.4 Some of the most notable PMMA implants are the quasi-integrated implants, which are still used occasionally to this day. These all display surface mounds that not only coordinate the alignment of the rectus muscles but transfer the movement of these extraocular muscles to a complementarily shaped prosthesis. Allen implant, lower left. Iowa implant, upper right. Universal implant, lower right. Conformers for the Allen and Iowa implants are seen at the upper left and middle, respectively. (Image from Sami et al. [15] © Elsevier)

implant was translated to motion of the prosthetic. As such, this was a great option to restore normal motion of the eye. Major complications included prosthesis edge show on extreme gaze, lower lid droop and exaggeration of the upper lid sulcus due to poor ability to support the prosthetic's weight [15].

The Iowa implant was also a PMMA implant with a similar concept to the Allen implant – four mounds on the anterior surface of the implant found a complementary contour on the posterior of the prosthesis, and four depressions in the implant created slots for the rectus muscles to weave through (Fig. 5.4) [7, 19]. However, engineered changes in its design made it better able to support the prosthesis, minimizing the pull on the lower lid, and eliminated problems with problems of prosthesis edge show and torsional end gaze movements [19]. The exposure rate was about 9% – usually occurring over the mounds of the implant due to localized pressure necrosis – with an accompanying extrusion rate of 4% [19]. The most recent buried-integrated implant was introduced to the market in 1987 as the Universal implant [7]. This imparted all of the benefits of the Iowa implant, but with slightly less prominent mounds in the hope to decrease the pressure necrosis responsible for causing exposure. However, due to the rise in popularity of a different family of implants – the porous implants – the Universal implant fell out of favor before its efficacy was fairly judged [7].

A variation on the theme of the quasi-integrated orbital implant were the magnetic implants, which were buried behind conjunctiva and connected magnetically to the prosthesis via very strong magnets. The first of these implants were used into 1949 by Troutman, and although motility was shown to be well maintained, the magnets were capable of compressing the conjunctival tissue, causing tissue breakdown and exposure [20]. Moreover, rusting of the magnets was a large concern, with risks for ferrous toxicity (Fig. 5.5) [7].

The Advent of Porous Orbital Implants

In the 1950s, porous ceramics, both biological and synthetic, emerged as a potential biomaterial. The appeal of these materials, in addition to being durable and resistant to wear, was their ability to integrate into the soft ocular tissues via fibrovascularization. The porous matrix allows the vascular connective tissue to permeate throughout the implant's core architecture, imparting three main benefits: migration prevention due to the mechanical anchoring of the implant, infiltration by the immune system providing infection surveillance, and enhanced healing capabilities of soft tissue injuries [17].

The first of these porous materials to be used regularly as an orbital implant was hydroxyapatite (HA) – a calcium phosphate mineral network which comprises the primary inorganic portion of animal bone. This was introduced into the literature in 1899 by Schmidt as a derivative from charred cancellous bovine bone [7]. Guist popularized their use in the 1930s, and "Guist's bone spheres" were lauded as being effective and comfortable alternative to Mules' glass spheres [21, 22]. Despite high

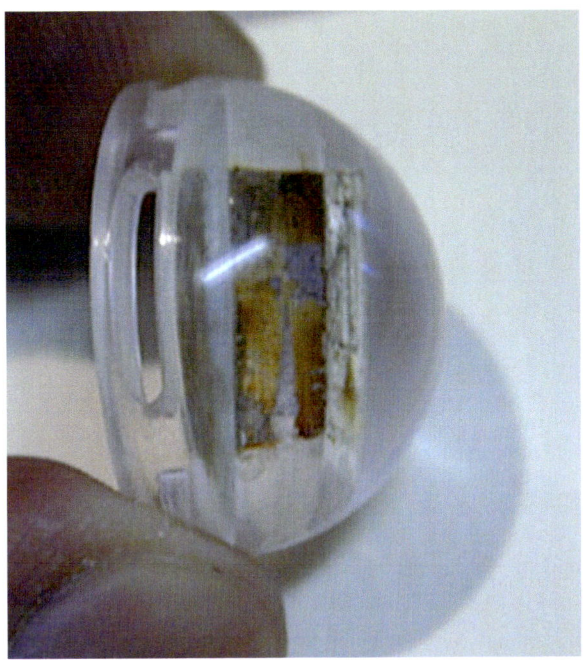

Fig. 5.5 Magnetic orbital implant demonstrating significant rusting. (Image from Sami et al. [15] © Elsevier)

praise, they were overshadowed by the excitement of the novel nonporous PMMA and silicone implants in the 1940s and bone implants were moved out of the spotlight for several decades. Eventually, the high exposure rates experienced with the use of polymer implants redirected some focus back to porous materials in an attempt to find implants that were more resistant to migration and able to spontaneously heal small exposures [23]. Furthermore, medical research on HA had been steadily progressing thanks to Per-Ingvår Branemark, who made the initial discovery in 1952 that HA integrates with bone and soft tissue [24].

Thus, the stage was set for the resurfacing of natural bone apatite, and in the 1970s a New Zealand professor named Anthony Molteno launched the Molteno M-Sphere, which is currently still in use, albeit much more rarely than before [25]. Derived from the deproteinized bone of calf fibulae, this mineralized matrix of cancellous bone imparted all of the aforementioned benefits of porous implants. They are also extremely light, decreasing tension on lower lid structures and minimizing the potential for deformity such as ectropion [26]. However, this material is not without major drawbacks. Molteno M-Sphere implants are rather brittle due to their high porosity and extremely expensive to manufacture [27]. HA has also been shown to incite a foreign body giant cell reaction, sometimes years after the introduction of the implant. Additionally, the surface of the implant is rough and abrasive, which is associated with conjunctival thinning and increased the potential for exposure, infection, and pyogenic granuloma formation. To compensate, these

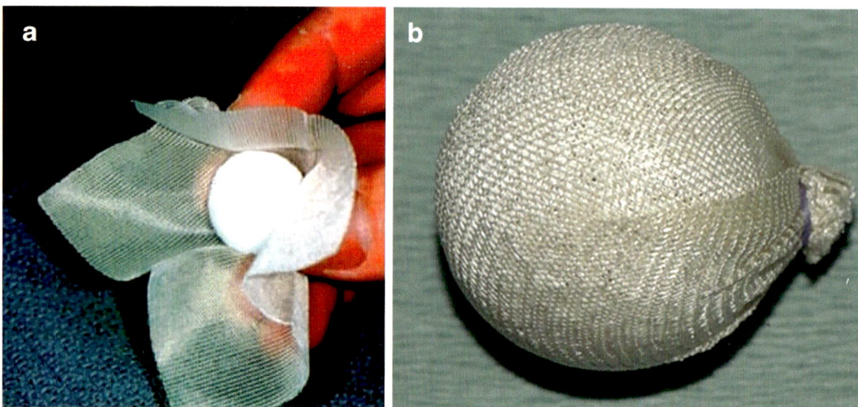

Fig. 5.6 Wrapping of an orbital implant in Vicryl mesh protects the soft tissues of the orbit from abrasion during insertion and provides a substrate to which extraorbital muscles may be sutured. (Image (a) from Jordan and Klapper [28]. © Springer. Image (b) from Baino and Potestio [17]. © Elsevier)

implants are often wrapped in Vicryl mesh or donor sclera during insertion [7]. Wrapping the implant also allows the intraocular muscles to be sutured to the otherwise too brittle material (Fig. 5.6). Finally, because the hydroxyapatite sphere is buried under the conjunctiva without any means of transmitting motion to the overlying prosthesis, motility with this early porous implant is often quite poor.

In an effort to develop a porous orbital implant that was also more durable, in 1985, Perry and Dutton independently introduced the use of HA spheres derived from sea coral (Bio-Eye, Fig. 5.7) [28–30]. These coralline structures are complex calcium phosphate matrices with interconnected pores [30]. Similar to the Molteno M-Sphere, these are very costly materials, as they must be harvested from natural reef-building marine corals; the damage caused to delicate marine ecosystems is also a cause for ethical concern [7]. Coralline HA is also abrasive and must be wrapped in a sheet of material that both prevents conjunctival thinning and allows attachment of the muscles. Newer versions of the Bio-Eye have been able to bypass this drawback by incorporating a polymer coating that makes them less abrasive and allows direct fixation of the extraocular muscles onto the implant. One notable trait of the Bio-Eye HA implants is that they have a lower porosity than the bovine cancellous bone derived HA [28]. This makes the coralline HA much stronger; Bio-Eye implants are able to withstand the force of a drill and therefore and more amenable to pegging. Pegging involved the use of a titanium peg, which was drilled into the implant and then fit into a corresponding groove on the back of the prosthesis [28]. This allowed the movement of the orbital implant to be translated into movement of the prosthesis. However, because this technique requires a break in the conjunctiva, it can promote infection and lead to higher rates of extrusion [31]. As such, many

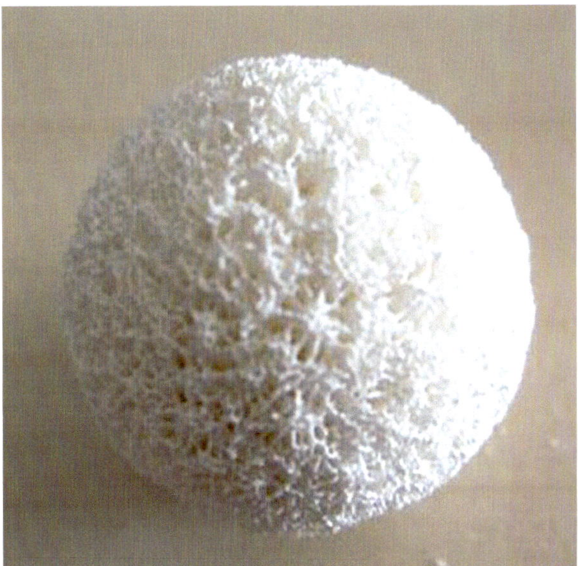

Fig. 5.7 The Bio-Eye orbital implant. (Image from Baino et al. [7] © Elsevier)

surgeons elect not to peg HA implants, even when they are durable enough to handle the procedure.

In the late 1970s, Teflon composites were the first artificial materials developed to be used as porous implants. Carbon/Teflon composites (Proplast I) and aluminum/Teflon composites (Proplast II) were developed and early experience showed satisfactory outcomes after implant use with no migration or extrusion [7, 32, 33]. However, due to a high rate of late-onset infections with Proplast I and poor vascularization due to pseudocapsule formation with Proplast II, these materials were abandoned in a matter of decades [34].

The next porous artificial material to be developed was polyethylene (PE), which started to be used as an orbital implant in the late 1980s [35, 36]. Although this material is less biocompatible than HA, it is still decently well tolerated by orbital soft tissue. The biggest appeal to PE is that it has a nonabrasive surface, meaning that exposure and extrusion are rare, even without wrapping the implant [7]. PE also allows the extraocular muscles to be sutured directly onto implant, further decreasing the need for wrapping (Fig. 5.8).

1990 saw the rise of synthetic HA, also known as FCI3 [37]. This material, generated in the laboratory, has a matrix structure virtually identical to that of coralline HA, but is much less costly to produce and spares the damage done to any coral reef ecosystems [28]. The largest disadvantages noted with these materials is that, unless tightly regulated, the HA may contain defects that can range from subpar porous

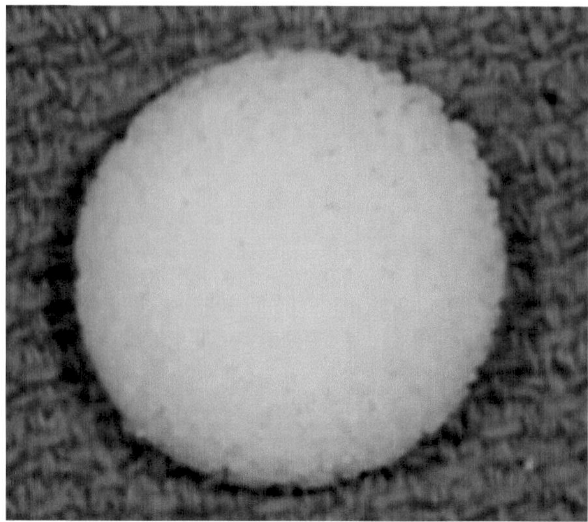

Fig. 5.8 A polyethylene (PE) orbital implant. (Image from Jordan and Klapper [28]. © Springer)

structure that limits fibrovascularization to contamination with caustic impurities [38, 39].

Finally, one of the most recent orbital implants to come to light is the use of porous alumina spheres. This orbital implant was approved by the FDA in 2000 and has garnered attention for being as biocompatible, if not more so, than HA [40]. This is due to the observation that fibroblasts and osteoblasts proliferate more rapidly on alumina than HA, as well as the fact that a protein coating is formed around the implant after insertion, which prevents it from being recognized and rejected as a foreign body and makes alumina is incredibly inert. Moreover, the surface texture of alumina is smoother than HA implants (Fig. 5.9) [41]. All of these factors serve to make alumina one of the least inflammatory implants to date.

Looking to the Future

The most commonly used orbital implants nowadays include silicone, hydroxyapatite, and polyethylene. However, to this day, the search continues to design an orbital implant that will perfectly address all of the pitfalls and shortcomings that have been presented thus far. Until then, remembering the innovations that have delivered us the implants as we known them today will guide us in this quest.

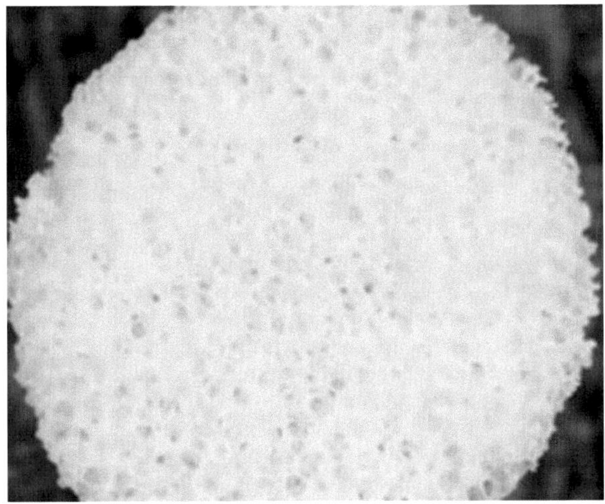

Fig. 5.9 A close-up view of an alumina orbital implant. (Image from Jordan and Klapper [28]. © Springer)

References

1. Reisberg DJ, Habakuk SW. A history of facial and ocular prosthetics. Adv Ophthalmic Plast Reconstr Surg. 1990;8:11–24.
2. Yousef YA. Enucleation surgery—orbital implants and surgical techniques. US Ophthalmic Rev. 2016;09(01):46–8.
3. Danz W Sr. Ancient and contemporary history of artificial eyes. Adv Ophthalmic Plast Reconstr Surg. 1990;8:1–10.
4. Pine KR, Sloan BH, Jacobs RJ. History of ocular prosthetics. In: Clinical ocular prosthetics. Cham: Springer; 2015. p. 283–312.
5. den Tonkelaar I, Henkes HE, van Leersum GK. Herman Snellen (1834–1908) and Muller's 'reform-auge'. A short history of the artificial eye. Doc Ophthalmol. 1991;77(4):349–54.
6. Martin O, Clodius L. The history of the artificial eye. Ann Plast Surg. 1979;3(2):168–71.
7. Baino F, Perero S, Ferraris S, et al. Biomaterials for orbital implants and ocular prostheses: overview and future prospects. Acta Biomater. 2014;10(3):1064–87.
8. Wood CA. A system of ophthalmic operations: being a complete treatise on the operative conduct of ocular diseases and some extraocular conditions causing eye symptoms. Chicago: Cleveland Press; 1911.
9. Luce CM. A short history of enucleation. Int Ophthalmol Clin. 1970;10(4):681–7.
10. Mules PH. Evisceration of the globe with artificial vitreous. 1884–1895. Adv Ophthalmic Plast Reconstr Surg. 1990;8:69–72.
11. Soll DB. The anophthalmic socket. Ophthalmology. 1982;89(5):407–23.
12. Gougelmann HP. The evolution of the ocular motility implant. Int Ophthalmol Clin. 1970;10(4):689–711.
13. Guyton JS. Enucleation and allied procedures: a review, and description of a new operation. Trans Am Ophthalmol Soc. 1948;46:472–527.
14. Culler AM. Orbital implants after enucleation; basic principles of anatomy and physiology of the orbit and relation to implant surgery. Trans Am Acad Ophthalmol Otolaryngol. 1952;56(1):17–20.

15. Sami D, Young S, Petersen R. Perspective on orbital enucleation implants. Surv Ophthalmol. 2007;52(3):244–65.
16. Soll DB. Evolution and current concepts in the surgical treatment of the anophthalmic orbit. Ophthalmic Plast Reconstr Surg. 1986;2(3):163–71.
17. Baino F, Potestio I. Orbital implants: state-of-the-art review with emphasis on biomaterials and recent advances. Mater Sci Eng C. 2016;69:1410–28.
18. Cutler NL. A positive contact ball and ring implant for use after enucleation. Arch Ophthalmol. 1947;37(1):73–81.
19. Spivey BE, Allen L, Burns CA. The Iowa enucleation implant: a 10-year evaluation of technique and results. Am J Ophthalmol. 1969;67(2):171–88.
20. Troutman RC. Five-year survey on use of a magnetic implant for improving cosmetic result of enucleation. AMA Arch Ophthalmol. 1954;52(1):58–62.
21. Allen TD. Guist's bone spheres. Am J Ophthalmol. 1930;13(3):226.
22. McCoy LL. Guist bone sphere. Am J Ophthalmol. 1932;15(10):960.
23. Bansal RK. Cadaver bone as orbital implant. Br J Ophthalmol. 1976;60(6):486–8.
24. Ratner BD, Hoffman AS, Schoen FJ, Lemons JE. Biomaterials science: an introduction to materials in medicine. Saint Louis: Elsevier Science; 2004.
25. Molteno AC, van Rensberg JH, van Rooyen B, Ancker E. "Physiological" orbital implant. Br J Ophthalmol. 1973;57(8):615–21.
26. Frueh BR. Bone implants after enucleation. Aust N Z J Ophthalmol. 1991;19(2):97.
27. Jordan DR, Hwang I, Brownstein S, et al. The molteno M-sphere. Ophthalmic Plast Reconstr Surg. 2000;16(5):356–62.
28. Guthoff R, Katowitz JA. Oculoplastics and orbit. Berlin, New York: Springer; 2007.
29. Dutton JJ. Coralline hydroxyapatite as an ocular implant. Ophthalmology. 1991;98(3):370–7.
30. Nunery WR, Heinz GW, Bonnin JM, Martin RT, Cepela MA. Exposure rate of hydroxyapatite spheres in the anophthalmic socket: histopathologic correlation and comparison with silicone sphere implants. Ophthalmic Plast Reconstr Surg. 1993;9(2):96–104.
31. Jordan DR, Chan S, Mawn L, et al. Complications associated with pegging hydroxyapatite orbital implants. Ophthalmology. 1999;106(3):505–12.
32. Shah S, Rhatigan M, Sampath R, et al. Use of proplast II as a subperiosteal implant for the correction of anophthalmic enophthalmos. Br J Ophthalmol. 1995;79(9):830–3.
33. Lyall MG. Proplast implant in Tenon's capsule after excision of the eye. Trans Ophthalmol Soc U K. 1976;96(1):79–81.
34. Whear NM, Cousley RRJ, Liew C, Henderson D. Post-operative infection of proplast facial implants. Br J Oral Maxillofac Surg. 1993;31(5):292–5.
35. Karesh JW, Dresner SC. High-density porous polyethylene (Medpor) as a successful anophthalmic socket implant. Ophthalmology. 1994;101(10):1688–95; discussion 1695–6.
36. Blaydon SM, Shepler TR, Neuhaus RW, White WL, Shore JW. The porous polyethylene (Medpor) spherical orbital implant: a retrospective study of 136 cases. Ophthalmic Plast Reconstr Surg. 2003;19(5):364–71.
37. Jordan DR, Bawazeer A. Experience with 120 synthetic hydroxyapatite implants (FCI3). Ophthal Plast Reconstr Surg. 2001;17(3):184–90.
38. Jordan DR, Hwang I, McEachren T, et al. Brazilian hydroxyapatite implant. Ophthalmic Plast Reconstr Surg. 2000;16(5):363–9.
39. Jordan DR, Pelletier CR, Gilberg TS, Brownstein S, Grahovac SZ. A new variety of hydroxyapatite: the Chinese implant. Ophthalmic Plast Reconstr Surg. 1999;15(6):420–4.
40. Jordan DR, Gilberg S, Mawn LA. The bioceramic orbital implant: experience with 107 implants. Ophthalmic Plast Reconstr Surg. 2003;19(2):128–35.
41. Salerno M, Reverberi A, Baino F. Nanoscale Topographical Characterization of Orbital Implant Materials. Materials (Basel). 2018;11(5):660.

Part II
Surgical Techniques

Chapter 6
Enucleation and Techniques of Orbital Implant Placement

Sara Tullis Wester

Background

While removal of the eye was performed by Sumerians and Egyptians thousands of years ago, the medical literature first described enucleation in the sixteenth century [1], and modifications over time have led to a significant improvement in patient outcomes. *Enucleation* refers to the removal of the eye and the anterior portion of the optic nerve from the orbit, with retention of the extraocular muscles to be attached to the implant. Due to the irreversibility and psychological impact of an enucleation, it is extremely important that the procedure be reserved for individuals with severe trauma, infection, pain, significant cosmetic deformity, or ocular tumors requiring surgical intervention. In addition, psychological support and guidance regarding the nature of the procedure and the postoperative course is exceedingly valuable to patients.

For optimal outcomes, it is important to recognize the complex interaction between the eye and surrounding orbital tissue. As in all surgical procedures, a well thought out and meticulous approach is needed to minimize the post operative risks of eyelid malposition, forniceal foreshortening, superior sulcus deformities, poor motility, poor eyelid closure, and implant migration or extrusion.

S. T. Wester (✉)
Bascom Palmer Eye Institute, Department of Oculoplastics, Miami, FL, USA
e-mail: swester2@med.miami.edu

T. E. Johnson (ed.), *Anophthalmia*,
https://doi.org/10.1007/978-3-030-29753-4_6

Indications

Enucleation or evisceration are often indicated in patients with a blind, painful eye. The choice between enucleation and evisceration can be controversial. In cases of suspected intraocular malignancy, inadequate scleral shell, or concern for sympathetic ophthalmia, enucleation is the procedure of choice. Evisceration does not provide an adequate specimen for pathological evaluation if there is any concern for malignancy, and ultrasound should be used to assess the posterior pole when direct visualization is prevented by anterior segment scarring to help guide decision making. In addition, when there is significant phthisis bulbi or inadequate scleral shell size, enucleation is advised.

While enucleation may be indicated for cosmetic rehabilitation in some cases, good cosmesis and motility can sometimes be achieved in patients without pain if the natural globe can be preserved and fitted with a scleral shell or cosmetic contact lens. In children particularly, the globe should be preserved whenever possible to provide a stimulus for orbital growth and development. In cases with persistent corneal sensation, a Gunderson flap may be indicated and will assist in tolerance of a scleral shell. For those with pain without cosmetic concerns, topical medications may often improve symptoms. Other therapies to restore comfort to a blind painful eye nonsurgically, such as retrobulbar alcohol injections, are controversial.

Due to the irreversible nature of the procedure, it is critical that a detailed informed consent is explained to the patient. Risks such as impaired motility, eyelid malpositions, infection, implant migration or extrusion, poor prosthetic fit, superior sulcus deformity, and the possibility of an asymmetric appearance are discussed. The procedure and postoperative period are reviewed extensively, including the temporary use of a conformer and the plan for prosthesis fitting by an ocularist (with samples shown to the patient if interested) at 5–6 weeks following surgery. In office drawings, which show implant placement and extraocular muscle attachment, can be helpful to some patients.

Surgical Procedure

Enucleation is most commonly performed with monitored anesthesia care and retrobulbar block, but in certain cases is performed under general anesthesia. Even when the eye to be removed is clinically notable by external examination, the operative side should obviously always be reconfirmed by reviewing clinic notes and the operative consent. The unoperated fellow eye should be protected with an ocular shield throughout the procedure, and it is helpful to let the patients know this eye will be covered to minimize anxiety or claustrophobia.

An eyelid speculum is placed, and a 360° conjunctival peritomy is performed adjacent to the corneoscleral limbus using blunt Westcott scissors, with care to preserve as much conjunctiva as possible and release Tenon's attachments to the sclera

(Fig. 6.1). A Steven's tenotomy scissor is passed into each quadrant and spread to separate Tenon's capsule from the sclera between the rectus muscles (Fig. 6.2). A smooth muscle hook is passed behind the rectus muscle insertion and care is taken to ensure the entire muscle is hooked and no adjacent Tenon's attachments have been hooked. A cotton tipped applicator can be useful for removing any attachments anteriorly (Fig. 6.3). The muscle is secured with a locking suture of double-armed 5-0 Vicryl™ near its insertion, with the first arm passed partial thickness through about one-half the width of the muscle and then the needle is passed back from the muscle edge full thickness about one-quarter to one-third the width of the muscle (Fig. 6.4). The muscle is then disinserted. This is done for each of the four recti muscles, and this should be done without significant disruption of the attachment of

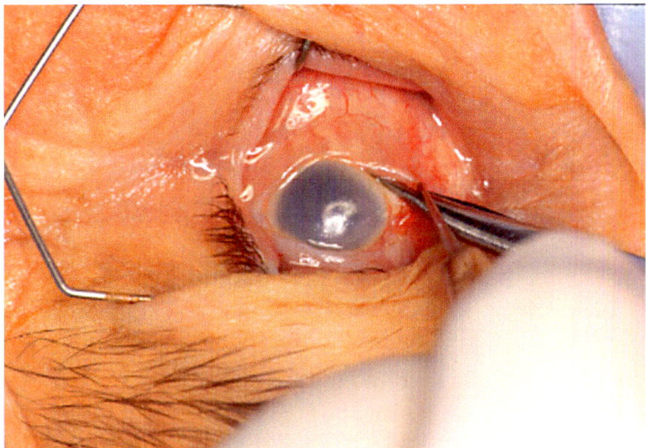

Fig. 6.1 An eyelid speculum is placed, and a 360° conjunctival peritomy is performed adjacent to the corneoscleral limbus using blunt Westcott scissors, with care to preserve as much conjunctiva as possible and release Tenon's attachments to the sclera

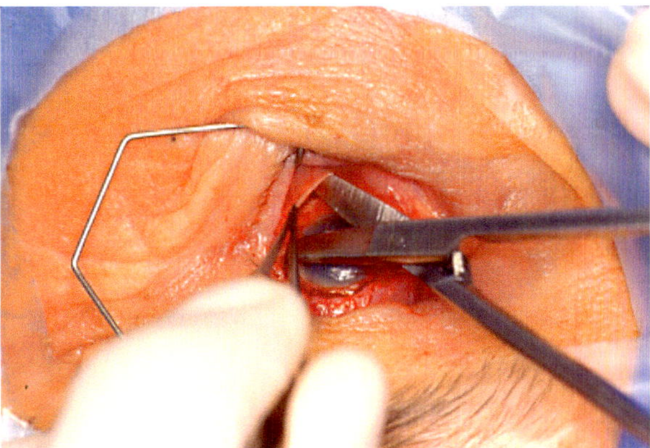

Fig. 6.2 A Steven's tenotomy scissor is passed into each quadrant and spread to separate Tenon's capsule from the sclera between the rectus muscles

the muscles to Tenon's capsule. The ends of the suture are clamped to the surrounding drape with a bulldog or hemostat. A 1- to 2-mm stump of medial rectus tendon is often left adherent to the sclera as this can be useful for traction later in the procedure. The inferior oblique muscle is isolated with a small muscle hook or by using a malleable retractor for exposure. It is cross-clamped with a hemostat before transection due to its vascularity. In certain cases, when the surgeon intends to attach the inferior oblique to the implant, a 5-0 Vicryl™ suture is used to secure it as well. The superior oblique muscle is identified and detached from the globe. Any remaining adherent tissues should be identified and separated from the globe with Stevens scissors as far posteriorly as possible (Fig. 6.5). Schepens and/or malleable retractors may assist in exposure at this point. In cases of multiple prior ocular surgeries,

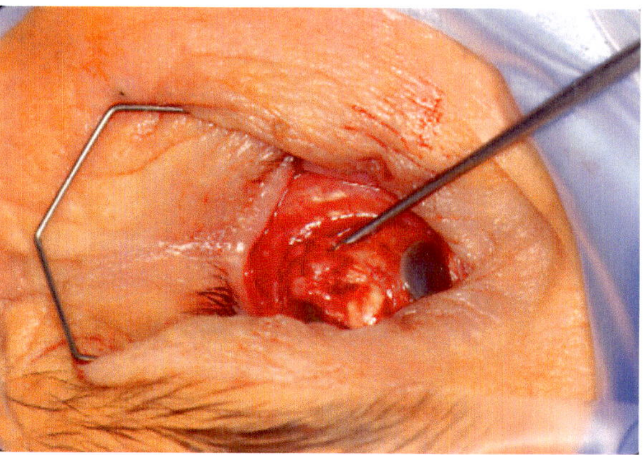

Fig. 6.3 A muscle hook is placed around each rectus muscle

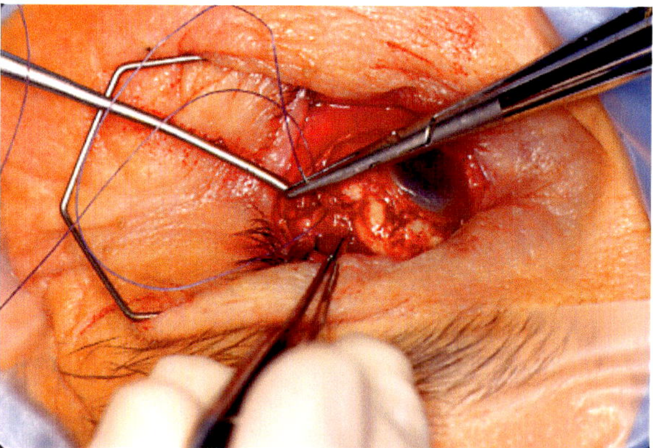

Fig. 6.4 The muscle is secured with a locking suture of double-armed 5-0 Vicryl near its insertion, with the first arm passed partial thickness through about one-half the width of the muscle, and then the needle is passed back from the muscle edge full thickness about one-quarter the width of the muscle

significant scarring and implants such as glaucoma drainage implants or scleral buckles may be encountered. Any external implants should be removed and submitted separately to pathology. Once all adhesions are lysed, the globe should be able to rotate in either direction quite easily. At this point, the medial rectus muscle insertion is grasped with a hemostat, and the globe is gently elevated. A large curved hemostat is passed behind the globe from the medial side. The optic nerve position is determined by strumming the nerve with the closed instrument. The tips are then opened and placed on either side of the optic nerve as far posteriorly as possible. The nerve is clamped for several minutes (Fig. 6.6). When traction is placed on the rectus muscles or the nerve is clamped, care should be taken to ensure the patient's blood pressure and heart rate are stable as some patients can experience bradycardia due to the oculocardiac reflex [2]. The hemostat is removed and a curved enucleation scissors is passed behind the globe in a similar fashion. The nerve is then

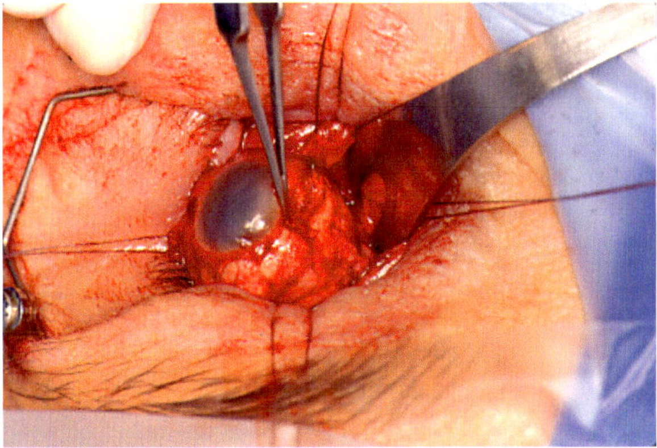

Fig. 6.5 Any remaining adherent tissues should be identified and separated from the globe with Stevens scissors as far posteriorly as possible

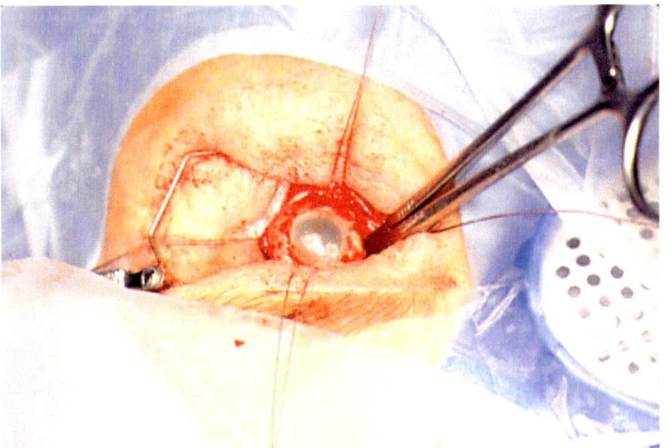

Fig. 6.6 The nerve is clamped for several minutes

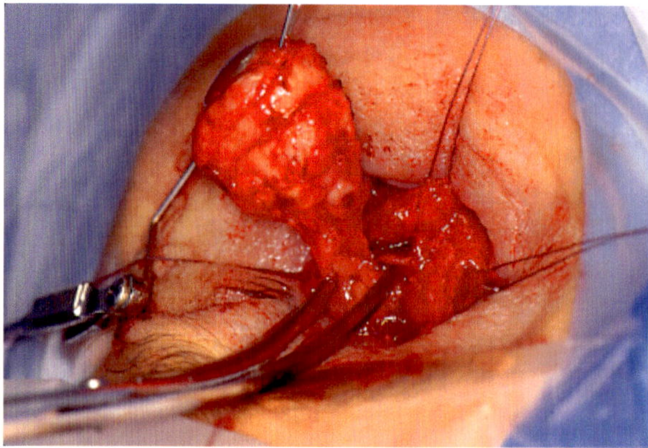

Fig. 6.7 The nerve is then transected, taking care to avoid trauma to the rectus muscles by retracting them away from the inserter, and the globe is removed

transected, taking care to avoid trauma to the rectus muscles by retracting them away from the scissors, and the globe is removed (Fig. 6.7). In cases of ocular tumors, the maximal amount of optic nerve possible should be transected.

Once the globe is removed, the socket is packed with either an acrylic sizer or a moistened gauze pad and pressure is applied for several minutes. Typically, eyes with chronic glaucoma and atrophic optic nerves may have less bleeding. When the gauze is removed, the socket is inspected and any residual bleeding is cauterized with bipolar cautery. In cases where patients are anticoagulated, it is often advisable to keep pressure on the socket while preparing the implant as this will help with hemostasis.

It should also be noted that in cases of severe ocular injury with either primary enucleation (which should be a very rare procedure due to the associated psychosocial impact to patients) or secondary enucleation soon after failed ruptured globe repair, all uveal tissue should be removed and the orbit should be carefully inspected.

At this point, attention is directed to the preparation of the implant. A variety of implants may be used, but it is important to review the evolution of orbital implants over time to understand some of the risks and benefits as well as variations in operative technique associated with different implant types.

Types of Implants

While the first orbital implant for enucleation was placed in the late 1800s [3], the ideal surgical implant is still controversial. Initial implants were typically glass, but over the past almost 150 years, myriad orbital implants have been developed in an attempt to improve the results of enucleation surgery. Interestingly, many of the implants developed over time have been associated with increased postoperative complications and are therefore no longer used. Although there are many different classifications of implant types [4, 5], for purposes of simplicity, many break implants into the categories of buried (may be nonintegrated, porous, or with biogenic wrapping), exposed-integrated, and quasi-integrated implants. Herein, we will briefly discuss orbital implants, but for a full review please see the Chapter on Orbital Implants.

Simple, buried spherical implants, such as silicone, glass, or polymethyl methacrylate (PMMA), are positioned within the muscle cone either anterior or posterior to the posterior Tenon's capsule. When the spherical implants are wrapped (see below), the muscles may be attached to the "muscles windows" created in the sclera. Of note, in young children who may receive multiple implants for progressive orbital and socket expansion (although this is not the authors' preferred technique for congenital anophthalmos), a wrapped silicone implant is preferred during the expansion phase to prevent fibrovascular ingrowth which makes implant exchange more difficult [5]. Motility in unwrapped, nonporous spherical implants is felt to be dependent on forniceal movement, as the smooth contour of the spherical implant cannot engage the overlying prosthesis. Due to suboptimal results with this, in cases where wrapping is not available, attachment of the extraocular muscles to the conjunctival fornices may enhance prosthesis motility. Cross-suturing of the extraocular muscles in front of the implant is less efficient in transmitting movement and is not advised as it may be associated with postoperative sphere migration [6, 7]. Some surgeons find silicone implants preferable due to a low extrusion rate (0.84% in 119 patients over a 10-year follow-up period) [8] and lower cost, but others have been frustrated by the implants' poor motility and higher risk of migration. This has led to the development of a variety of different implant types (exposed integrated implants, tantalum mesh spheres, and quasi-integrated implants such as the Allen, Iowa, and Universal). Interestingly, however, these implants have had other complications such as high extrusion and migration rates [9], exposure and eyelid malpositions [10]. Several additional modifications were made to these implants (Iowa implant II [11, 12] and Universal implant [13, 14]) to improve outcomes [15], but around this time porous implants were introduced and became more widely used.

Porous implants were first used in the late nineteenth century using the mineral framework of bovine cancellous bone, but were for the most part replaced after WWII by more biologically inert spheres [16, 17]. In 1989, however, the Bio-eye coralline hydroxyapatite (HA) orbital implant (Bio-Eye; Integrated Orbital Implants, San Diego, CA), which is a biocompatible integrated orbital implant derived from a specific genus of marine coral, received FDA approval. Since then, numerous other porous implants have been developed (such as synthetic HA and synthetic porous polyethylene implants). The benefits of these porous implants included fibrovascular ingrowth, which was thought to reduce the risk of migration, extrusion, and infection. Interestingly, coralline HA orbital implants have been shown to have more rapid vascularization than synthetic [18]. Some of the reported complications of HA implants, however, include cost, conjunctival thinning, exposure (although easier to treat than in silicone exposure cases and less common when the implants are wrapped [19]), discharge and/or chronic infection [20], pyogenic granuloma, and discomfort [21, 22]. Synthetic porous polyethylene implants (MEDPOR; Stryker Corporation, Kalamazoo, MI) are less biocompatible and have less vascular integration than HA, but they are usually well tolerated and have a smoother surface allowing for easier implantation. Several studies have been performed to compare outcomes between HA and PP implants with conflicting results [23, 24]. Some authors have cited increased exposure risk with HA implants, as well as more pronounced postoperative edema and erythema [25]. Others have found higher extrusion rates with porous polyethylene (although the porous polyethylene were unwrapped and compared to wrapped hydroxyapatite implants) [26]. Several studies, however, have found similar results between porous polyethylene and hydroxyapatite [23, 27] and most therefore suggest that implant choice be governed by patient factors, surgeon experience, ease of use, and cost.

Newer technologies have been released which preclude the need for scleral wrapping by allowing for direct suturing of the muscles to the implant, and will be discussed further in the Orbital Implant Chapter. In addition, there are ongoing studies of potential biomaterials with better vascular in-growth, anti-bacterial effects, and increased motility potential among other things as the "perfect implant" has not yet been found [5]. Regardless of implant type, meticulous surgical technique is essential to minimize complications.

Implant Placement

Preparation of Implant

Once the globe is removed and all bleeding points are cauterized, the largest sphere implant that will fit into Tenon's capsule without undue tension at closure of the anterior Tenon's capsule and conjunctiva (typically 20, 21, or 22 mm but anywhere between 18 and 22 mm diameter) is determined using a sizer (Fig. 6.8). Wrapping the implant in preserved sclera obtained from a whole cadaver eye (Fig. 6.9) facilitates the introduction of the rough-surfaced porous sphere and for all spherical implants (porous and non-porous) provides a covering on which to suture the extraocular muscles. When scleral wrapping is performed, it is important to remember that this will add approximately 1–2 mm of diameter to the implant when considering appropriate implant size. Other possible donor tissue may be used as wrapping material, such as bovine pericardium or acellular dermis. Thorough screening and appropriate precautions must be taken when implanting any donor material to reduce the risk of transmission of infectious disease. In addition, autogenous tissue (fascia, posterior auricular muscle, or periosteum) or synthetic materials such as polyglactin may be used to wrap the implants and eliminate the theoretical risk of infection transmission with donor material. Autogenous tissue harvest adds surgical time, however, which must be weighed against the exceedingly low risk of infectious disease transmission given appropriate screening and processing of donor tissue.

If sclera is used as the wrapping material, the implant is injected into the sclera after relaxing incisions are made on the anterior aspect of the donor sclera where the cornea was excised (Fig. 6.10). The sclera is then closed over the implant using 4-0

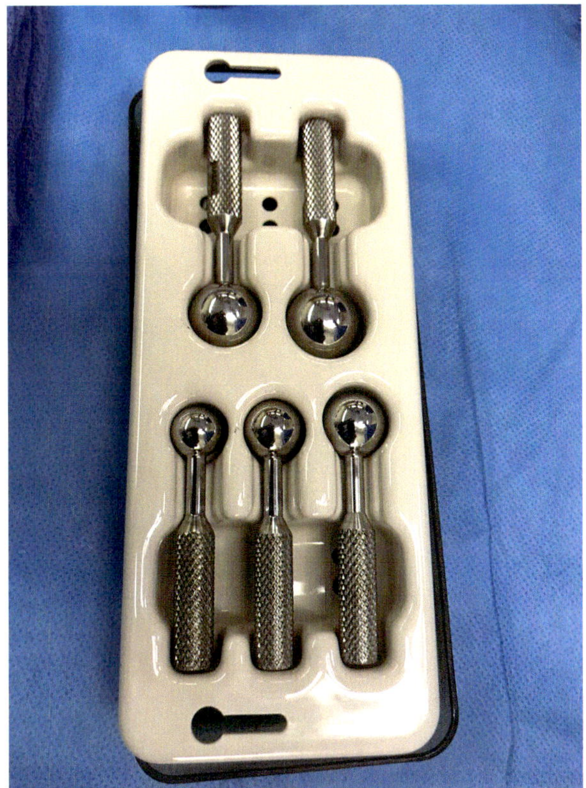

Fig. 6.8 The appropriate implant size is determined using a sizer

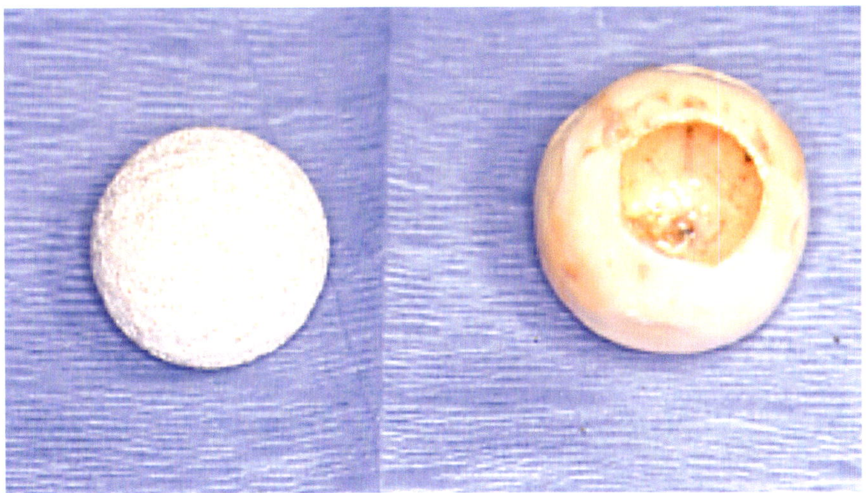

Fig. 6.9 The implant is wrapped in preserved sclera obtained from a whole cadaver eye

Vicryl™ suture in an interrupted fashion. Occasionally, redundant sclera is excised when a smaller than average implant is used so as to allow the implant to sit tightly in the sclera. Four "windows" are then marked in the sclera, each measuring approximately 2.5 × 5 mm, a few millimeters anterior to the equator of the sclera-wrapped implant and cut using Stevens scissors or a blade at the proposed 12, 3, 6, and 9 o'clock meridians (Fig. 6.11). Some individuals measure the spiral of Tillaux precisely to determine where the muscle windows should be placed, but most do not deem this necessary.

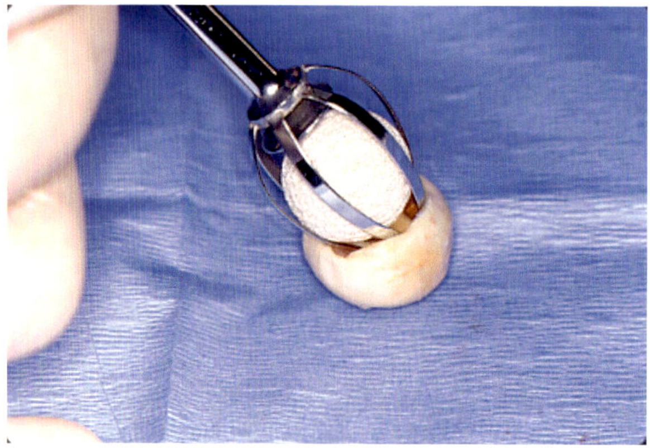

Fig. 6.10 The implant is injected into the sclera after relaxing incisions are made on the anterior aspect of the donor sclera where the cornea was excised

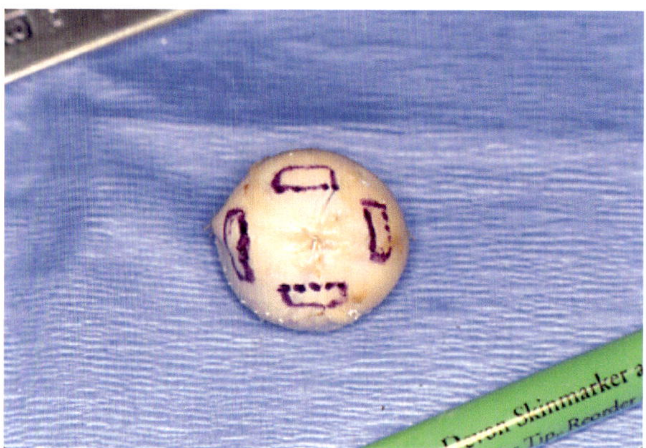

Fig. 6.11 Four "windows" are then marked in the sclera, each measuring approximately 2.5 × 5 mm, a few millimeters anterior to the equator of the sclera-wrapped implant and cut using Stevens scissors or a blade at the proposed 12:00, 3:00, 6:00, and 9:00 o'clock meridians

Placement of Implant

Attention is then directed to placement of the implant. The intraconal fat can be visualized through the vent created in the posterior Tenon's capsule after transecting the optic nerve. The wrapped implant is injected through this opening and placed within the Tenon's capsule using a sphere introducer (Fig. 6.12) with the exposed portion of the implant oriented posteriorly to promote fibrovascular ingrowth from the orbit.

If an introducer is not available, one can use the tip of a sterile glove to slide the implant in (cutting the tip of the finger off to allow removal of the glove material once the implant is in position). A Schepens or a malleable retractor may be used to help prevent the cactus effect while placing the implant [28]. Although rarely necessary, scissors may be used to enlarge the rent in posterior portion of Tenon's capsule to accommodate the implant.

The rectus muscles are sutured to the anterior lip of the corresponding scleral windows with the double-armed 5-0 Vicryl™ sutures in a mattress fashion. One of the rectus muscles is sutured to the scleral wrapping (Fig. 6.13). This step approximates the cut edge of the rectus muscle to the exposed portion of the porous material to promote fibrovascular ingrowth and improve motility. Models such as the MEDPOR smooth surface tunnel implant (MEDPOR SST; Stryker Corporation, Kalamazoo, MI) may allow for direct suturing of the muscles to the implant.

When no wrapping or pre-cut implants are available, the double-armed 5-0 Vicryl™ sutures secured to the ends of the rectus muscles may be passed through the anterior layer of Tenon's capsule and conjunctiva into the corresponding conjunctival fornices to transmit greater motility to the prosthesis.

The anterior Tenon's capsule is closed horizontally with interrupted 5-0 Vicryl™ sutures with the knots buried (Fig. 6.14). It is extremely important for the surgeon

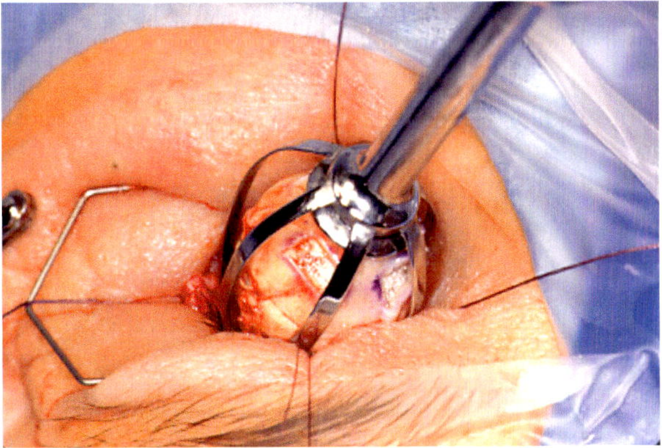

Fig. 6.12 The implant is injected through the opening in posterior Tenon's capsule using a sphere introducer

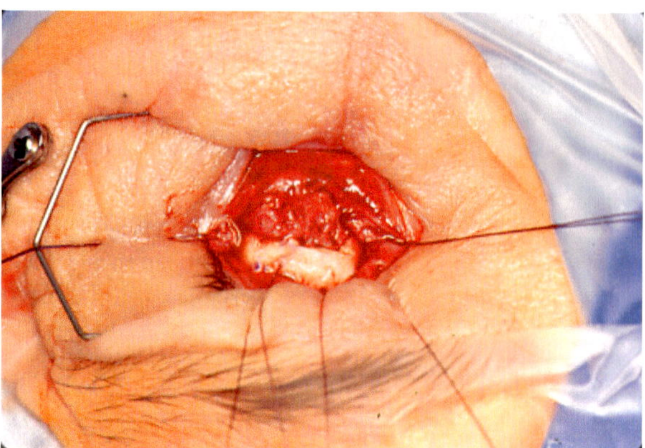

Fig. 6.13 One of the rectus muscles is shown sutured to the scleral wrapping

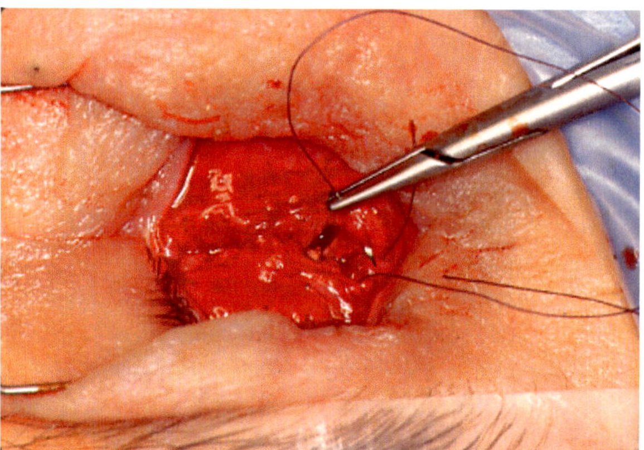

Fig. 6.14 The anterior Tenon's capsule is closed horizontally with interrupted 5-0 Vicryl sutures with the knots buried

to realize how critical this step is and ensure that Tenon's closure be meticulous to minimize the risk of implant extrusion. The conjunctival edges are approximated with a running 6-0 plain gut suture. Care is taken to grasp the end of the conjunctiva so that no conjunctival tissue is buried, as this can pre-dispose to cyst formation. Sterile ophthalmic antibiotic ointment is placed in the socket, an acrylic conformer is inserted (Fig. 6.15), and a pressure dressing is applied. One 6-0 plain gut suture may be placed through the eyelid in a suture tarsorrhaphy fashion to reduce the risk of conformer loss in the early postoperative period, which can be associated with prolonged chemosis and/or eyelid malpositions.

At the conclusion of the case, 0.5% Marcaine is injected to the inferior and superior fornices for postoperative pain relief. The patient is counseled that it is normal to have pain for several days after surgery, and limited amounts of postoperative opioid medications may be given for 3–4 days. After this point, however, the major-

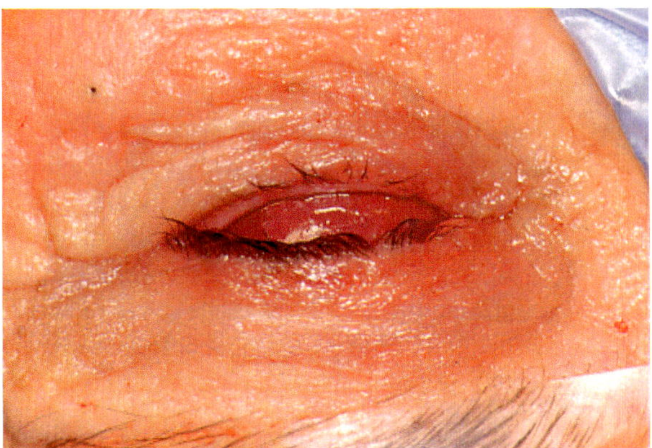

Fig. 6.15 Sterile ophthalmic antibiotic ointment is placed in the socket, an acrylic conformer is inserted

ity of patients are pain-free, and those with residual pain should find sufficient pain relief with acetaminophen. It is best to avoid prolonged opioid medication use, as the risks associated with the use of this medication are significant and cannot be underestimated. Patients with postoperative pain that does not improve should be evaluated to assess for postoperative bleeding or other complications. In rare cases, postoperative ketorolac intramuscular or intravenous injections are given for pain.

The pressure dressing is removed 7 days postoperatively, and antibiotic ointment is continued for 2–3 weeks. Six weeks after surgery, the patient is fitted with a standard customized ocular prosthesis. In the interim, the conformer is left in place to maintain the fornices and prevent socket contraction. Polycarbonate glasses are recommended to protect the contralateral eye.

Peg Placement

Once the implant is incorporated into the orbital tissues (approximately 6 months after implantation), some orbital surgeons advocate the use of a peg that inserts into the implant and integrates with the ocular prosthesis to transmit the full range of implant motility [29, 30]. Despite the potential motility benefits, peg placement is associated with a high rate of complications [31]. Appropriate candidates for pegged implants must understand the increased follow-up visits and socket care as well as the increased complications of pyogenic granuloma, conjunctival overgrowth, extrusion, spontaneous loosening of the peg sleeve, pain, clicking, and chronic discharge [32] associated with their use. In addition, peg placement requires coordination with the ocularist to couple the prosthesis for optimal outcome. The high rate of complications associated with pegs has led many to discontinue their use. For peg placement using the peg-and-sleeve system, the implant is placed primarily without simultaneous peg placement. The peg should not be placed until the implant is completely vascularized (which can be assessed by gadolinium-enhanced magnetic resonance imaging or bone scan). In order to ensure accurate peg placement, the surgeon first marks the center of the implant with the patient sitting in the upright position. Subsequently, local or retrobulbar anesthesia is administered and a 3-mm incision through conjunctiva, Tenon's capsule, and the scleral wrapping is made with a size 15 Bard-Parker blade in the central portion of the socket to expose the porous implant. An air-powered drill, with a 3-mm-diameter cutting burr, is held perpendicular to the implant surface, to drill an 11–13mm hole into the implant. A straight needle can be placed into the hole to ensure that it is perpendicular. The hole is irrigated with antibiotic solution to remove any residual debris and for anti-infective purposes. The sleeve is then screwed into the hole until the surface of the screw is flushed with the anterior surface of the implant. A temporary flat-headed peg is inserted into this sleeve, which is then exchanged about 6 weeks later with a rounded peg. It is important that the peg hole has the appropriate depth, size, placement, and angle to ensure a tight fit of the peg, minimizing the risks of implant infection, exposure, and migration. Titanium modifications of the original peg and sleeve system have been developed and are associated with lower complications when compared to their plastic counterpart [33, 34]. Once the peg is placed, the ocular prosthesis can be modified by the ocularist to couple with the round head of the peg in a ball-and-socket fashion to transmit the movement of the implant directly to the prosthesis [35].

Complications

Proper surgical technique significantly reduces the risk of postoperative complications after enucleation surgery. The most common complications postoperatively are related to eyelid malpositions and volume deficit which often develop over many years. Over time, a heavy prosthesis can lead to laxity of the lower eyelid, which may require a lower eyelid tightening procedure. While the description of this surgical approach is beyond the scope of this chapter, many advocate placing an additional suture when a lateral tarsal strip procedure is performed on an anophthalmic socket to help support the eyelid against the prosthetic weight. In the event of volume deficit (either early due to inadequate implant size or a later complication due to orbital fat atrophy), the surgeon and ocularist may first try to improve this with a larger prosthesis. It is important to note, however, that lower eyelid malpositions may often be caused by a heavy, oversized prosthesis.

In cases of significant volume deficit manifesting in superior sulcus deformity or enophthalmos that persists despite adequate modification of the prosthesis, volume augmentation procedures may be indicated. One helpful way to demonstrate this to patients in the clinic is to place your finger below the implant (outside of the lower eyelid) which simulates replacement of volume and improvement in this deformity. Options for treatment of volume deficits include nonsurgical (orbital filler or fat injections, eyelid fat or filler injections) or surgical (placement of a larger orbital implant, placement of a subperiosteal orbital floor implant, or dermis–fat graft).

Forniceal contracture is another complication of enucleation surgery. This is best avoided by minimizing tension on the fornix at the time of initial surgery. In some cases (when the central incision is well healed and the contracture is not severe), this may be treated with customized pressure conformers made by an ocularist. Late or severe forniceal contracture may necessitate additional surgery such as a mucous membrane grafting procedures to lengthen the fornices.

Other risks of surgery include implant infection, migration, and extrusion. Infections should be treated with topical and systemic antibiotics depending on the degree and type of infection.

Extrusion is more commonly seen in cases of infection. The underlying infection must be treated and the implant must be removed and/or replaced. In the absence of infection, small defects may heal with conservative management, while larger defects are more complicated. In some cases, surgical repair can be achieved with conjunctival or tarsoconjunctival flaps, dermal-fat grafts, periosteal grafts, hard palate grafts, and scleral or fascial patch grafts. In the case of large exposures, implant removal is often necessary as secondary infection may develop (or these may actually represent low-grade infections). A secondary implant can be placed once the infection has resolved completely.

Implant migration is less common with porous implants, but can be seen when muscles are imbricated in front of a spherical, nonporous, unwrapped implant. In some of these cases, the orbital implant should be removed and replaced to allow for better prosthesis fit.

In summary, while enucleation is sometimes considered to be a simple procedure, it alters the quite complex orbital anatomy and thus must be treated as a complex procedure and approached with meticulous care. When performed in this fashion, it can provide significant patient and physician satisfaction as it may relieve severe pain and improve the overall ocular aesthetic with excellent results.

References

1. Luce CM. Complication of enucleation. Trans Pa Acad Ophthalmol Otolaryngol. 1973;26(2):102–6.
2. Munden PM, Carter KD, Nerad JA. The oculocardiac reflex during enucleation. Am J Ophthalmol. 1991;111(3):378–9.
3. Mules PH. Evisceration of the globe with artificial vitreous. 1884–1895. Adv Ophthalmic Plast Reconstr Surg. 1990;8:69–72.
4. Sami D, Young S, Petersen R. Perspective on orbital enucleation implants. Surv Ophthalmol. 2007;52(3):244–65.
5. Baino F, Potestio I. Orbital implants: state-of-the-art review with emphasis on biomaterials and recent advances. Mater Sci Eng C Mater Biol Appl. 2016;69:1410–28.
6. Trichopoulos N, Augsburger JJ. Enucleation with unwrapped porous and nonporous orbital implants: a 15-year experience. Ophthalmic Plast Reconstr Surg. 2005;21(5):331–6.

7. Allen L. The argument against imbricating the rectus muscles over spherical orbital implants after enucleation. Ophthalmology. 1983;90(9):1116–20.
8. Nunery WR, et al. Extrusion rate of silicone spherical anophthalmic socket implants. Ophthalmic Plast Reconstr Surg. 1993;9(2):90–5.
9. Beard C. Remarks on historical and newer approaches to orbital implants. Ophthalmic Plast Reconstr Surg. 1995;11(2):89–90.
10. Fan JT, Robertson DM. Long-term follow-up of the Allen implant. 1967 to 1991. Ophthalmology. 1995;102(3):510–6.
11. Allen L, Ferguson EC, Braley AE. A quasi-integrated buried muscle cone implant with good motility and advantages for prosthetic fitting. Trans Am Acad Ophthalmol Otolaryngol. 1960;64:272–86.
12. Allen L, Spivey BE, Burns CA. A larger Iowa implant. Am J Ophthalmol. 1969;68(3): 397–400.
13. Anderson RL, et al. The universal orbital implant: indications and methods. Adv Ophthalmic Plast Reconstr Surg. 1990;8:88–99.
14. Jordan DR, et al. A preliminary report on the Universal Implant. Arch Ophthalmol. 1987;105(12):1726–31.
15. Spivey BE, Allen L, Burns CA. The Iowa enucleation implant. A 10-year evaluation of technique and results. Am J Ophthalmol. 1969;67(2):171–88.
16. Allen TD. Guist's bone spheres. Am J Ophthalmol. 1930;13:226–30.
17. McCoy L. Guist bone sphere. Am J Ophthalmol. 1932;15:960–3.
18. Celik T, et al. Vascularization of coralline versus synthetic hydroxyapatite orbital implants assessed by gadolinium enhanced magnetic resonance imaging. Curr Eye Res. 2015;40(3):346–53.
19. Oestreicher JH, Liu E, Berkowitz M. Complications of hydroxyapatite orbital implants. A review of 100 consecutive cases and a comparison of Dexon mesh (polyglycolic acid) with scleral wrapping. Ophthalmology. 1997;104(2):324–9.
20. Galindo-Ferreiro A, et al. Chronic orbital inflammation associated to hydroxyapatite implants in anophthalmic sockets. Case Rep Ophthalmol. 2017;8(3):574–80.
21. Jordan DR, Brownstein S, Jolly SS. Abscessed hydroxyapatite orbital implants. A report of two cases. Ophthalmology. 1996;103(11):1784–7.
22. Remulla HD, et al. Complications of porous spherical orbital implants. Ophthalmology. 1995;102(4):586–93.
23. Sadiq SA, et al. Integrated orbital implants--a comparison of hydroxyapatite and porous polyethylene implants. Orbit. 2008;27(1):37–40.
24. Ramey N, et al. Comparison of complication rates of porous anophthalmic orbital implants. Ophthalmic Surg Lasers Imaging. 2011;42(5):434–40.
25. Yousuf SJ, Jones LS, Kidwell ED Jr. Enucleation and evisceration: 20 years of experience. Orbit. 2012;31(4):211–5.
26. Tabatabaee Z, et al. Comparison of the exposure rate of wrapped hydroxyapatite (Bio-Eye) versus unwrapped porous polyethylene (Medpor) orbital implants in enucleated patients. Ophthalmic Plast Reconstr Surg. 2011;27(2):114–8.
27. Chao DL, Harbour JW. Hydroxyapatite versus polyethylene orbital implants for patients undergoing enucleation for uveal melanoma. Can J Ophthalmol. 2015;50(2):151–4.
28. Sagoo M, Rose G. Mechanisms and Treatment of Extruding Intraconal Implants: Socket Aging and Tissue Restitution (the "Cactus Syndrome"). Arch Ophthalmol. 2007;125(12):1616–20.
29. Shields CL, Shields JA, De Potter P. Hydroxyapatite orbital implant after enucleation. Experience with initial 100 consecutive cases. Arch Ophthalmol. 1992;110(3):333–8.
30. Guillinta P, et al. Prosthetic motility in pegged versus unpegged integrated porous orbital implants. Ophthalmic Plast Reconstr Surg. 2003;19(2):119–22.
31. Jordan DR, et al. Complications associated with pegging hydroxyapatite orbital implants. Ophthalmology. 1999;106(3):505–12.

32. Jordan DR. Spontaneous loosening of hydroxyapatite peg sleeves. Ophthalmology. 2001;108(11):2041–4.
33. Shoamanesh A, Pang NK, Oestreicher JH. Complications of orbital implants: a review of 542 patients who have undergone orbital implantation and 275 subsequent PEG placements. Orbit. 2007;26(3):173–82.
34. Jordan DR, Klapper SR. Surgical techniques in enucleation: the role of various types of implants and the efficacy of pegged and nonpegged approaches. Int Ophthalmol Clin. 2006;46(1):109–32.
35. Custer PL. Enucleation: past, present, and future. Ophthalmic Plast Reconstr Surg. 2000;16(5):316–21.

Chapter 7
Evisceration

Brian C. Tse and Thomas E. Johnson

Introduction

Evisceration is the surgical removal of the intraocular contents while leaving the scleral shell in place with the extraocular muscles attached. Compared to enucleation, evisceration offers the advantages of being a shorter and less traumatic procedure. Thus, it is a useful procedure in patients who may be in poor health or medically unstable, where shorter operating times are imperative. Additionally, there is usually less bleeding during an evisceration when compared to enucleation, which is an important consideration in an acutely inflamed orbit or in patients who are unable to discontinue blood thinners prior to surgery. Postoperative fornices are usually deeper than in enucleation and may lead to easier prosthesis fitting [1]. Finally, evisceration offers theoretical advantages of better motility and improved cosmesis, since the extraocular muscles and orbital suspensory ligaments are untouched during the procedure. However, evisceration does leave a small risk of developing sympathetic ophthalmia in the contralateral eye and may lead to the inadvertent orbital spread of a previously undetected intraocular malignancy. In patients with phthisical eyes, an adequately sized orbital implant can be difficult if not impossible to place at the time of surgery, leading to postoperative orbital volume deficit and poor cosmesis.

B. C. Tse (✉) · T. E. Johnson
Bascom Palmer Eye Institute, University of Miami Miller School of Medicine, Miami, FL, USA
e-mail: b.tse@med.miami.edu

T. E. Johnson (ed.), *Anophthalmia*,
https://doi.org/10.1007/978-3-030-29753-4_7

Preoperative Considerations

Evisceration is being used with increased frequency to treat blind painful eyes because of the procedure's benefits compared to enucleation listed above. Traditionally, evisceration is most commonly performed in eyes with endophthalmitis or corneal ulceration that cannot be controlled medically and globe integrity is at risk. In patients with fungal endophthalmitis, however, where scleral invasion may occur early in the disease process, enucleation should remain a consideration. In general, in eyes with questionable scleral integrity (scleral laceration or staphyloma) or inadequate sclera (phthisis bulbi), enucleation should be performed.

An absolute contraindication for evisceration is the presence of an intraocular tumor [2]. If an intraocular tumor is detected, or even suspected, preoperatively, enucleation should be performed. B-scan ultrasonography should be performed by an experienced ultrasonographer in all patients undergoing evisceration. If there is concern for an anterior tumor, ultrasound biomicroscopy should be performed. If the ultrasound findings are equivocal, additional imaging with computed tomography or magnetic resonance imaging can be obtained. In cases of suspected retinoblastoma, CT scan should never be performed. If an intraocular cannot be definitively ruled out prior to surgery, enucleation should be performed instead of evisceration. Eagle has posited that in the reported cases where evisceration was done in eyes with intraocular tumors, there seemed to be a trend of inadequate preoperative workup, underscoring the importance of this step [3].

Surgical Technique

The surgery can be performed under general anesthesia or retrobulbar block along with monitored anesthesia care. A lid speculum is placed, and a 360° conjunctival peritomy is performed. Gentle dissection with Stevens scissors is carried out between the sclera and Tenon's capsule in each of the four quadrants between the rectus muscles. A number 11 Bard-Parker™ blade is used to make a paracentesis, entering the anterior chamber at the corneoscleral limbus. Keratectomy is performed using Westcott or cataract scissors. If the indication for evisceration is endophthalmitis, an abundant amount of purulent material will often present during keratectomy. Cultures should be taken at this point, and antibiotic therapy can later be adjusted depending on culture results. An evisceration spatula is then used to gently separate the scleral spur and uveal contents off the scleral wall 360° just behind the iris plane. The spatula is run along the inside of the sclera from the anterior lip toward the posterior pole, detaching the uveal contents from the sclera, clock hour by clock hour. Attempt should be made with a larger evisceration spatula to remove the uveal contents intact, but this may not be possible. The surgeon should make every effort to remove all of the uveal tissue to minimize the risk of sympathetic ophthalmia. The inside of the sclera is next scrubbed with cotton tip applicators soaked in absolute ethanol in order to denature and remove residual uvea. Care is taken to avoid the alcohol from coming into contact with the conjunctiva. After several sweeps with the absolute ethanol, copious irrigation is then performed with an antibiotic solution such as gentamicin to remove any residual alcohol. Posterior sclerotomies can be performed at this time to allow for placement of a large implant and facilitate vascularization of a porous implant. If the sclera looks healthy and non-infected, an acrylic or porous orbital implant is placed in the sclera, and the sclera is closed over the implant using 5-0 Vicryl™ or Mersilene™ sutures. Tenon's capsule is then closed with interrupted sutures of 5-0 Vicryl™, taking care to bury the knots. The conjunctiva is closed with a running 6-0 plain gut suture. Subconjunctival injection of an antibiotic is then placed. Finally, a proper-sized conformer and a firm pressure patch are placed, with the pressure patch staying in place for 1 week.

If the sclera appears necrotic, as often happens with pseudomonas or streptococcal infections, necrotic sclera can be trimmed, and the sclera is packed with betadine-soaked gauze. The gauze is then removed and replaced a few days after the procedure. The tissues eventually are allowed to heal by secondary intention. A secondary implant can be placed once the infection is completely cleared and inflammation has subsided, usually about 3 months.

Implant Placement

An area of controversy concerns the placement of a primary implant after evisceration in the setting of endophthalmitis. Advocates of a two-staged approach (evisceration followed by delayed secondary orbital implant insertion) argue that primary placement of an implant in this infected setting would result in a high incidence of implant extrusion [4]. Proponents of a one-staged procedure point to decreased recovery time, lower cost, fewer surgical procedures, less patient anxiety, and decreased hospitalization time [5, 6].

Dresner and Karesh evaluated 11 patients who underwent evisceration for endophthalmitis with placement of a primary implant [7]. They found that 10 of 11 patients had an uneventful postoperative course with successful prosthesis fitting. One patient with *Pseudomonas aeruginosa* endophthalmitis had an implant exposure. Ozgur and coworkers reported the results of 25 patients with endophthalmitis treated with evisceration and primary implant placement. With a mean follow-up of 25.4 months, they found three patients (12%) developed implant exposure and one patient (4%) developed a pyogenic granuloma [5]. Additionally Tawfik and Budin reported 67 patients with endophthalmitis who underwent evisceration with primary implant placement and found 63 successfully retained their implant [6]. These studies concluded that primary implant placement with evisceration patients with endophthalmitis is an acceptable treatment. These findings are in concert with other studies that have shown that primary implant placement is safe in the majority of cases when antibiotic therapy is used in the perioperative period. However, in patients in whom there is concern for or documentation of more virulent infections (i.e., *Pseudomonas aeruginosa*, *Streptococcus*, or *Bacillus cereus*), consideration should be given to delaying implant placement, as there may be greater risk of extrusion. Some advocate for secondary implant placement only after the initial infection has been cleared.

Another debate centers on the type of implant (porous or nonporous) to be placed after enucleation or evisceration in the setting of endophthalmitis. Originally it was thought that nonporous implants should be used after evisceration or enucleation in endophthalmitis cases because of the risk of implant infection. Recent studies have found that porous implants such as hydroxyapatite and porous polyethylene can be safely implanted. Abel and Meyer described 22 patients with advanced endophthalmitis or panophthalmitis who underwent enucleation with primary implant placement, 11 with hydroxyapatite and 11 with silicone implants [8]. All were treated during surgery with intravenous antibiotics. No patients had persistent orbital cellulitis, and none developed meningitis. Only two patients with silicone implants had implant extrusions. There appears to be a trend toward the placement of porous polyethylene implants over nonporous implants [9].

Sympathetic Ophthalmia

Another area of controversy surrounding evisceration is the risk of sympathetic ophthalmia occurring after evisceration. Sympathetic ophthalmia is a rare condition occurring after penetrating ocular injury (traumatic or surgical) and presents as a granulomatous panuveitis with potentially devastating visual consequences, especially in a monocular patient [10]. Incidence of sympathetic ophthalmia has previously been reported as 0.03/100,000 [11]. The inciting antigen for sympathetic ophthalmia is likely uveal in nature, and thus, many believe that there is a theoretical risk of sympathetic ophthalmia after evisceration, as residual pigmented melanocytes may remain in the sclera and could be a nidus for inflammation [12, 13].

No uniform consensus exists regarding evisceration and sympathetic ophthalmia, owing mostly to the rarity of the disease. Levine and colleagues in a small case series of 51 eviscerated patients did not have any cases of sympathetic ophthalmia. In the same paper, a survey of oculoplastic, uveitis, and ophthalmic pathologists examined 841 eviscerated patients and found only 5 anecdotal cases of sympathetic ophthalmia that were recalled by respondents; no pathology was available for any of these cases [14]. While the incidence of sympathetic ophthalmia after evisceration is low, the surgeon should keep in mind the theoretical increased risk after evisceration compared to enucleation. These risks should be considered alongside improved cosmetic outcome and the clinical scenario during the clinical decision-making process.

References

1. Park Y, Paik J, Yang S. The results of evisceration with primary porous implant placement in patients with endophthalmitis. Korean J Ophthalmol. 2010;24:279–83.
2. Rath S, Honavar SG, Naik MN, et al. Evisceration in unsuspected intraocular tumors. Arch Ophthalmol. 2010;128(3):372–9.
3. Eagle RC. Inadvertent evisceration of a largely necrotic uveal melanoma: diagnosis confounded by orbital inflammation. Combined Meeting of the Eastern and Pan American Ophthalmic Pathology Societies. Orlando, 1999.
4. Shore JW, Dieckert JP, Levine MR. Delayed primary wound closure use to prevent implant extrusion following evisceration for endophthalmitis. Arch Ophthalmol. 1988;106(9):1303–8.
5. Ozgur OR, Akcay L, Dogan OK. Primary implant placement with evisceration in patients with endophthalmitis. Am J Ophthalmol. 2007;143:902–4.
6. Tawfik HA, Budin H. Evisceration with primary implant placement in patients with endophthalmitis. Ophthalmology. 2007;114:1100–3.
7. Dresner SC, Karesh JW. Primary implant placement with evisceration in patients with endophthalmitis. Ophthalmology. 2000;107:1661–4.
8. Abel AD, Meyer DR. Enucleation with primary implant insertion for treatment of recalcitrant endophthalmitis and panophthalmitis. Ophthal Plast Reconstr Surg. 2005;21:220–6.
9. Hui J. Outcomes of orbital implants after evisceration and enucleation in patients with endophthalmitis. Curr Opin Ophthalmol. 2010;21:375–9.
10. du Toit N, Motala MI, Richards J, et al. The risk of sympathetic ophthalmia following evisceration for penetrating eye injuries at Groote Schuur Hospital. Br J Ophthalmol. 2008;92:61–3.
11. Kilmartin DJ, Dick AD, Forrester JV. Prospective surveillance of sympathetic ophthalmia in the UK and the Republic of Ireland. Br J Ophthalmol. 2000;84:259–63.
12. Bilyk JR. Enucleation, evisceration, and sympathetic ophthalmia. Curr Opin Ophthalmol. 2000;11:372–85.
13. Gasch AT, Foster CS, Grosskreutz CL, et al. Postoperative sympathetic ophthalmia. Int Ophthalmol Clin. 2000;40:69–84.
14. Levine MR, Pou CR, Lash RH. Evisceration: is sympathetic ophthalmia a concern in the new millennium? Ophthalmic Plast Reconstr Surg. 1999;15:4–8.

Chapter 8
Exenteration and Multidisciplinary Approaches

Catherine J. Choi

Indications

Orbital exenteration is most commonly performed with the goal of achieving local disease control in malignancies and severe infections. Examples of primary orbital tumors that may lead to exenteration include adenoid cystic carcinoma, rhabdomyosarcoma, retinoblastoma, and mucoepidermoid carcinoma [1–8]. Eyelid or ocular adnexal tumors, such as melanoma, basal cell carcinoma, squamous cell carcinoma, and sebaceous cell carcinoma, as well as sinonasal tumors such as esthesioneuroblastoma may also lead to exenteration in cases of extensive invasion into the orbit [1–8]. In case of malignancies, the inherent characteristics of orbital anatomy and orbital tissues make it challenging to obtain distinct tumor margins for complete resection once intraorbital tumor infiltration is present. In such cases, exenteration may be the only viable option for ensuring complete resection and for decreasing the risk of metastasis [1–4]. When advanced metastatic disease is already present, exenteration is sometimes offered as a palliative measure to relieve intractable pain of significant mass effect [1–8].

Local disease control via exenteration for nonmalignant condition is indicated in severe life-threatening orbital fungal infections such as *mucormycosis* and aspergillosis with risk of intracranial extension [1–8] and rare cases of severe periocular necrotizing fasciitis (group A β-hemolytic *Streptococcus*) unresponsive to medical therapy and debridement [9]. Congenital deformities or benign tumors and trauma with severe disfigurement and irreversible vision loss may also be candidates for exenteration [10, 11].

For all of the above malignant and nonmalignant conditions, exenteration is a radical surgery that is offered as a last-resort option. Needless to say, the permanent

C. J. Choi (✉)
Ophthalmic Plastic and Reconstructive Surgery, Department of Ophthalmology, Bascom Palmer Eye Institute, University of Miami Miller School of Medicine, Miami, FL, USA
e-mail: catherine.j.choi@kp.org

T. E. Johnson (ed.), *Anophthalmia*,
https://doi.org/10.1007/978-3-030-29753-4_8

vision loss and facial disfigurement come with significant physical and emotional burden for the patient and his or her family. In cases of some elderly or severely debilitated patients with complex medical comorbidities or limited life expectancy, a realistic discussion regarding the expected benefit of exenteration for the particular pathology in question should be held.

Preoperative Evaluation

Every patient must be evaluated with a complete ocular examination. Special attention is directed to the eyelid and adnexal structures, including the nasolacrimal system and adjacent sinonasal anatomy depending on the underlying etiology. Any lymphadenopathy or facial sensory deficits can provide additional clues with regard to the extent of disease. These findings can be confirmed on orbital imaging with CT and/or MRI. If not already available at this stage, an incisional biopsy is obtained for a definitive pathological diagnosis on permanent section prior to consideration of subsequent steps.

A multidisciplinary approach may be needed if involvement of the intracranial space or sinonasal cavity is noted. A combined approach with neurosurgery and/or otolaryngology is sometimes chosen to allow for complete resection of adjacent structures in addition to orbital exenteration. For malignant lesions, the team may also include radiation oncology and medical oncology for coordination of neoadjuvant or adjuvant chemotherapy and radiation. For infectious etiologies, tailored medical therapy guided by infectious disease specialists is essential.

A comprehensive preoperative evaluation can determine the extent of exenteration to be performed: total, eyelid-sparing, or subtotal. Diffusely infiltrating disease involving significant areas of eyelid skin and conjunctiva, as well as orbital structures, is best treated with total exenteration. A posteriorly located disease with no surface or skin involvement, on the other hand, can be approached via the eyelid-sparing technique. Rarely, pathology with more localized involvement of the orbit can be treated with subtotal exenteration with partial removal of orbital contents.

Operative Technique

Antiplatelet and anticoagulation agents are discontinued prior to surgery in the absence of major medical contraindications.

- *Incision: total exenteration vs. eyelid-sparing exenteration*

Under general anesthesia, an injection of local anesthetic with epinephrine (i.e., 2% lidocaine with 1:100,000 epinephrine) is given for hemostasis. A tarsorrhaphy

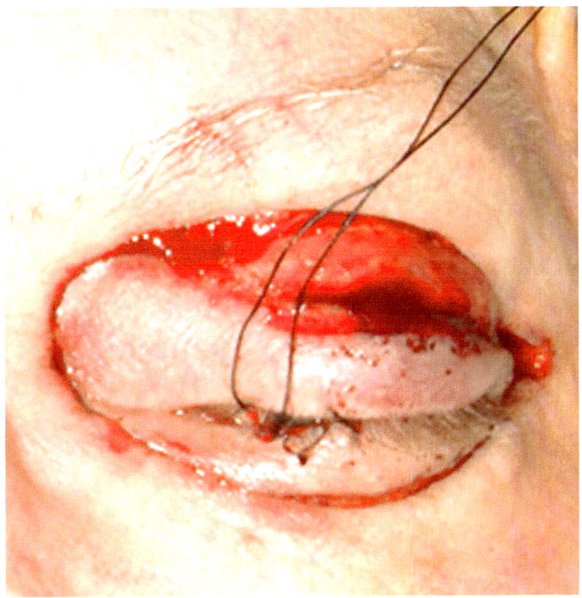

Fig. 8.1 Intraoperative photo demonstrating suture tarsorrhaphy and incision for a partial eyelid-sparing exenteration

can be placed through the central lid margins to help with traction. For total exenteration, a #15 blade or monopolar cutting cautery is used to incise the skin 2–3 mm outside the arcus marginalis down to periosteum. In an eyelid-sparing exenteration, the skin incision is made outside the upper and lower eyelid lash lines (Fig. 8.1). Dissection is then carried out in either the pre-orbicularis plane or the pre-tarsal plane toward the orbital rim, which is then incised as above.

- *Dissection*

A subperiosteal dissection is carried out with a Freer elevator toward the orbital apex. The extent of the posterior dissection depends on the location of the primary pathology (subtotal vs. total exenteration). Controlled, gentle dissection is used near the delicate medial wall, inferomedial floor, and the neurovascular bundles (supraorbital, supratrochlear, anterior and posterior ethmoidal, zygomaticofacial, and zygomaticotemporal), in combination with sharp dissection around the firm attachments of medial and lateral canthal tendons, trochlea, lateral orbital tubercle, and the origin of the inferior oblique muscle. The nasolacrimal sac-duct junction and the supraorbital and infraorbital fissure contents are transected. Dissection in the area of primary pathology is typically performed last in order to allow for uncomplicated dissection of all other areas and improved access and visualization of the area of interest, which may involve bony erosion or abnormal anatomy. Bleeding during the dissection can be controlled with cautery, bone wax, vascular ligation clips, or pro-hemostatic agents.

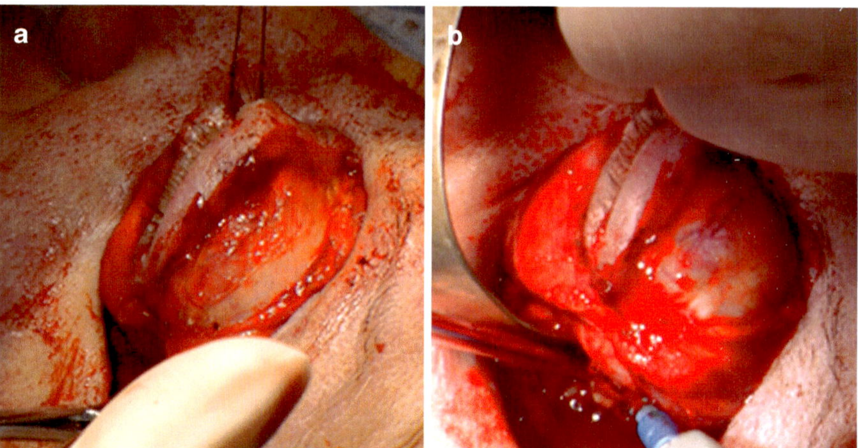

Fig. 8.2 (**a**) A large hemostat placed around the apical structures of the orbit following complete subperiosteal dissection. (**b**) Monopolar cutting cautery is used to transect the apical tissues above the hemostat

- *Removal of orbital contents*

Following adequate dissection, one or two large hemostats are placed posteriorly across the apical structures (Fig. 8.2a). It should be noted that some patients may develop significant bradycardia during this maneuver, and the anesthesiologist should be informed ahead of time for appropriate monitoring. Using scissors or monopolar cutting cautery, the apical tissues are transected above the hemostat and the orbital contents removed in toto (Fig. 8.2b). Any arterial bleeding from the ophthalmic artery is controlled with cautery or surgical clips. If posterior extension of the main lesion or pathology is suspected, intraoperative frozen sections of the remaining apical tissues can be taken to clear the margin. Concurrent bony resection may be necessary in the setting of bony erosion, which may involve a multidisciplinary approach (e.g., craniotomy, maxillectomy).

- *Reconstruction of exenterated socket*

A number of techniques are available for primary reconstruction of an exenterated socket: healing by secondary intention, skin graft, dermal substitute, myocutaneous advancement flap, or free flap [8, 12–14].

Healing by Second Intention

Healing by second intention is the simplest option in which the exenterated socket is left to granulate on its own. At the end of surgery, the bare bone of the exenterated socket is covered with iodoform gauze and antibiotic ointment. This dressing is then changed on a regular basis (every 2 days) as granulation tissue forms and slowly epithelializes over 3–4 months. Despite perhaps having the shortest surgical time and good tissue color match with the rest of facial skin, the surface is typically irregular and can mask recurrence in cases of malignancy. The lengthy healing time is also generally uncomfortable for the patient and too long for those in need of adjuvant radiation.

Split-Thickness Skin Graft

Lining the exenterated socket with split-thickness skin graft allows for faster healing and a smooth surface [12]. Non-hair-bearing skin of the thigh is a commonly used donor site. A dermatome is used to harvest an even-thickness (0.3–0.6 mm) 3 × 5 inch graft. The split-thickness skin graft is then fed through a 1:1 or 1:2 ratio mesher, which cuts the graft in a mesh-like pattern allowing it to be stretched to cover a larger surface area. The perforations also serve as premade vents that prevent formation of hematomas under the graft (Fig. 8.3a, b). The graft is molded to the socket and sutured to the edges of the circumferential incision around the orbit with interrupted and running dissolvable sutures. Complete contact between the graft and the recipient bed is ensured by lining the graft with antibiotic ointment, non-adherent dressing, and pressure packing (e.g., surgical sponges, gauze, iodoform dressing). A firm pressure patch is fashioned over the packing and maintained for 5–7 days. The donor site for the skin graft is covered with non-adherent dressing.

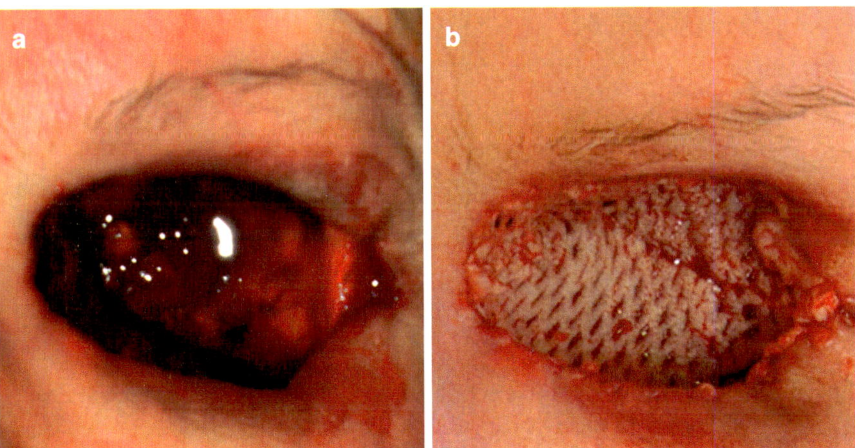

Fig. 8.3 (**a**) Exenterated socket following removal of orbital contents. (**b**) A split-thickness skin graft lining the exenterated socket

Dermal Substitute

Using a commercially available dermal substitute avoids the need for a skin graft and the associated donor site morbidity. An example of such product is an acellular extracellular matrix scaffold made of biodegradable cross-linked bovine tendon collagen and glycosaminoglycan layered on a silicone membrane (Integra®) [13, 14]. The dermal substitute is positioned over the exenterated socket and sutured to the skin edges. The scaffold provides a supportive environment for rapid granulation and epithelialization. The silicone membrane is removed by 3–4 weeks, and healing is typically complete by 6–8 weeks. While effective, the major limitation of such product is the cost.

Myocutaneous Advancement Flap or Free Flap

When exenteration is combined with concurrent resection of adjacent structures (e.g., maxillectomy) leading to large soft tissue and bony defects, there may not be any contiguous bony surface to cover with a skin graft or dermal substitute. In such cases, myocutaneous advancement flaps or free flaps are used to cover the resection bed [7, 8]. Options for local transposition flaps include the temporalis, frontalis, galea-frontalis flap, and the temporoparietal fascial flap [7, 8]. Some commonly utilized free flap sources include the radial forearm, latissimus dorsi, rectus abdominis, lateral arm, or anterolateral thigh [7, 8]. In contrast to reconstructive strategies discussed above, exenterated sockets covered by flaps cannot be fitted with a prosthesis and typically have a bulky, less aesthetically satisfactory outcome. The relative thickness of the flap can also mask tumor recurrence, and close surveillance via imaging is therefore needed.

Potential Complications

Potential complications of exenteration may arise from specific surgical techniques as well as from the nature and extent of the underlying pathology. Some of the most notable complications include hematoma formation, postoperative infection, cerebrospinal fluid leak, sino-orbital fistula, and recurrence.

Hematoma Formation Sources of bleeding include the ophthalmic artery, ethmoidal arteries, and neurovascular bundles coursing through the superior and inferior orbital fissures and other perforating foramens. Hematoma can form under a skin graft or a flap in the setting of poor hemostasis and cause graft failure or delayed healing. The hematoma should be promptly evacuated, the source of bleeding controlled, and any necrotic tissue debrided. Limited areas of graft dehiscence or flap failure can be left to heal by secondary intention, but larger areas may require repeat grafting.

Postoperative Infection True surgical site infection is rare with appropriate sterile technique. In cases of an underlying infectious etiology leading to exenteration (invasive fungal or bacterial infection), concurrent local and/or systemic administration of antifungal or antibiotic agent is usually given. If frank purulence is noted in the exenterated socket, gram stain and cultures should be obtained to guide therapy and any necrotic tissue debrided. A povidone-iodine wet-to-dry dressing can be applied for further debridement and wound care.

Cerebrospinal Fluid (CSF) Leak Penetration of dura with subsequent CSF leak can happen via the cribriform plate, orbital roof, or the greater wing of the sphenoid. Small CSF leaks can close spontaneously, but larger leaks may require direct repair using tissue graft and/or tissue adhesive in conjunction with neurosurgery.

Sino-orbital Fistula Full thickness penetration of orbital walls with direct communication into the adjacent sinuses can result in fistulas. The defect in the orbital wall can be from unnecessarily forceful dissection at the time of surgery, direct bony erosion from the primary pathology, or from tissue breakdown secondary to adjuvant radiation therapy. While small fistulas can be observed and the edges allowed to granulate, large fistulas can lead to chronic discharge from the sinus mucosa and difficulty with breathing and phonation. Options for closure of fistulas include additional skin graft or vascularized tissue flap.

Recurrence In cases of malignancy, the risk of tumor recurrence secondary to positive surgical margins or residual areas of microscopic disease requires ongoing surveillance for all patients. While a thorough margin clearance via frozen sections at the time of surgery decreases the potential for this complication, it does not guarantee complete tumor clearance or prevent microscopic metastasis (Fig. 8.4).

Postoperative Care

Appropriate postoperative care of an exenterated socket depends on the method of reconstruction used. For healing by secondary intention, the socket can be packed with wet-to-dry dressing of 4 × 4 gauze soaked in 10% povidone-iodine solution to allow for debridement of dried blood and keratin debris, while the granulation tissue forms over the bony surface. As noted above, this can be a lengthy process that requires daily wound care by the patient or the caregiver over 3–4 months.

If a split-thickness skin graft was placed, the pressure packing can be removed 5–7 days after surgery and a wet-to-dry dressing with a 50:50 mixture of 10% povidone-iodine solution and hydrogen peroxide initiated. The frequency of dressing change is gradually decreased until the socket is fully epithelialized. Dermal substitute-based reconstruction should be managed according to the manufacturer's instructions for optimal healing. In the setting of adjuvant radiation therapy, the socket will be more prone to epithelial breakdown, and additional dressing change or treatment with antibiotic ointment and topical emollient may be necessary.

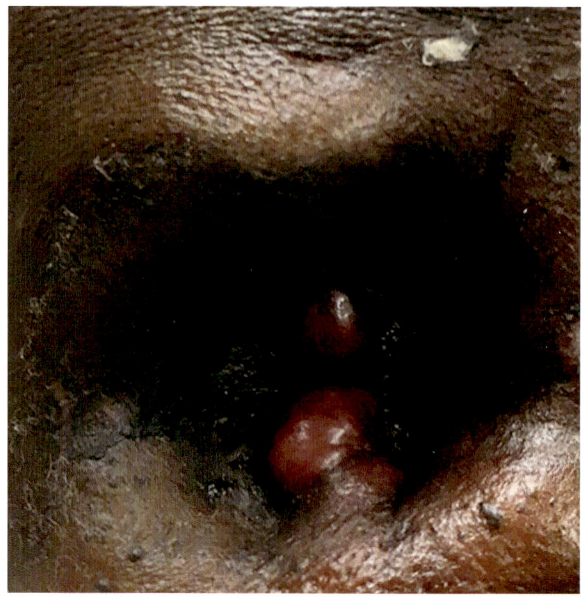

Fig. 8.4 Patient with a history of eyelid-sparing exenteration for invasive squamous cell carcinoma presenting with large nodular growths, concerning for recurrence

In cases of myocutaneous advancement flap or free flap, maintaining flap perfusion and survival is the primary goal of postoperative management. Early detection of any hypo-perfused areas with timely debridement of any necrotic tissue is recommended.

After the socket has been completely epithelialized, the patient can be fitted with an oculofacial prosthesis. The traditional method of prosthesis construction involves taking an impression of the orbit with a plaster cast to make a mold, with which a silicone template is made and painted to resemble the other eye. The prosthesis can be attached to thicker glasses frame to help camouflage the prosthesis-skin interface or directly attached to periorbital skin with skin adhesive or magnetic posts (see chapter on osseointegrated prosthesis) [15]. More recently, advancements in 3D-printing technology are being applied to making custom-printed prostheses at a lower cost than the traditional methods. Along with the prosthesis, all patients are required to wear polycarbonate glasses to protect the remaining eye, with lifelong monocular precautions.

References

1. Bartley GB, Garrity JA, Waller RR, et al. Orbital exenteration at the Mayo Clinic: 1967–1986. Ophthalmology. 1989;96:468–74.
2. Shields JA, Shields CL, Demirci H, Honavar SG, Singh AD. Experience with eyelid-sparing orbital exenteration: the 2000 Tullos O. Coston Lecture. Ophthal Plast Reconstr Surg. 2001;17(5):355–61.

3. Levin PS, Dutton JJ. A 20-year series of orbital exenteration. Am J Ophthalmol. 1991;112:496–501.
4. Kiratli H, Koç İ. Orbital exenteration: institutional review of evolving trends in indications and rehabilitation techniques. Orbit. 2018;37(3):179–86.
5. Nagendran ST, Lee NG, Fay A, Lefebvre DR, Sutula FC, Freitag SK. Orbital exenteration: the 10-year Massachusetts Eye and Ear Infirmary experience. Orbit. 2016;35(4):199–206.
6. Ben Simon GJ, Schwarcz RM, Douglas R, Fiaschetti D, McCann JD, Goldberg RA. Orbital exenteration: one size does not fit all. Am J Ophthalmol. 2005;139(1):11–7.
7. Tse D. Color atlas of oculoplastic surgery. 2nd ed. Philadelphia: Lippincott Williams & Wilkins; 2012.
8. Zhang Z, Ho S, Yin V, Varas G, Rajak S, Dolman PJ, et al. Multicentred international review of orbital exenteration and reconstruction in oculoplastic and orbit practice. Br J Ophthalmol. 2018;102(5):654–8.
9. Elner VM, Demirci H, Nerad JA, Hassan AS. Periocular necrotizing fasciitis with visual loss pathogenesis and treatment. Ophthalmology. 2006;113(12):2338–45.
10. Rose GE, Wright JE. Exenteration for benign orbital disease. Br J Ophthalmol. 1994;78(1):14–8.
11. Thach AB, Johnson AJ, Carroll RB, Huchun A, Ainbinder DJ, Stutzman RD, Blaydon SM, Demartelaere SL, Mader TH, Slade CS, George RK, Ritchey JP, Barnes SD, Fannin LA. Severe eye injuries in the war in Iraq, 2003-2005. Ophthalmology. 2008;115(2):377–82.
12. Mauriello JA Jr, Han KH, Wolfe R. Use of autogenous split-thickness dermal graft for reconstruction of the lining of the exenterated orbit. Am J Ophthalmol. 1985;100(3):465–7.
13. Rafailov L, Turbin RE, Langer PD. Use of bilayer matrix wound dressing in the exenterated socket. Orbit. 2017;36(6):397–400.
14. Ozgonul C, Diniz Grisolia AB, Demirci H. The use of Integra® dermal regeneration template for the orbital exenteration socket: a novel technique. Ophthal Plast Reconstr Surg. 2018;34(1):64–7.
15. Nerad JA, Carter KD, LaVelle WE, Fyler A, Brånemark PI. The osseointegration technique for the rehabilitation of the exenterated orbit. Arch Ophthalmol. 1991;109(7):1032–8.

Chapter 9
Orbital Implants and Wrapping Materials

Andrew J. Rong and Thomas E. Johnson

Introduction

The development of enucleation techniques by Farrell and Bonnet in the mid-1800s offered surgeons novel means for removing the globe. Prior to the introduction of the orbital implant, the residual orbital deficit was left to fill by granulation, with a conformer placed into the socket to prevent contracture [1, 2]. Due to the cosmetic and functional downsides resulting from the volume deficit, the glass implant was introduced by Mules in 1884 in a seminal paper titled "Evisceration of the globe, with artificial vitreous": In this paper, he writes:

> …I might introduce a light hollow glass sphere or artificial vitreous into the cavity of the denuded sclera which, whilst preserving the shape of the globe and causing no irritation, would perfect the stump for the adaptation of an artificial eye. [3]

During early implantation surgeries, the goal of the surgeon was simply to fill the orbital volume and to prevent extrusion of the implanted material. This latter goal proved difficult, and in Mules case, despite being attributed with creating the first modern orbital implant, five of his nine glass implants would ultimately extrude—a complication that was partially attributed to poor antiseptic technique [2, 4].

The next half century saw an explosion in surgical techniques and implant design. Due to the high rates of implant extrusion, Frost and Lang improved the surgical technique by closing Tenon's capsule around the implant as a means of preventing extrusion [5]. This method still lies at the core of modern enucleation and evisceration surgery and proved efficient as a barrier to implant extrusion. As antiseptic technology and surgical techniques improved, implant design also evolved. Surgeons

A. J. Rong (✉)
Oculoplastic Surgery, Bascom Palmer Eye Institute, Miami, FL, USA
e-mail: ajr211@med.miami.edu

T. E. Johnson
Bascom Palmer Eye Institute, University of Miami Miller School of Medicine, Miami, FL, USA

T. E. Johnson (ed.), *Anophthalmia*,
https://doi.org/10.1007/978-3-030-29753-4_9

began experimenting with various implant materials, creating implants made from gold, silver, and autogenous materials. In the 1930s, Wheeler began incorporating the rectus muscles into his orbital implants, designing a grooved implant in which these muscles could be attached, and providing additional implant stability [6]. The inclusion of recti muscles into orbital implant surgery spurred the next iteration of implant design, placing both an importance on preventing implant extrusion and a new emphasis on prosthetic motility [7]. In the 1940s, Cutler's "positive contact ball and ring implant" became the first iteration of the peg, highlighting the modern principles of socket reconstruction and cosmesis [8].

The modern implant is built from lessons learned from these innovative surgeons. The importance of implant retention, volume replacement, and adequate prosthetic motility lie at the foundation of anophthalmic socket reconstruction. This chapter will review the special considerations the ophthalmic surgeon must weigh when choosing an orbital implant following enucleation and evisceration surgeries.

Implant Size

Following enucleation or evisceration of the globe, which on the average fills 6–7 ml of the orbital volume, the surgeon faces a variety of options regarding orbital implant preference. One of the first considerations is size of the implant. This was a concern even during the inception of implant design, as Mules describes choosing an implant:

> best suited to the case… until the sphere will with difficulty enter the cavity. This difficulty only refers to introducing the globe; when it is in, the sclera should unite quite easily without any tension, and leave no awkward angles; therefore the largest sphere fulfilling these conditions is the best… [9]

Insufficient implant sizing can result in orbital volume deficiency leading to a superior sulcus deformity (Fig. 9.1), enophthalmos, ptosis, and poor fitting prosthesis. Too large of an implant can also lead to a poor fitting prosthesis and may lead to implant exposure and poor motility. Thus, proper sizing of the implant by the surgeon is integral.

There are a variety of methods in determining the size of an orbital implant. The numbers used to categorize implants refer to the sphere's diameter, with implants commonly ranging from 12 to 23 mm in size. Some surgeons primarily use the patient's age to base implant size, where a 20 mm implant is essentially placed in all adult patients [10]. Other authors prefer a 22 mm implant placed deep in the orbit for the majority of their cases [11]. Others yet have developed equations to calculate the ideal implant size ($V_{implant}$) by using a graduated cylinder to measure total orbital tissue loss (V_{tissue}) and subtracting from this number the ideal prosthetic volume (2 ml) and implant wrap volume (V_{wrap}) to determine ideal implant volume [12].

$$\left(V_{\text{implant}}\right) = \left(V_{\text{tissue}}\right) - \left(V_{\text{wrap}}\right) - 2\text{ml}$$

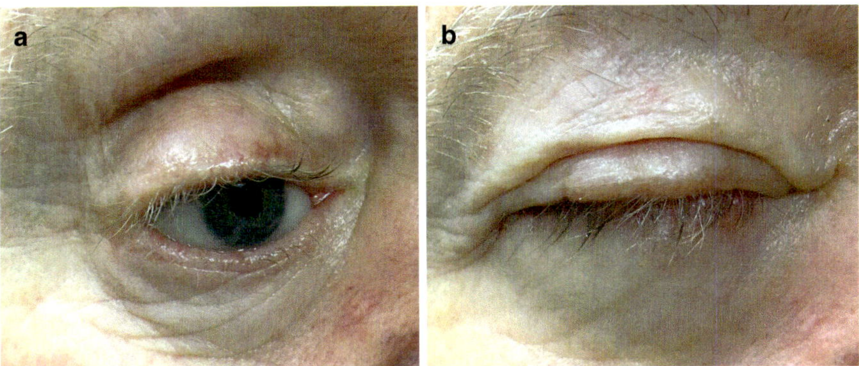

Fig. 9.1 (**a**) Superior sulcus deformity in an anophthalmic patient due to orbital volume deficiency. (**b**) Resolution of the superior sulcus deformity postorbital implant exchange and subperiosteal wedge placement

We prefer using an intraoperative sizer placed deep in the orbit to choose the largest implant that can still easily be covered by Tenon's capsule and conjunctiva. This typically lies between a 20 and 22 mm implant in adults. Mathematically, a 20–22 mm implant fills a volume of 4.2–5.6 ml, and as the "ideal" prosthetic eye fills another 2 ml, the total 6–7 ml average orbital volume deficit is adequately filled with this size implant [12, 13].

Special Considerations

Implant sizing in children is more variable due to their having an immature orbit which undergoes rapid growth from birth to about 5 years of age. The orbit then slowly continues to grow before finally reaching its full adult size at around 15 years of age [14]. Generally, 16 mm implants may be used in infants less than 6 months of age, 18 mm implants in children less than 4 years of age, and the 20 mm implant for older ages [10, 15]. Another option is the use of an orbital tissue expander such as the OSMED SPHERE™ orbital expander (FCI Ophthalmics, Issy-Les-Moulineaux, Cedex, France), which slowly increases in size once implanted, providing the stimulus for orbital soft tissue and bony growth during childhood.

Implant Material

The ideal characteristics for an implant material include the following: it should be bioinert, easy to work with, and inexpensive. Previous iterations of implant material have included glass (Fig. 9.2), gold (Fig. 9.3), cartilage, fat, bone, silk, wool, aluminum, cork, ivory, and paraffin [3, 4, 8, 16]. These materials have since fallen

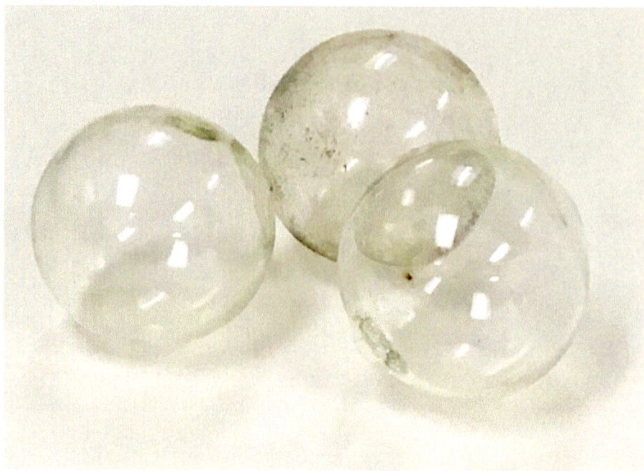

Fig. 9.2 Hollow glass orbital implant. (Courtesy of the Museum of Vision, American Academy of Ophthalmology)

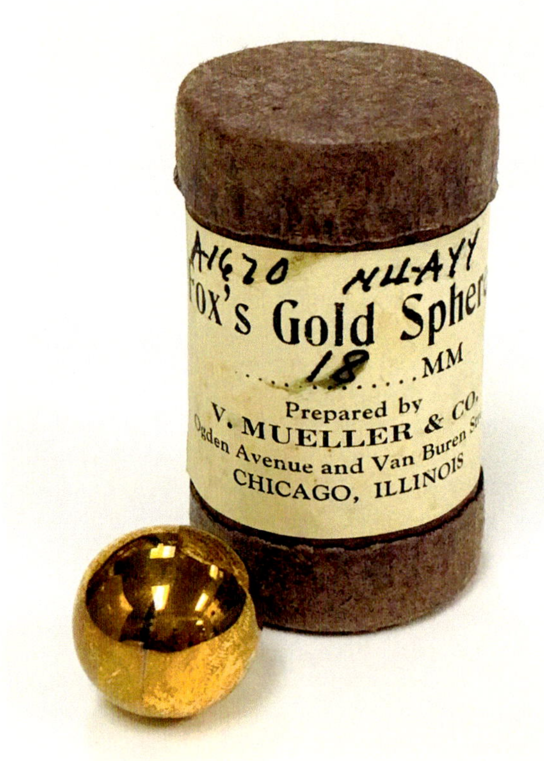

Fig. 9.3 Fox's gold sphere. (Courtesy of the Museum of Vision, American Academy of Ophthalmology)

out of favor due to a variety of reasons and will not be included in the discussion below.

Nonporous Implants

Nonporous implants have been the "traditional" implants and may be placed with or without wrapping material. Due to the length of time these implants have been around, they are typically cheaper to purchase. Despite their lower cost, these implants have been shown to have similar if not lower exposure rates compared to their newer porous counterparts, but have higher rates of implant migration due to lack of fibrovascular ingrowth [17]. Nonporous implants cannot be coupled with a peg system, but overall motility of unpegged porous versus nonporous implants has been found to be comparable in numerous studies [18, 19]. Nonporous implants remain popular, with a 2003 poll of American Society of Ophthalmic Plastic and Reconstructive Surgeons (ASOPRS) showing that 20% of respondents primarily use nonporous (silicone or polymethyl methacrylate) implants [20].

Silicone

Silicone is commonly used in medicine as an implantation material, such as in breast augmentation surgery. In ophthalmology, silicone is used during intraocular lens implantation, glaucoma tube placement, and in retinal detachment surgery.

Orbital silicone implants are much cheaper to purchase compared to porous implants. Interestingly, despite this lower cost, studies comparing orbital asymmetry using hydroxyapatite versus silicone implants showed that the more expensive HA implant produced no better orbital volume symmetry compared to the silicone implant [21]. Furthermore, some authors have introduced new techniques of suturing muscles directly onto the silicone sphere with minimal complications. This technique obviates the need for wrapping material and, in conjunction with the already low cost of silicone implants, argues for the increased use of this material, especially in regions where healthcare resources are scarce [22].

Polymethyl Methacrylate

Polymethyl methacrylate (PMMA), otherwise known as acrylic, is still a commonly used implant material following enucleation/evisceration surgeries (Fig. 9.4). It is well tolerated in the orbit and may be prefabricated into a sphere or molded into various specialized configurations. Historically, PMMA has been used as the material of choice for the quasi-integrated completely buried implants such as the Allen implant, the Iowa implant, and the Universal implant, which have all largely fallen out of favor [23]. PMMA implants are also relatively inexpensive.

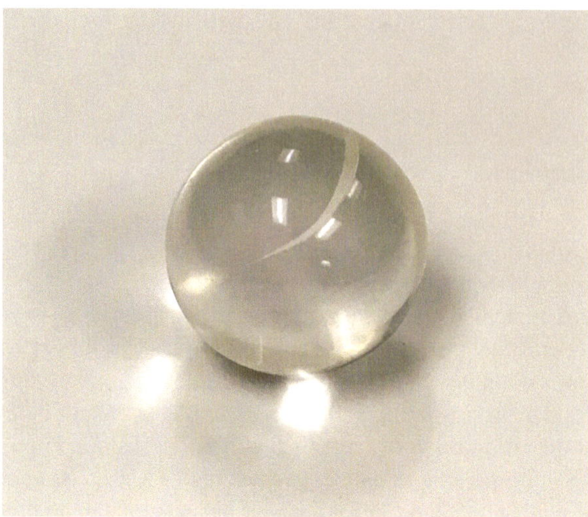

Fig. 9.4 Polymethyl methacrylate (PMMA) implant. (Courtesy of the Museum of Vision, American Academy of Ophthalmology)

Porous Implants

Porous implants are currently the most popular choice for orbital implant material, replacing the solid nonporous implants of the past. Porous implants allow for biointegration, promoting fibrovascular ingrowth into the micropores, theoretically decreasing the risk of infection and implant migration [24, 25]. These types of implants also allow the surgeon to place a peg, coupling the implant with an ocular prosthesis thereby improving prosthetic motility.

Porous implants are typically more expensive to purchase than their older, nonporous counterparts. The implant's pores, though providing numerous benefits to vascular integration, have a rough surface that can cause chronic irritation to the overlying conjunctiva. Once these porous implants become infected, they oftentimes must be explanted as the bacterial infection is commonly found deep in the avascular center of the implant [25, 26].

Porous Hydroxyapatite

Hydroxyapatite (HA) is a coralline-derived implant that first received FDA approval (BioEye™; Integrated Orbital Implants, San Diego, CA) in 1989 and represented the first generation of porous implant (Fig. 9.5) [27, 28]. Vascular ingrowth occurs slowly and, if wrapped in sclera, starts at the scleral windows and progresses centrally [29]. At 3 months, the periphery of the implant becomes vascularized, but the center of the implant does not fully vascularize until around 7 months post implantation [30, 31].

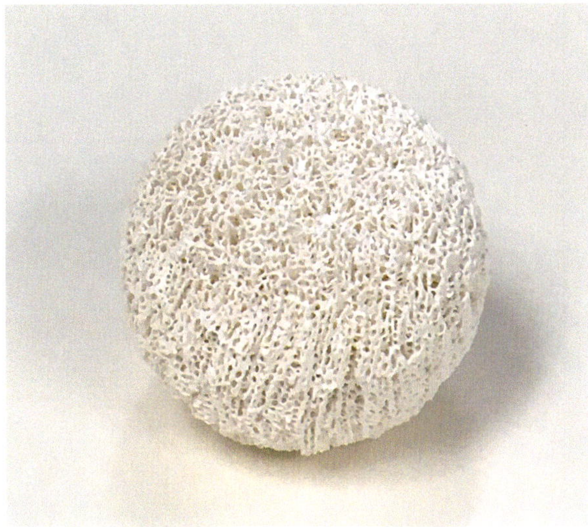

Fig. 9.5 Porous hydroxyapatite (HA). (Courtesy of the Museum of Vision, American Academy of Ophthalmology)

Despite the benefits of fibrovascular ingrowth, reports began to surface that HA had higher rates of implant extrusion and inflammation rates compared to older silicone spheres [30]. Indeed, following the introduction of HA, numerous reports of prolonged orbital inflammation to the material emerged with increasing reports of implant exposure [32, 33]. Due to these issues, improvements in surgical technique and implant wrapping have largely addressed these concerns [15, 30]. The largest series by Yoon et al. from 1990 to 2005 reported a wrapped HA implant exposure rate of 2.1% [15].

Currently, there are numerous companies that produce a hydroxyapatite implant. BioEye™ produces the original coralline HA implant. BioEye™ has also produces the Coated BioEye™ HA implant, which became available in 2003 and purports to be smoother and allow direct suturing of the muscle to the implant. The M Sphere™ (Molteno Ophthalmic Limited, Dunedin, New Zealand) is derived from the mineral portion of mammalian bone devoid of its organic components. This implant has a similar pore size as the BioEye implant and similar vascular ingrowth capabilities but is more fragile than the original BioEye implant [34]. The newer-generation synthetic HA implants (FCI; Issy-Les-Moulineaux, Cedex, France) have similar physical and biologic characteristics to the BioEye implant and are not coralline-derived [35, 36].

Porous Polyethylene

Porous polyethylene (PP) is a synthetic material that is an alternative material to HA, offering several advantages (Fig. 9.6). Its porous design, much like in HA implants, offers fibrovascular ingrowth, providing similar qualities that prevent

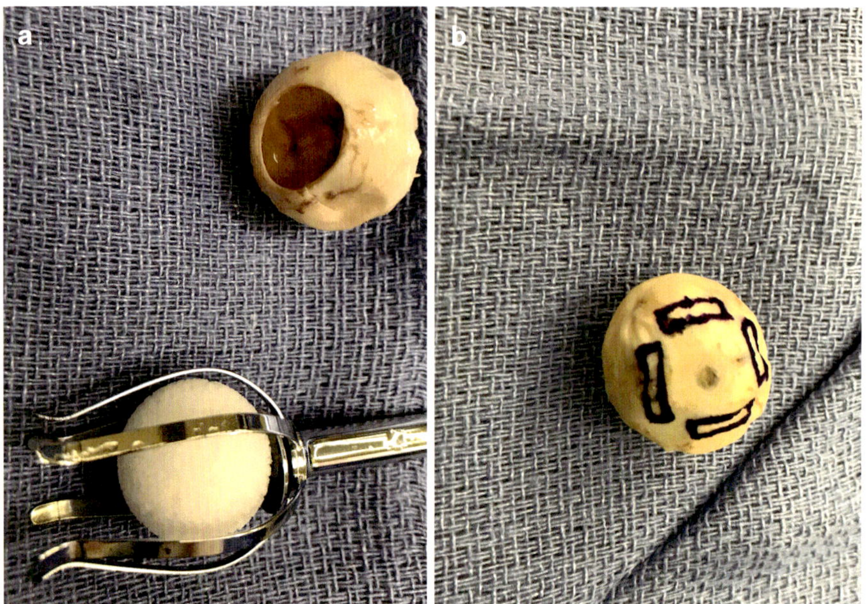

Fig. 9.6 (**a**) Porous polyethylene (PP) implant in a sphere introducer in preparation for placement into a scleral shell. (**b**) Porous polyethylene housed within a scleral wrap with rectus muscle windows cut out

implant migration and infection. The material causes less inflammation and has a smoother surface compared to HA, allowing it to be well tolerated in the orbit and conjunctiva without the necessity of using an overlying wrapping material [37]. PP is generally a cheaper material to purchase compared to HA while having similar rates of implant extrusion [20, 26]. Unlike hydroxyapatite, porous polyethylene is a softer material which allows for the rectus muscles to be directly sutured to the implant without the need for wrapping material. Pegging, if desired, may be also performed by hand drill instead of a power drill as is required in the case of HA.

Due to these benefits, porous polyethylene has become a popular implant material. A 1992 ASOPRS survey showed that 56% of oculoplastic surgeons preferred the use of HA implants [38], but following the introduction of PP, the same survey performed 10 years later showed a shift toward a preference for porous polyethylene implants (43%) compared to a 26% preference for HA [20]. However, both materials are widely used, and the choice comes down to a surgeon's preference.

Currently, PP implants are made by MEDPOR (Stryker, Kalamazoo, MI, USA) and SU-POR (Poriferous LLC, Newnan, GA, USA). Newer implants include the MEDPOR smooth surface tunnel (SST), SST-EZ, PLUS SST, PLUS SST-EZ, and the SU-POR Cor-Tec sphere. These implants have components which promote increased fibrovascular ingrowth, a porous anterior surface, and prefabricated tunnel and suture holes for the placement of rectus muscles without the need to use a wrapping material. The MEDPOR and SU-POR conical implants have a conical shape, filling more posterior volume compared to the standard spherical implant. These newer-generation implants may incur higher costs compared to the spherical porous polyethylene implants.

Aluminum Oxide

Aluminum oxide is an alternative porous implant material that was FDA approved in 2000 as the Alumina™ implant (FCI, Issy-Les-Moulineaux, France). This material has been long used in otolaryngology and orthopedics due to its bioinert characteristics. Like other porous implants, it provides the same benefits associated with fibrovascular ingrowth and has a more uniform pore structure when compared to HA implants [39]. The material does not dissolve over time and, following placement into the body, forms an overlying protein layer, decreasing the immune foreign body response against it [39].

Special Considerations

Prior to placement of a porous implant, many surgeons soak the material in an antibiotic solution as prophylaxis against infection. However, Badilla et al. showed that implants soaked in a dye solution for 5 minutes had insufficient dye reaching the center of the implant [40]. The authors instead suggest placing the implant in a large 40–60 ml syringe with 20 ml of solution, blocking the exit port, and alternately compressing and withdrawing plunger for 1 minute to adequately saturate the entire implant [40]. Notably, it is unclear if improved implant saturation provides a clinical benefit of infection prevention.

In cases of trauma where there is higher potential for infection, the authors prefer use of a PMMA sphere. If the rectus muscles are found, a wrapping material may be used to cover the implant to allow for attachment of the rectus muscles; if there is loss of the rectus muscles, the PMMA implant is placed deep into the orbit, and a multilayered Tenon's closure is performed.

In cases of infection such as in a corneal ulcer or endophthalmitis, the decision to place an implant is made on a case-to-case basis. If an implant is placed, the authors prefer a wrapped PMMA sphere, as it may be easily explanted if an infection develops. Additionally, its nonporous structure prevents bacteria from becoming sequestered in the otherwise central avascular core of a porous implant.

Wrapping Materials

Following determination of which implant type to use, the surgeon must determine whether to directly place the implant into the orbit or to first encase it in a wrapping material. The use of this material varies between surgeons; a 2003 survey showed that the majority (60%) of ASOPRS surgeons do not wrap their orbital implants [20]. This preference is likely related to the increased utility of PP implants, where the rectus muscles can be directly attached to the implant. In the case of nonporous implants, the use of a wrap is necessary to facilitate rectus muscle attachment. Even in cases where porous implants are utilized, the use of wrapping material allows for improved ease of extraocular muscle attachment. Furthermore, despite the numerous benefits described following the introduction of porous implants in the 1990s, one major complication is implant exposure, especially anteriorly where the implant surface and conjunctiva meet [41]. In order to prevent exposure, surgeons began wrapping porous implants to create a smoother anterior surface and improved insertion into the orbit. The wrapping material protects the conjunctiva from underlying inflammation and erosion.

Currently the most popular wrapping materials include donor sclera (Fig. 9.6) and polyglactin 910 (Vicryl™, Ethicon, Somerville, NJ) mesh. The most popular wrap material is donor sclera (25% of ASOPRS respondents in 2003), which has been found to have implant exposure rates of 1.1–11% [20, 42]. In countries where donor sclera is readily accessible, the material is characteristically easy to work with, provides a smooth barrier for implant insertion, and provides a good anchor for muscle attachment. In patients with poor wound healing, such as those exposed to radiation from retinoblastoma, studies have shown that unwrapped PP implants yielded a 24% exposure rate versus <1% in patients receiving sclera-wrapped implants [43]. Rather surprisingly, histologic studies have shown that the sclera overlying an implant may act as a barrier for fibrovascular ingrowth, preventing proper vascularization of a porous implant and theoretically increasing the risk for tissue breakdown [16]. Furthermore, concerns of disease transmission from donor sclera such as HIV can be used to argue against the use of this material [44]. Notably, despite these theoretical risks, there have not been reports of disease transmission with the use of donor sclera. We prefer the use of donor sclera as our first choice wrapping material due to its aforementioned advantages.

Other authors prefer polyglactin 910 mesh due to its inexpensive cost, ease of use, and rapid fibrovascular ingrowth [45]. When used, this material has been found to have an implant exposure rate of 2.1–9.4% [42]. Although polyglactin 910 has been found to have improved fibrovascular ingrowth due to its mesh sheeting, its absorbable characteristics give it the potential to cause breakdown of the conjunctiva, especially if the underlying implant surface is irregular [45]. However, histopathological analysis has shown that upon its absorption, the implant surface becomes surrounded by a fibrocellular barrier that prevents exposure [45]. Other similar absorbable wraps include polyester urethane and polyglycolic acid which both promote vascular ingrowth and provide barrier characteristics against implant extrusion.

Less commonly used wrapping materials include autologous temporalis fascia, fascia lata, posterior auricular muscle, and rectus abdominis sheath wraps [20].

The overall benefit of utilizing wrapping material remains unclear as reports provide conflicting data on whether wraps prevent conjunctival erosion. In the case of porous implants, some authors report benefit [16, 46], while others report no added benefit to its use [47, 48]. In the case of nonporous implants, extrusion rates may be prevented with implant wrapping, with some studies demonstrating as low as a 0.6% extrusion rate following use of donor sclera wrap [46]. However, utilizing an implant wrap adds both increased material cost and operative time to the procedure.

Pegging

Implanting a peg into an orbital implant is typically performed to provide improved prosthetic motility and allow direct transfer of force from the implant onto the ocular prosthesis. Ideally, the increased motility provides a more realistic appearance to the prosthetic, allowing for the fine darting eye movements that occur during conversation. In the 1992 survey of ASOPRS members, 73% of respondents performed the pegging procedure, but as surgeons noted the complications of pegging including implant exposure, chronic discharge, pyogenic granuloma formation, and infection, the practice grew less popular [20, 38]. A 2003 ASOPRS survey showed that the popularity of pegging plunged to only 8% of implants performed [20].

If the surgeon decides to place a peg, a porous implant such as hydroxyapatite, porous polyethylene, or aluminum oxide must be used. It typically takes around 6 months for an implant to completely vascularize before a pegging procedure can be performed; the status of an implant's vascularization may be checked with magnetic resonance imaging to confirm complete vascular integration of the orbital implant. Notably, if a patient has poor vascular function, illness, infection, or a barrier to implant vascularization, then the surgeon must consider the increased risks of this procedure, as poor implant vascularization can lead to peg or implant extrusion(Fig. 9.7).

Previous iterations of peg material include nonsleeved PMMA or sleeved polycarbonate systems which had peg extrusion rates of 20% [15]. By switching to titanium pegs, the rates of complications including peg extrusion, pyogenic granuloma, and discharge were lowered [15, 49]. In our practice, we no longer perform pegging procedures given the aforementioned complications and find that patients still attain excellent motility results. Furthermore, studies have shown that after prioritizing the health of the remaining eye, anophthalmic patients were most bothered by watering, crusting, and discharge in their prosthetic eye [50]. As pegging may increase these unwanted symptoms, the authors believe patients also attain high postoperative satisfaction following simple unpegged orbital implant placement.

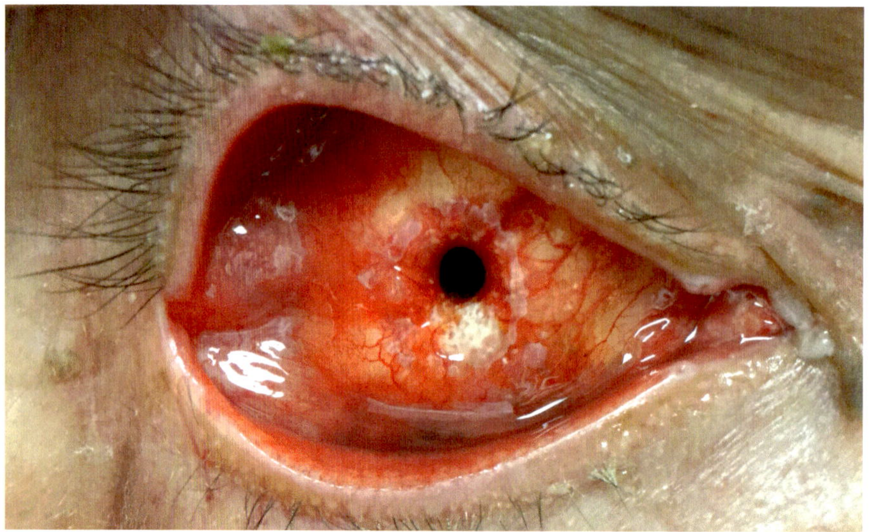

Fig. 9.7 Extruded peg with early implant exposure

References

1. Burch FE. Evisceration of the globe with scleral implant and preservation of the cornea. Trans Am Ophthalmol Soc. 1939;37:272–82.
2. Luce CM. A short history of enucleation. Int Ophthalmol Clin. 1970;10(4):681–7.
3. Mules PH. Evisceration of the globe with artificial vitreous. 1884–1895. Adv Ophthalmic Plast Reconstr Surg. 1990;8:69–72.
4. Berens C. Enucleation with implantation of foreign substances into Tenon's capsule: a technique in which no sutures are buried. Am J Ophthalmol. 1937;20(3):293–6.
5. Lang W. On the insertion of artificial globes into Tenon's capsule after excising the eye. Trans Ophth Soc UK. 1887;7:286.
6. Wheeler JM. Implantation of hollow grooved body into orbit for filling: late after enucleation of eyeball. Arch Ophthalmol. 1938;20(5):709–12.
7. Allen JH, Allen L. A buried muscle cone implant. Development of a tunneled hemispherical type. Arch Ophthalmol. 1950;43(5):879–90.
8. Cutler NL. A positive contact ball and ring implant for use after enucleation. Arch Ophthalmol. 1947;37(1):73–81.
9. Mules PH. Evisceration of the eye, and its relation to the bacterial theory of the origin of sympathetic disease. Br Med J. 1886;1(1310):246–7.
10. Shields CL, Shields JA, De Potter P, Singh AD. Problems with the hydroxyapatite orbital implant: experience with 250 consecutive cases. Br J Ophthalmol. 1994;78(9):702–6.
11. Kaltreider SA, Newman SA. Prevention and management of complications associated with the hydroxyapatite implant. Ophthalmic Plast Reconstr Surg. 1996;12(1):18–31.
12. Custer PL, Trinkaus KM. Volumetric determination of enucleation implant size. Am J Ophthalmol. 1999;128(4):489–94.
13. Tyers AG, Collin JR. Baseball orbital implants: a review of 39 patients. Br J Ophthalmol. 1985;69(6):438–42.
14. Bentley RP, Sgouros S, Natarajan K, Dover MS, Hockley AD. Normal changes in orbital volume during childhood. J Neurosurg. 2002;96(4):742–6.
15. Yoon JS, Lew H, Kim SJ, Lee SY. Exposure rate of hydroxyapatite orbital implants a 15-year experience of 802 cases. Ophthalmology. 2008;115(3):566–72 e2.

16. Remulla HD, Rubin PA, Shore JW, Sutula FC, Townsend DJ, Woog JJ, et al. Complications of porous spherical orbital implants. Ophthalmology. 1995;102(4):586–93.
17. Trichopoulos N, Augsburger JJ. Enucleation with unwrapped porous and nonporous orbital implants: a 15-year experience. Ophthalmic Plast Reconstr Surg. 2005;21(5):331–6.
18. Colen TP, Paridaens DA, Lemij HG, Mourits MP, van Den Bosch WA. Comparison of artificial eye amplitudes with acrylic and hydroxyapatite spherical enucleation implants. Ophthalmology. 2000;107(10):1889–94.
19. Custer PL, Trinkaus KM, Fornoff J. Comparative motility of hydroxyapatite and alloplastic enucleation implants. Ophthalmology. 1999;106(3):513–6.
20. Su GW, Yen MT. Current trends in managing the anophthalmic socket after primary enucleation and evisceration. Ophthalmic Plast Reconstr Surg. 2004;20(4):274–80.
21. Lyle CE, Wilson MW, Li CS, Kaste SC. Comparison of orbital volumes in enucleated patients with unilateral retinoblastoma: hydroxyapatite implants versus silicone implants. Ophthalmic Plast Reconstr Surg. 2007;23(5):393–6.
22. Wells TS, Harris GJ. Direct fixation of extraocular muscles to a silicone sphere: a cost-sensitive, low-risk enucleation procedure. Ophthalmic Plast Reconstr Surg. 2011;27(5):364–7.
23. Spivey BE, Allen L, Burns CA. The Iowa enucleation implant. A 10-year evaluation of technique and results. Am J Ophthalmol. 1969;67(2):171–88.
24. Karsloglu S, Serin D, Simsek I, Ziylan S. Implant infection in porous orbital implants. Ophthalmic Plast Reconstr Surg. 2006;22(6):461–6.
25. Chuo JY, Dolman PJ, Ng TL, Buffam FV, White VA. Clinical and histopathologic review of 18 explanted porous polyethylene orbital implants. Ophthalmology. 2009;116(2):349–54.
26. Custer PL, Trinkaus KM. Porous implant exposure: incidence, management, and morbidity. Ophthalmic Plast Reconstr Surg. 2007;23(1):1–7.
27. Dutton JJ. Coralline hydroxyapatite as an ocular implant. Ophthalmology. 1991;98(3):370–7.
28. Perry AC. Integrated orbital implants. Adv Ophthalmic Plast Reconstr Surg. 1990;8:75–81.
29. Shields CL, Shields JA, De Potter P, Singh AD. Lack of complications of the hydroxyapatite orbital implant in 250 consecutive cases. Trans Am Ophthalmol Soc. 1993;91:177–89; discussion 89–95.
30. Nunery WR, Heinz GW, Bonnin JM, Martin RT, Cepela MA. Exposure rate of hydroxyapatite spheres in the anophthalmic socket: histopathologic correlation and comparison with silicone sphere implants. Ophthalmic Plast Reconstr Surg. 1993;9(2):96–104.
31. Klapper SR, Jordan DR, Brownstein S, Punja K. Incomplete fibrovascularization of a hydroxyapatite orbital implant 3 months after implantation. Arch Ophthalmol. 1999;117(8):1088–9.
32. Rosner M, Edward DP, Tso MO. Foreign-body giant-cell reaction to the hydroxyapatite orbital implant. Arch Ophthalmol. 1992;110(2):173–4.
33. Goldberg RA, Holds JB, Ebrahimpour J. Exposed hydroxyapatite orbital implants. Report of six cases. Ophthalmology. 1992;99(5):831–6.
34. Jordan DR, Hwang I, Brownstein S, McEachren T, Gilberg S, Grahovac S, et al. The molteno m-sphere. Ophthalmic Plast Reconstr Surg. 2000;16(5):356–62.
35. Jordan DR, Munro SM, Brownstein S, Gilberg SM, Grahovac SZ. A synthetic hydroxyapatite implant: the so-called counterfeit implant. Ophthalmic Plast Reconstr Surg. 1998;14(4):244–9.
36. Celik T, Yuksel D, Kosker M, Kasim R, Simsek S. Vascularization of coralline versus synthetic hydroxyapatite orbital implants assessed by gadolinium enhanced magnetic resonance imaging. Curr Eye Res. 2015;40(3):346–53.
37. Karesh JW, Dresner SC. High-density porous polyethylene (Medpor) as a successful anophthalmic socket implant. Ophthalmology. 1994;101(10):1688–95; discussion 95–6.
38. Hornblass A, Biesman BS, Eviatar JA. Current techniques of enucleation: a survey of 5,439 intraorbital implants and a review of the literature. Ophthalmic Plast Reconstr Surg. 1995;11(2):77–86; discussion 7–8.
39. Jordan DR, Mawn LA, Brownstein S, McEachren TM, Gilberg SM, Hill V, et al. The bioceramic orbital implant: a new generation of porous implants. Ophthalmic Plast Reconstr Surg. 2000;16(5):347–55.
40. Badilla J, Dolman PJ. Methods of antibiotic instillation in porous orbital implants. Ophthalmic Plast Reconstr Surg. 2008;24(4):287–9.

41. Buettner H, Bartley GB. Tissue breakdown and exposure associated with orbital hydroxyapatite implants. Am J Ophthalmol. 1992;113(6):669–73.
42. Li T, Shen J, Duffy MT. Exposure rates of wrapped and unwrapped orbital implants following enucleation. Ophthalmic Plast Reconstr Surg. 2001;17(6):431–5.
43. Christmas NJ, Van Quill K, Murray TG, Gordon CD, Garonzik S, Tse D, et al. Evaluation of efficacy and complications: primary pediatric orbital implants after enucleation. Arch Ophthalmol. 2000;118(4):503–6.
44. Seiff SR, Chang JS Jr, Hurt MH, Khayam-Bashi H. Polymerase chain reaction identification of human immunodeficiency virus-1 in preserved human sclera. Am J Ophthalmol. 1994;118(4):528–30.
45. Jordan DR, Allen LH, Ells A, Gilberg S, Brownstein S, Munro S, et al. The use of Vicryl mesh (polyglactin 910) for implantation of hydroxyapatite orbital implants. Ophthalmic Plast Reconstr Surg. 1995;11(2):95–9.
46. Jongman HP, Marinkovic M, Notting I, Koetsier L, Swart W, Schalij-Delfos NE, et al. Donor sclera-wrapped acrylic orbital implants following enucleation: experience in 179 patients in the Netherlands. Acta Ophthalmol. 2016;94(3):253–6.
47. Suter AJ, Molteno AC, Bevin TH, Fulton JD, Herbison P. Long term follow up of bone derived hydroxyapatite orbital implants. Br J Ophthalmol. 2002;86(11):1287–92.
48. Blaydon SM, Shepler TR, Neuhaus RW, White WL, Shore JW. The porous polyethylene (Medpor) spherical orbital implant: a retrospective study of 136 cases. Ophthalmic Plast Reconstr Surg. 2003;19(5):364–71.
49. Jordan DR, Klapper SR. A new titanium peg system for hydroxyapatite orbital implants. Ophthalmic Plast Reconstr Surg. 2000;16(5):380–7.
50. Rokohl AC, Koch KR, Trester M, Trester W, Pine KR, Heindl LM. Concerns of anophthalmic patients wearing cryolite glass prosthetic eyes. Ophthalmic Plast Reconstr Surg. 2018;34(4):369–74.

Chapter 10
Osseous Integration After Exenteration

Zakeya Mohammed Al-Sadah and Mohammed Salman AlShakhas

- Historical prospective
- Implant healing biology
- Factors affecting osseointegration
- Principle of implant surgery: preoperative planning, surgical technique, postoperative care, and follow-up
- Osseointegration in irradiated patients
- Advantages and disadvantages of osseointegrated implants
- Complications of orbital implants

Historical Perspective

A Swedish physician and researcher, Professor P.I. Brånemark, discovered osseointegration in the 1960s during insertion of hollow thread-shaped titanium chambers into a rabbit's tibia. He found it hard to separate the titanium chambers once healing occurred and that bone was in intimate contact with the implant and had grown into thin spaces within the implant [1]. He reached the conclusion that bone was integrated with the titanium implant. However, it was not possible to study histologically the implant-bone interface without bone decalcification or removal of the implant. It was only after the development of the Sage-Schliff (saw and

Z. M. Al-Sadah (✉)
Ophthalmic Plastic and Reconstructive Surgery, Department of Ophthalmology, Bascom Palmer Eye Institute, University of Miami Miller School of Medicine, Miami, FL, USA
e-mail: zxa133@med.miami.edu

M. S. AlShakhas
Department of Oral and Maxillofacial Surgery, University of Alabama at Birmingham, Birmingham, AL, USA

T. E. Johnson (ed.), *Anophthalmia*,
https://doi.org/10.1007/978-3-030-29753-4_10

grind) technique in 1982 [2], when osseointegration was confirmed at higher magnification [3].

In further experimental studies, Brånemark succeeded in rehabilitating canines after dental extraction with an implant-supported prosthesis. This study demonstrated the ability of the implant to withstand the functional load of mastication without negative impact [1]. He then applied this finding in human subjects and placed the first dental implant in an edentulous patient in 1965. A 10-year-long clinical study was published in 1977, and osseointegration was accepted by the Swedish academy of dentistry [3]. The research by Brånemark was not recognized outside Scandinavia until his data was presented in the seminal Toronto conference in 1982 [4].

The application of osseointegration was then further expanded outside the oral cavity to include the craniofacial area. The first bone-anchored hearing aid (BAHA) was introduced by Tjellström et al. in 1977 [5] which improved comfort and quality utilizing a hearing aid. The first implant-retained ear prosthesis was successfully performed by Tjellström et al. in 1981 [6] after resection of basal cell carcinoma. This implant-fixed prosthesis offered excellent cosmesis and improved retention making it superior to the traditional fixation methods used for prosthesis retention after exenteration (Fig. 10.1). Those traditional fixation methods include eye glasses or frames, adhesives, and tissue undercuts. The traditional methods have the issues of instability, lack of secure attachment to the face, and the fact that adhesives would weaken with time, requiring frequent application of glue or double-sided tape to keep the prosthesis in place. In addition, skin irritation from the adhesives limits the patient's activity and affects their self-confidence and overall quality of life [7].

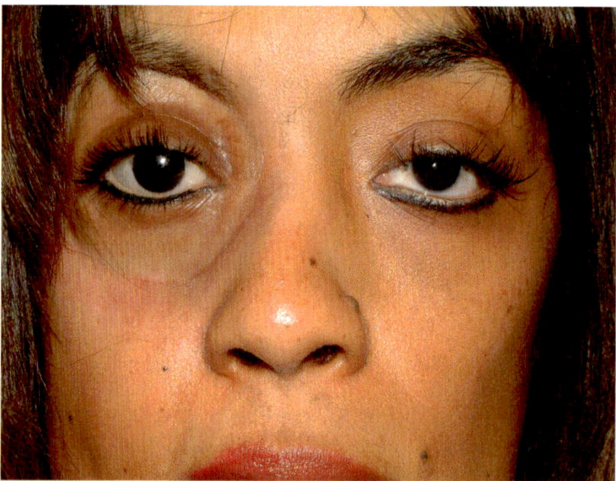

Fig. 10.1 Post-exenteration implant-retained upper facial prosthesis. (Published with kind permission of Dr. Allison K. Vest. All rights reserved)

Definition and Biology of Osseointegration

The first definition of osseointegration was published in 1981 as "a direct contact between a loaded implant surface and bone at the light microscopic level of resolution" [8]. Shortly, the definition of osseointegration evolved from a pure histological description and was replaced with "a direct structural and functional connection between ordered living bone and the surface of a load-carrying implant" in 1985 [3]. In 1991, Zarb and Alberktsson introduced a more comprehensive clinical and goal-oriented definition as "a process whereby clinically asymptomatic rigid fixation of alloplastic materials Is achieved and maintained in bone during functional loading" [9].

Osseointegration is not a distinct singular biological process; however, it is a combination of bone regeneration and remodeling processes similar in many aspects to the healing process observed in fractures [10, 11]. Peri-implant osteogenesis can be categorized as contact osteogenesis (bone formation from implant surface toward the host bone) and distance osteogenesis [10] (from host bone toward implant surface). Both involve three basic mechanisms: osteoconduction, de novo osteogenesis, and later remodeling [10, 12].

Osteoconduction term implies formation of bone along a biologically compatible conduit or scaffold. Osteoconduction starts with the initial tissue contact to the implant. When blood contacts the titanium implant, it results in the breakdown and formation of fibrin matrix around the implant and migration of differentiating osteogenic cells toward the implant. Critical to this process is platelet degranulation and release of growth and chemotactic factors creating a high concentration along the implant surface, favoring migration toward the implant surface [10, 12].

De novo bone formation starts with the formation of a matrix resembling the cement lines seen in bone histology separating old and newly formed bone. This matrix is secreted by the osteoprogenitor cell adhering to implant surface, and this interface is described to be of 0.2–0.5 micrometer thickness [13]. This formation is followed by collagen fiber deposition and later calcification [10]. Both osteoconduction and de novo bone formation contribute to formation of contact osteogenesis. However, together with distance osteogenesis, woven bone formation around the implant will contribute to biological fixation during and after a few weeks post operatively, differing from primary stability achieved mechanically at the time of surgery through friction of the implant with bone [10, 12, 13].

Remodeling occurs to replace the rapidly deposited woven bone with dense lamellar bone. Woven bone is formed in a rapid fashion resulting in less density of collagen fibers and random architectural orientation. Lamellar bone offers superior mechanical properties due to the higher density of collagen and higher mineralization. Remodeling is a continuous process most importantly governed by strain and mechanical forces at the healing sites as described by Wolff's law [10, 13].

Factors Influencing Success of Osseointegration

Implant Material

Two materials are currently used in osseointegrated implants: commercially pure titanium (cp-Ti) in oral and craniofacial application and titanium alloy (Ti6Al4V) in orthopedics [14]. Titanium and its alloys particularly show high biocompatibility, high strength, and resistance to corrosion [12]. Titanium spontaneously forms an oxide layer upon exposure to air. Most importantly, this oxide layer is stable and maintained under various physiological conditions. This stability renders titanium exceptionally corrosion resistant. In addition, cp-Ti has a modulus of elasticity closer to bone than other metals making it mechanically favorable [15, 16].

Implant Design and Surface Characteristics

The surface of the implant influences the biology of osseointegration, strength of bone-implant interface, and loading forces distribution [17]. The surface design substantially influences the osteoconduction phase of osseointegration. It affects the level of platelet activation and more importantly the adhesion of fibrin matrix along the implant surface [10]. Surface roughness also increases implant surface area providing larger bone-implant interface [12]. In addition, experimental and clinical data indicate that increasing roughness of an implant would enhance and accelerate bone integration. In contradistinction, implants with smooth surface are found to have poor soft and hard tissue interface in addition to weaker biomechanical interface strengths [18].

Bone Quality

Higher bone density provides superior mechanical strength and resistance to loading forces secondary to higher bone-implant contact. The cortical bone has ten times more mechanical strength than cancellous bone and provides support by preventing micromotion and implant failure. Elasticity is another mechanical property influenced by bone density. Similarly, implants are found to have up to ten times the modulus of elasticity of the least dense bone. Mismatch in elasticity can result in implant failure at bone-implant interface due to dimensional changes and microstrains [17, 19].

Surgical Technique

Preoperative Evaluation

An ideal orbit for osseointegration has a thick healthy bone, a 4–5 mm of soft tissue thickness, and minimal dead space [20]. A multidisciplinary team consisting of an oculoplastic surgeon, a radiation oncologist, a medical oncologist, an anaplastologist, and a psychologist is needed for a thorough evaluation and careful planning along with coordinated post-operative care for the best results. Constant psychological evaluation should be performed, and realistic expectations and results should be always discussed with the patient continuously throughout the process [7, 20]. Specialized software can help plan and guide the whole procedure. A reconstructed 3D format of the CT images can help visualize the residual bony tissue for implant installation and its thickness after exenteration [7, 20]. This will help design and create a surgical guide for the position, number, trajectory, and angle of the implant for optimal implant position to support the prosthesis (Fig. 10.2). It will also help digitally design the prosthesis and customize the abutments needed for the prosthesis retention. The aim of the surgery is to have appropriate angles and spacing of the implant to allow manipulation of the prosthesis and eventually have a transparent, subtle transition line of the prosthesis [7, 20]. The use of stereotactic image guidance intraoperatively has also been described to help in implant placement specially in thin, poor-quality bone [21].

The complex 3D anatomy of the orbit and the varying thickness of different orbital bones make planning of the procedure and placement of the implant more challenging. The thicker lateral and superolateral orbital bone makes it more favorable for implant placement [7, 20]. Sometimes bone grafting should be considered if there was an extensive bony loss after exenteration. Healthy and adequate soft tissue around the implants is crucial for a healthy prosthetic placement and maintenance. Sometimes in cases of malignancy and when tumor surveillance is needed, a different method of prosthetic fixation should be used [22].

A decision is made whether to place the implants as a one-stage or a two-stage procedure. In the one-stage procedure, recommended only in the non-radiated bone, everything is inserted in one procedure including the implant and the abutment. The implants are left in place for 3–4 months for healing and for the osseointegration process to take place during which time the fabrication and fitting of the prosthesis can be performed. On the other hand, the two-stage prosthesis requires a 4–6-month interval between the insertion of the implant and the abutment to allow the osseointegration process to take place. One month after inserting the abutment, the prosthesis is fabricated and fitted. The two-stage procedure is preferred for all orbital cases, especially with those patients with irradiated bone and in pediatric patients and those patients with poor bone quality [7, 20]. Whenever possible, a 4 mm implant is

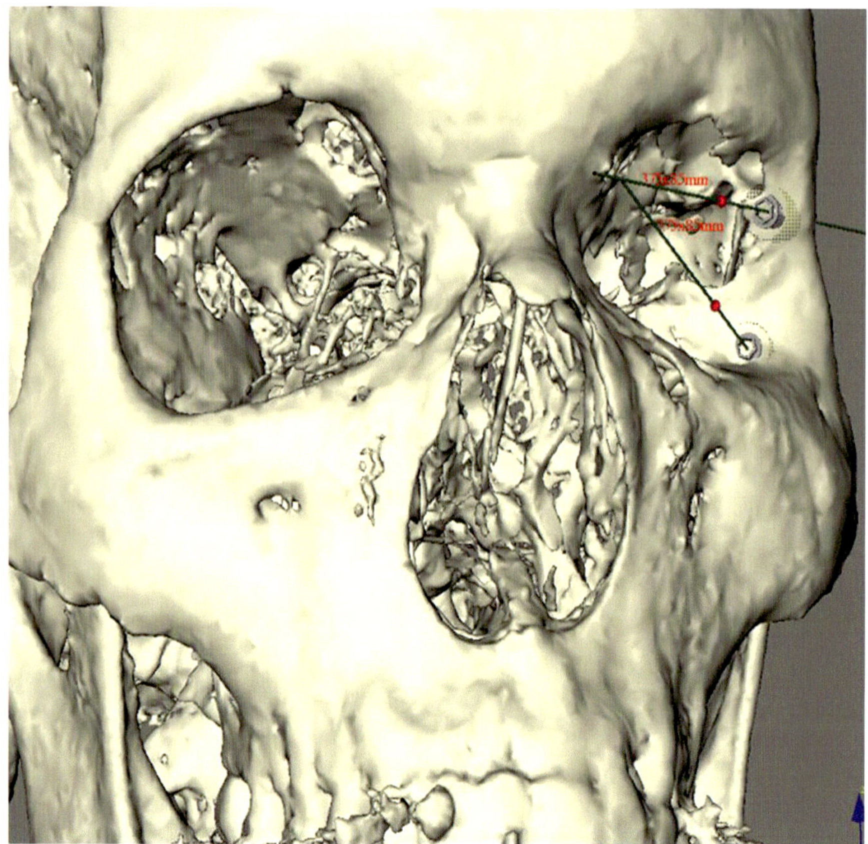

Fig. 10.2 Preoperative digital planning of a post-exenteration patient for implants to support an orbital prosthesis. (Published with kind permission of Dr. Edmond Bedrossian. All rights reserved)

used if the bone volume allows it [20]. Sleeper implants, which are extra implants placed simultaneously with the primary implants at the time of the surgery, are recommended in the irradiated bone cases due to higher rates of failure.

It is also important to determine the type of prosthetic attachment to be used, because it will affect the number of the implants. Generally, two options are available, the bar and clip versus the magnetic attachments. The bar construction is preferred due to stronger retention forces and MRI compatibility due to the lack of ferromagnetic material. Only when space is limited or cleaning under the cap difficult the magnetic attachment is recommended. In those cases, the magna cap (attached to the implant) is preferred over the magnabutment (directly mounted on the implant). With magnabutment, there is an inability to apply counter torque forces [23].

For a successful reconstruction by osseointegration, the mechanical system has to attach to an anchoring component that is fabricated by an inert material with an appropriate matching geometrical shape and dimension. The use of three points of fixation is advised for optimum implant placement. Care should be taken to minimally manipulate the surface of the implant to preserve its microarchitecture with careful preparation of the implant site for optimal osteointegration results. Minimum mobility of the skin around the abutment at the penetration site is required and achieved by preparing the skin in such a way that it adheres firmly and directly to underlying the periosteum.

Procedure Description

The surgical site preparation should be handled in atraumatic fashion. Most cases are performed under general anesthesia in the operating theater. After prepping and draping the patient in the usual sterile fashion for oculoplastic surgery, the planned areas of implants are marked with a marking pen. A template can be used for successful results. A mixture of 2% lidocaine with 1:100000 epinephrine is injected in the planned areas for a better control of hemostasis. Incisions are made a few millimeters behind the marked areas using a 15 blade. Dissection is carried down until the periosteum is exposed and incised (Fig. 10.3). A Freer elevator is used to expose the bone. Direct evaluation of the bone quality, health, and thickness is performed. Good quality bone and adequate bone thickness are crucial for implant placement to avoid undue convergence of the implant. Preparation of the surgical site for the implant consists of initial drilling at the marked site with a small round or spade-shaped burr (Fig. 10.4) followed by sequential parallel twist drills to increase the width and depth of the recipient site. This step takes place under copious irrigation and intermittent pressure to allow irrigation and decrease heat generation. A guide

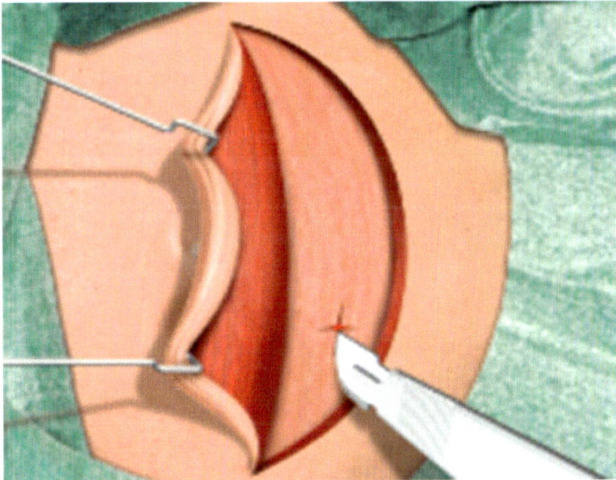

Fig. 10.3 Incision is made few millimeters behind the marked area, and dissection is carried down to expose periosteum. (Published with kind permission of COCHLEAR™ VISTAFIX®. All rights reserved)

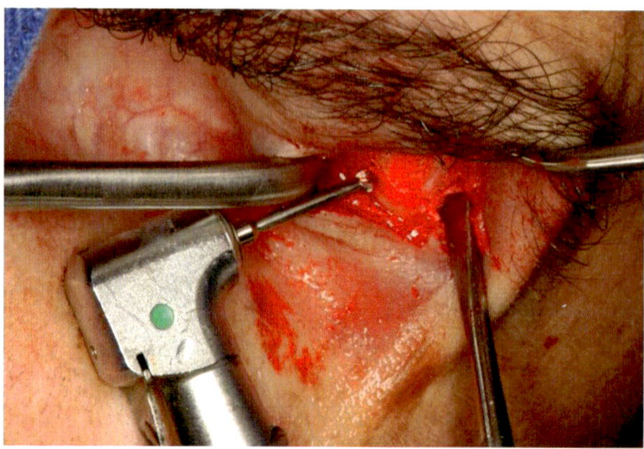

Fig. 10.4 Initial drilling at the marked site with a small round burr. (Published with kind permission of Dr. Edmond Bedrossian.)

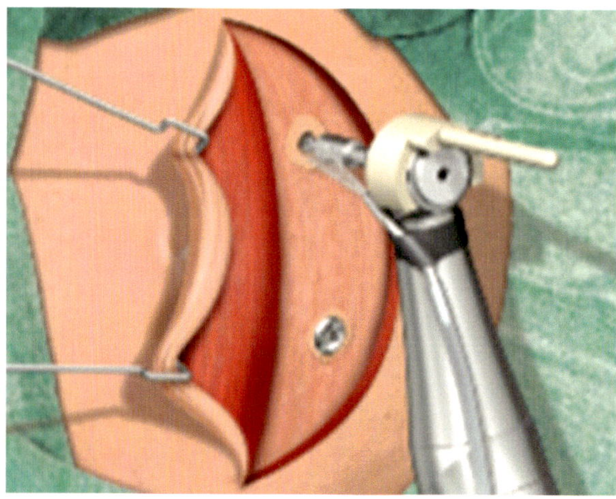

Fig. 10.5 Drilling is initiated with a guide drill and 3 mm spacer with continuous irrigation using manual drip. (Published with kind permission of COCHLEAR™ VISTAFIX®.)

drill with 3 mm spacer is used initially to create the osteotomies (Fig. 10.5). The drilling has to be performed perpendicular to the bone as it will affect the trajectory of the implant. It is important to move the burr up and down to ensure that the cooling solution reaches tip of the drill as excessive heat will jeopardize the osseointegration by damaging the bone. Over-widening of the osteotomy is also avoided as it will result in instability of the implant. If soft tissue is encountered, drilling is stopped at 3 mm depth. However, if bone volume is found adequate, the spacer is removed, and drilling is continued to a 4 mm depth. Depending on the depth reached with the counter drill, the osteotomy is widened with a countersink drill (Fig. 10.6).

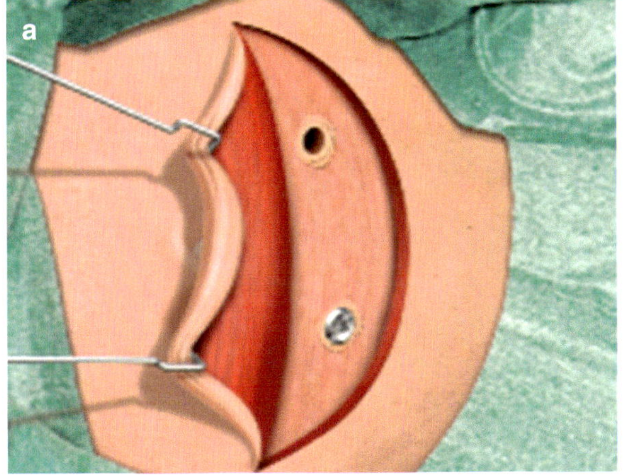

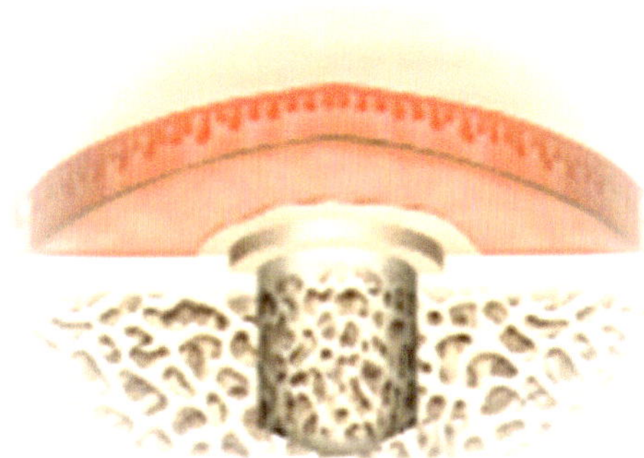

Fig. 10.6 (**a**) and (**b**) Widening drill is used to create a countersink in the bone. (Published with kind permission of COCHLEAR™ VISTAFIX®. All rights reserved)

A very low torque setting is recommended (20 Ncm) for implant insertion, and it can be increased as needed. Generally speaking, 2–3 implants are adequate to support the prosthesis and are placed at least 15 mm apart [23, 24]. If sleeper implants are planned, additional 3–4 implants are used. Some surgeons proposed the use of three extra (sleeper) implants in case of complications or failure of the first set of implants. The implant is inserted in the 3-mm-deep osteotomy after checking its depth and trajectory (Fig. 10.7). Abutments are placed, and the tissues are allowed to heal and osseointegration of the implant to take place for 3–4 months, followed by fabrication and fitting of the prosthesis (Fig. 10.8). This would conclude the one-stage osseointegration procedure. In general, local thin skin flaps to cover the implant are preferred over thick flaps since there will be less skin movement around the base of the abutment after healing due to the tight adhesions of the skin to the periosteum. Additionally the use of thin flaps helps prevent bacterial infections. Healing by secondary intention (granulation tissue) is not preferred due to the delay

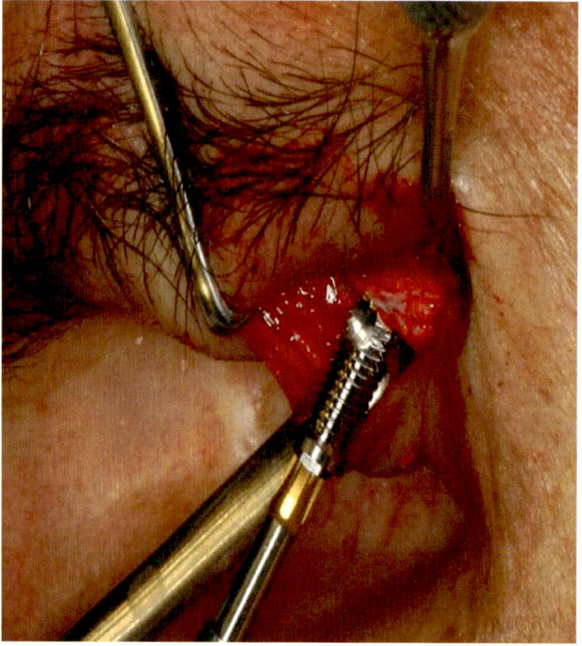

Fig. 10.7 Insertion of the implant into the osteotomy site. (Published with kind permission of Dr. Edmond Bedrossian.)

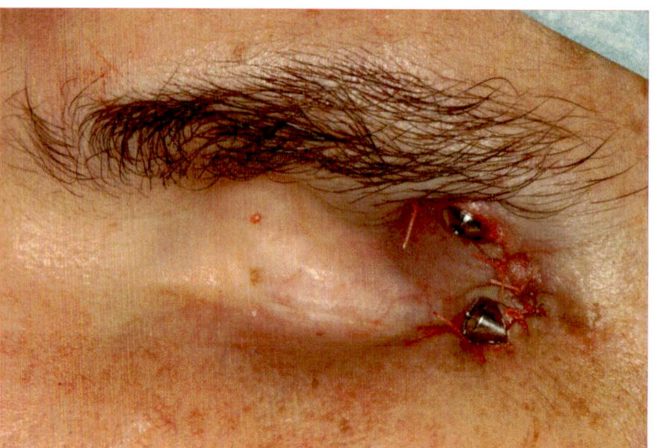

Fig. 10.8 Placement of healing abutments as the final step in the one-stage procedure. (Published with kind permission of Dr. Edmond Bedrossian.)

in healing. The edges of the flap are sutured to the trimmed periosteum to hold it in place. A 4 mm punch biopsy can be used to create holes in the skin around the implant sites. Permanent abutments are placed, but the use of healing abutments is recommended during the period of osseointegration, and permanent ones can be inserted later to allow tissue healing. Generally, 3–4 mm abutments are used, and they are placed onto the head of the implant and screwed partially down to secure it. The abutment holder is then removed by snapping it off. The internal screw is tightened into the implant using a hexagon screwdriver while holding the abutment in place using an abutment clamp to avoid any movement of the implant or the abutment. Plastic healing caps are placed on each abutment that is designed to hold a dressing in place to avoid postoperative hematomas. A light, even pressure dressing with antibiotic ointment is applied. The dressing has to be non-adherent to avoid tissue damage and patient discomfort, with light pressure to avoid hematoma formation. The pressure has to be even to avoid blood flow obstruction and tissue necrosis. It is cosmetically important to also fix both the medial canthal position and the eyebrow position after exenteration for precise prosthesis placement [24]. With the release of the arcus marginalis during exenteration, the brow tends to drop to a lower position than normal, and even further descent occurs as the healing process and scar formation with contracture of the tissues take place. Fixing the brow higher will provide better cosmesis, give a better transition between the normal tissue and the prosthesis, and prevent the descended brow from covering the abutments [24]. The two-stage implant procedure usually takes place 3 months after the initial procedure in non-irradiated orbits and after 6 months in irradiated orbits. The periosteum is folded over the flange of the implant, and cover screws are used after the implant insertion and covered with the soft tissue in the first stage. A minimum of three implants are exposed by thinning the soft tissue above the implant and exposing the cover screws or using 4 mm biopsy punch, and cover screws are removed (Fig. 10.9). The edges of the flap are sutured to the periosteum on the second stage, percutaneous abutments are connected, and a dressing is placed. If sleeper implants are used, they are left for possible use in the future in case of implant failure (Fig. 10.10).

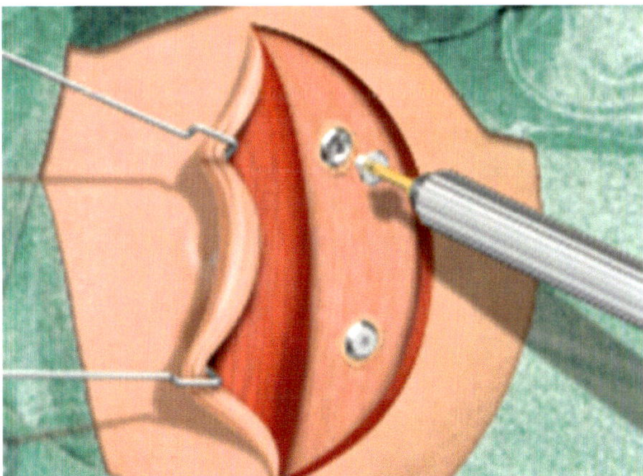

Fig. 10.9 Removal of cover screws using a screw driver after adequate exposure in the two-stage procedure. (Published with kind permission of COCHLEAR™ VISTAFIX®. All rights reserved)

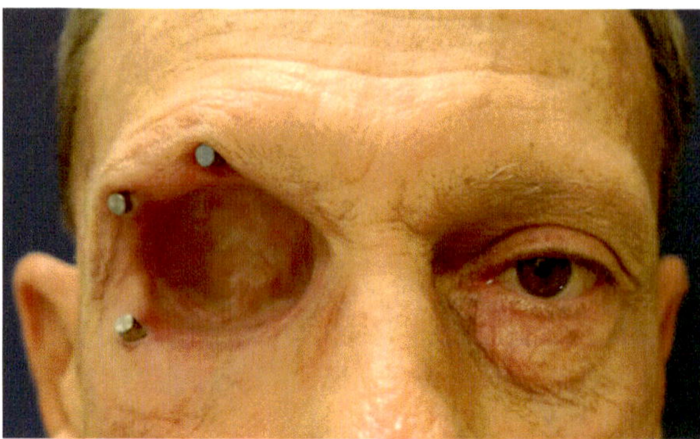

Fig. 10.10 Osseointegrated implants post-exenteration. (Published with kind permission of Dr. Thomas E, Johnson.)

Primary Stability

This term refers to the mechanical stability achieved at the initial stage of implant placement by engagement of the implant with bone. Stability is paramount to success, and micromotion >150 micrometers is detrimental to success as it favors cell differentiation toward fibroclasts over osteoblasts, leading to the failure of osseointegration. Primary stability depends mostly on the amount of cortical bone engagement and the quantity of surrounding bone. An increase in implant length and width will also add stability when clinically possible [25].

Post-op Care

The patient is seen 1 week postoperatively for suture and dressing removal. The site is cleaned and aerated, and a new dressing is applied. The patient is seen again after another week where the dressing and healing caps are removed in the two-stage procedure. The site is left open, and the patient is instructed to clean and apply antibiotic ointment onto the sites daily. It is normal to have skin debris which can be cleaned with a cotton-tip applicator. Vigorous cleaning should be avoided since it leads to irritation of the skin.

It is recommended in the one-stage procedure to avoid loading the implant until osteointegration is complete to avoid implant failure (Tables 10.1 and 10.2).

Success of Orbital Implant Osseointegration

Osseointegration success must be measured with clinical, radiographic, and functional parameters. In a craniofacial implant, success is measured in two ways. An overall success rate is determined by dividing the number of functioning implants

Table 10.1 Postoperative follow-up schedule for the one-stage osseointegration procedure

One-stage procedure	
Implant installation and abutment connection	
Surgical follow-up	*Time after surgery*
Change dressing and remove sutures, if healed	1 week
Remove final dressing	2–3 weeks
Osseointegration period	Minimum of 12 weeks
Clean the implant area	Daily by patient
Check by treatment team	3 weeks
Making and fitting the process	
Make an impression of the defect area	12 weeks after surgery, given that the soft tissue is sufficiently healed
Fabricate the prosthesis	3–4 days

Table 10.2 Postoperative follow-up schedule for the one-stage osseointegration procedure

Two-stage procedure	
First stage: Implant installation	
Surgical follow-up	*Time after surgery*
Remove sutures, if healed	1 week
Osseointegration period	Minimum of 12 weeks
Second stage, abutment connection	
Surgical follow-up	*Time after surgery*
Change dressing and remove sutures, if healed	1 week
Remove final dressing and healing cap	2–3 weeks
Clean the implant area	Daily by patient
Post-surgery check by treatment team	2–6 weeks depending on healing
Making and fitting the prostheses	
Make an impression of the defect area	2–6 weeks after surgery
Fabricate the prosthesis	3–4 days

by the total number of inserted implants. Alternatively, some authors used the overall functioning fixture survival rate by calculating the rate of functioning implants divided by the number of exposed implant at second stage [26].

The success rate of osseointegration in the orbit is unpredictable due to wide variation in published case series. Abu-Serriah et al. reviewed the outcome of treating 44 implants in 12 patients and reported a functioning fixture success rate of 72%, with half of cases followed up for 2–3 years [27]. Roumanas et al. inserted 47 implants in 15 patients and showed a 53% success rate with mean follow-up of 49 months. In 2005, a multicenter survey conducted by Toljanic et al. at 25 different centers found an overall success rate of 73.2% with a mean follow-up period of 52 months [28]. In this survey, several factors such as radiation usage and implant location failed to show statistical significance as risk factors for failure. Furthermore, Visser et al. showed an excellent success rate of 95.7% after placing a total of 34 implants with mean follow-up of 88 months [29].

Several authors speculated about the causes of higher rate of failure of orbital implants compared to those placed in other craniofacial areas. Late failure was found to be more common, and the number of lost implants increased with longer follow-up duration. Several causes were suggested by Nishimura et al., including nonaxial loading, poor care of orbital implant due to monocular vision, lack of depth perception, orbital rim poor capacity for remodeling, and poor bone quantity [26, 28, 30].

Radiotherapy and Osseointegration

Effect of Radiation on Bone

Radiation causes cellular damage through DNA breakage and free radical formation. In bone, radiation induces hypoperfusion initially through edema and increased basement membrane permeability. Subsequent lamina narrowing and vessel occlusion follow by means of fibrosis and hyalinization of the lumen. Another important change after irradiation is the increased proportion of osteoclasts to osteoblasts in irradiated bone [31].

Osteoradionecrosis is a chronic complication of radiation and is defined as a bone exposure in the area of radiation in the absence of tumor recurrence. In 1983, Marx explained the pathophysiology of osteoradionecrosis with the "hypoxic-hypocellular-hypovascular" theory for which he based his recommendation for hyperbaric oxygen therapy. More recently, Delanian and Lefaix developed a different theory called the "fibroatrophic theory" which is based on fibroblastic dysregulation and recommended treatment with fibroblast proliferation inhibitors and free radical scavengers [32, 33].

Dose of Radiotherapy

There is no consensus in the literature on what maximum radiation dosage would prevent successful placement of an implant, nor does it set a gold standard for how much time should be allowed to elapse after radiation treatment prior to implant placement. A systematic review of six published studies showed that implant failure rate is three times higher in the maxilla than in other bony sites [34]. It also found a fourfold higher failure rate for implants placed after >55 Gy treatment doses compared with doses <55 Gy [34]. Granstrom didn't find that the total dose of radiation accurately predicted complication rates. Therefore, he proposed measuring radiation dose with radiation cumulative effect which is reflected by the total number of radiotherapy sessions. In effect, he showed that dose range of 48–65 G corresponding to 20 CRE can result in a good success rate [35].

Success of Osseointegration in Irradiated Bone

The need for radiation therapy is evaluated preoperatively, since it will affect the timing of the implant placement. It was initially thought that radiation therapy was a contraindication for placement of osseointegrated implants [36]. The first clinical demonstration of success of osseointegration post-radiotherapy was published in 1988 in nine patients, with an implant survival rate of 86% [37]. A review of the literature by Visser et al. showed that success rate after irradiation varies and appears to be site dependent in the craniofacial area and that success of osseointegration in the orbit ranged from 45% to 96% [29]. Failure occurred most commonly during the first year due to lack of osseointegration [27].

The ideal timing of implant placement in relation to radiotherapy is controversial. Placing an osseointegrated implant prior to radiotherapy at the time of surgery offers favorable surgical exposure, decreases the total number of surgical interventions, and provides implant with healing time before radiotherapy takes place. However, osseointegrated implants exposed to radiotherapy have been shown to cause backscatter radiation, increasing the radiation dose 15% to surrounding (1–2 mm) bone leading to loss or failure of the implant [38].

An early study recommended a 12-month delay in implant placement post-irradiation [39]. Another study showed lower implant failure rates when placed after a 13–24-month period [40]. However, other authors have found that implant failure is proportional to the time after irradiation due to the accumulative dose effect [35]. More recent clinical studies of orbital implant success by Schoen [41] showed a 100% success rate in non-irradiated bone, a 90% success rate in pre-implant radiotherapy, and an 85% success rate in post-implant radiotherapy, supporting the preference of inserting the implant prior to irradiation.

Hyperbaric Oxygen Therapy

The use of hyperbaric oxygen (HBO) therapy was originally recommended for prevention and treatment of osteoradionecrosis [42]. If HBO is elected, treatment is considered pre- and post-implant insertion using the Marx protocol consistent with a 20/10 dive treatment. This consists of a 90-minute dive to 2.5 ATA per day for 20 days. On day 21 the implant operation is performed, and, starting on day 22, the patient will have ten more HBO treatments. The skin-penetrating abutments should be taken out, but the implants can be left in place under intact skin if a patient has already had implants inserted and is scheduled for irradiation [42]. However, an ongoing controversy regarding the efficacy of HBO use and potential harm is discussed in literature. Advocating HBO therapy, Granstrom [35] published a review article supported by his own the experience in Sweden since 1981 placing implants in irradiated patients. The same author conducted a case-controlled control study, and the results showed a statistically significant improvement of implant survival in irradiated patients who received adjunctive HBO (92% compared to 56% without HBO) [43]. Furthermore, a multivariate analysis of 107 patients with 631 implants showed a statistical significance favoring HBO, except in temporoparietal area, where HBO did not improve the outcome [44].

In contradistinction, Donoff [45] found no strong scientific evidence for the use of HBO lacking published randomized clinical trials. He emphasized that most of the implant issues and decreased success rates are due to soft tissue-related issues rather than bone-related issues. In addition, he speculated a possible role of HBO in increasing cancer resistance to radiotherapy. Nonetheless, Feldmeier [46] reviewed the theoretical basis for this hypothesis and found poor correlation between tumor growth mechanism and HBO angiogenesis. Additionally, Sun et al. cultured human oral cancer cell line in mice and monitored the effect of HBO on tumor activity and found no significant different between HBO and controls [47].

Advantages of Osseointegration [7, 20, 23]

- Higher retention rate with higher accuracy, durability, and stability of the prosthesis
- Incorporates readily into the patient's body image; increases self-confidence, comfort, and satisfaction; and enhances quality of life due to improved self-image leading to greater activity
- Improved aesthetics with the ability to use thinner and feathered prosthesis (Fig. 10.11)
- Ease of removal and maintenance
- Ability to remove the prosthesis and perform tumor surveillance

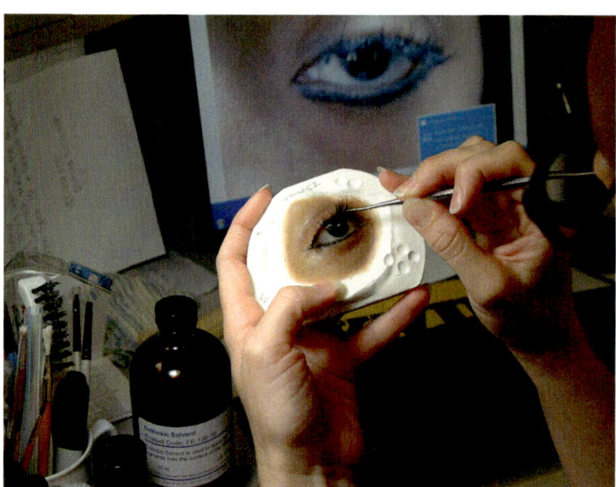

Fig. 10.11 Fabrication of post-exenteration, implant-retained upper facial prosthesis. (Published with kind permission of Dr. Allison K. Vest. All rights reserved)

Disadvantages of Osseointegration [7, 20, 23]

- A specialized multidisciplinary team is required for both the procedure and the prosthesis.
- A long time is needed between the primary surgery and the placement of the prosthesis.
- The need to change the silicone implant every 2–5 years because of normal wear and discoloration secondary to environmental factors like sunlight, smoking, and absorption of skin secretions and debris.
- Daily maintenance for skin and abutments is required.
- Multiple visits to both the surgeon and the ocularist are required for maintenance and adjustment and to ensure adequate stability of the implant/abutment.

Management of Possible Complications

It is crucial to understand that implant failure does not mean prosthesis failure, as the remainder of the implants or the sleeper implants can be used for prosthesis retention.

Soft Tissue Reaction and Infection

Soft tissue reactions and infections were found to be the most common complications in the orbital implants (3–60%), with no decrease in the incidence over the years after implant insertion [48]. It was also found that these complications were more common in younger patients which is possibly explained by the stronger immune systems of younger patients in addition to hormonal changes. In addition, in some studies soft tissue reaction occurred regardless of patient compliance with implant hygiene instructions, but the presence of skin reaction did not affect the implant success rate. The skin reaction is avoided intraoperatively by minimizing skin mobility through debulking of the flaps, hairless flap preparation by scraping off hair follicles which maintains a clean implant site and limits irritation, and trimming the periosteum to only its inner layer and suturing the flaps to the periosteum. Minimizing the flap mobility by fixating it to the periosteum leads to a lower incidence of skin irritation [49]. Skin reaction can be avoided by careful hygiene instructions and usage of a topical antibiotic +/− steroid ointment as well as avoidance of vigorous cleaning. Long-standing infections should be cultured and treated. Skin irritation can also occur if two implants are placed too close to each other and can be avoided by leaving a minimum of 15 mm between implants [49].

Soft Tissue Growth Up Against the Bar the Bar

Caused by inadequate tissue debulking, further debulking may be indicated [49].

Osseointegration Failure

The implant should be removed, and the implant site should be curetted and filled with blood coagulates which will cause healing in about 1 year. If a sleeper implant is present, it can be exposed and used. If not, adjacent bone is used for a new implant placement [49].

References

1. Brånemark P-I. Osseointegration and its experimental background. J Prosthet Dent. 1983;50:399–410.
2. Donath K, Breuner G. A method for the study of undecalcified bones and teeth with attached soft tissues*. J Oral Pathol Med. 1982;11:318–26.
3. Albrektsson T, Chrcanovic B, Jacobsson M, Wennerberg A. Osseointegration of implants: a biological and clinical overview. JSM Dent Surg. 2017;3(2):1022.
4. Albrektsson T. On implant prosthodontics: one narrative, twelve voices – 1. Int J Prosthodont. 2018;31(Suppl):s11–4.
5. Tjellström A, Yontchev E, Lindström J, Brånemark PI. Five years' experience with bone-anchored auricular prostheses. Otolaryngol Head Neck Surg. 1985;93:366–72.
6. Tjellströum A, Lindströum J, Nyléan O, Albrektsson T, Brårnemark PI, Birgersson B, Nero H, Sylvéan C. The bone-anchored auricular episthesis. Laryngoscope. 1981;91:811–5.
7. DeSerres JJ, Budden CR, Wolfaardt JF, Wilkes GH. Long-term follow-up of osseointegrated orbital prosthetic reconstruction. J Craniofac Surg. 2017;28(8):1901–5.
8. Albrektsson T, Brånemark PI, Hansson HA, Lindström J. Osseointegrated titanium implants: requirements for ensuring a long-lasting, direct bone-to-implant anchorage in man. Acta Orthop Scand. 1981;52:155–70.
9. Zarb GA, Albrektsson T. Osseointegration – a requiem for the periodontal ligament? (editorial). Int J Periodontics Restorative Dent. 1991;11:88.
10. Davies JE. Understanding peri-implant endosseous healing. J Dent Educ. 2003;67:932–49.
11. Albrektsson T, Johansson C. Osteoinduction, osteoconduction and osseointegration. Eur Spine J (2001) 10(Suppl 2): S96. https://doi.org/10.1007/s005860100282.
12. Mavrogenis AF, Dimitriou R, Parvizi J, Babis GC. Biology of implant osseointegration. J Musculoskelet Neuronal Interact. 2009;9:61–71.
13. Kuzyk P, Schemitsch E. The basic science of peri-implant bone healing. Indian J Orthop. 2011;45:108–10.
14. Shah FA, Trobos M, Thomsen P, Palmquist A. Commercially pure titanium (cp-Ti) versus titanium alloy (Ti6Al4V) materials as bone anchored implants – is one truly better than the other? Mater Sci Eng C. 2016;62:960–6.
15. Parr GR, Gardner LK, Toth RW. Titanium: the mystery metal of implant dentistry. Dental materials aspects. J Prosthet Dent. 1985;54:410–4.
16. Prasad S, Ehrensberger M, Gibson MP, Kim H, Monaco EA. Biomaterial properties of titanium in dentistry. J Oral Biosci. 2015;57:192–9.

17. Misch CE. Contemporary implant dentistry – E-book. London: Elsevier Health Sciences; 2007.
18. Puleo DA, Thomas MV. Implant surfaces. Dent Clin North Am. 2006;50:323–38, v.
19. Misch CE, Qu Z, Bidez MW. Mechanical properties of trabecular bone in the human mandible: implications for dental implant treatment planning and surgical placement. J Oral Maxillofac Surg. 1999;57:700–6; discussion 706–8.
20. Wei LA, Brown JJ, Hosek DK, Burkat CN. Osseointegrated implants for orbito-facial prostheses: preoperative planning tips and intraoperative pearls. Orbit. 2016;35:55–61.
21. Meltzer N, Garcia J, Byrne P, Boahene D. Image-guided titanium implantation for craniofacial prosthetics. Arch Facial Plast Surg. 2009;11(1):58–61.
22. Hu S, Arnaoutakis D, Kadakia S, Vest A, Sawhney R, Ducic Y. Osseointegrated implants and prosthetic reconstruction following skull base surgery. Semin Plast Surg. 2017;31(4):214–21.
23. Sinn DP, Bedrossian E, Vest AK. Craniofacial implant surgery. Dent Clin North Am. 2011;55(4):847–69. Available from: https://doi.org/10.1016/j.coms.2011.01.005.
24. Greig AVH, Jones S, Haylock C, Joshi N, McLellan G, Clarke P, et al. Reconstruction of the exenterated orbit with osseointegrated implants. J Plast Reconstr Aesthet Surg. 2010;63(10):1656–65.
25. Malchiodi L, Balzani L, Cucchi A, Ghensi P, Nocini P. Primary and secondary stability of implants in postextraction and healed sites: a randomized controlled clinical trial. Int J Oral Maxillofac Implants. 2016;31:1435–43.
26. Abu-Serriah MM, McGowan DA, Moos KF, Bagg J. Outcome of extra-oral craniofacial endosseous implants. Br J Oral Maxillofac Surg. 2001;39:269–75.
27. Abu-Serriah MM, McGowan DA, Moos KF, Bagg J. Extra-oral craniofacial endosseous implants and radiotherapy. Int J Oral Maxillofac Surg. 2003;32:585–92.
28. Toljanic JA, Eckert SE, Roumanas E, et al. Osseointegrated craniofacial implants in the rehabilitation of orbital defects: an update of a retrospective experience in the United States. J Prosthet Dent. 2005;94:177–82.
29. Visser A, Raghoebar GM, van Oort RP, Vissink A. Fate of implant-retained craniofacial prostheses: life span and aftercare. Int J Oral Maxillofac Implants. 2008;23:89–98.
30. Nishimura RD, Roumanas E, Moy PK, Sugai T, Freymiller EG. Osseointegrated implants and orbital defects: U.C.L.A. experience. J Prosthet Dent. 1998;79:304–9.
31. Pacheco R, Stock H. Effects of radiation on bone. Curr Osteoporos Rep. 2013;11:299–304.
32. Delanian S, Lefaix J-L. The radiation-induced fibroatrophic process: therapeutic perspective via the antioxidant pathway. Radiother Oncol. 2004;73:119–31.
33. Dhanda J, Rennie L, Shaw R. Current trends in the medical management of osteoradionecrosis using triple therapy. Br J Oral Maxillofac Surg. 2018;56:401–5.
34. Esposito M, Hirsch J-M, Lekholm U, Thomsen P. Biological factors contributing to failures of osseointegrated oral implants, (II). Etiopathogenesis. Eur J Oral Sci. 1998;106:721–64.
35. Granström G. Placement of dental implants in irradiated bone: the case for using hyperbaric oxygen. J Oral Maxillofac Surg. 2006;64:812–8.
36. Granström G, Bergström K, Tjellström A, Brånemark PL. A detailed analysis of titanium implants lost in irradiated tissues. Int J Oral Maxillofac Implants. 1994;9:1–20.
37. Jacobsson M, Tjellströum A, Albrektsson T, Thomsen P, Turesson I. Integration of titanium implants in irradiated bone histologic and clinical study. Ann Otol Rhinol Laryngol. 2016;97:337–40.
38. Mian TA, Van Putten MC, Kramer DC, Jacob RF, Boyer AL. Backscatter radiation at bone-titanium interface from high-energy X and gamma rays. Int J Radiat Oncol Biol Phys. 1987;13:1943–7.
39. Jacobsson M, Tjellströum A, Albrektsson T, Thomsen P, Turesson I. Integration of titanium implants in irradiated bone histologic and clinical study. Ann Otol Rhinol Laryngol. 1988;97:337–40.
40. Niimi A, Ueda M, Keller EE, Worthington P. Experience with osseointegrated implants placed in irradiated tissues in Japan and the United States. Int J Oral Maxillofac Implants. 1998;13:407–11.

41. Schoen PJ, Raghoebar GM, van Oort RP, Reintsema H, van der Laan BF, Burlage FR, Roodenburg JL, Vissink A. Treatment outcome of bone-anchored craniofacial prostheses after tumor surgery. Cancer. 2001;92:3045–50.
42. Marx RE. A new concept in the treatment of osteoradionecrosis. J Oral Maxillofac Surg. 1983;41:351–7.
43. Granström G, Tjellström A, Brånemark P-I. Osseointegrated implants in irradiated bone: a case-controlled study using adjunctive hyperbaric oxygen therapy. J Oral Maxillofac Surg. 1999;57:493–9.
44. Granström G. Osseointegration in irradiated cancer patients: an analysis with respect to implant failures. J Oral Maxillofac Surg. 2005;63:579–85.
45. Donoff RB. Treatment of the irradiated patient with dental implants: the case against hyperbaric oxygen treatment. J Oral Maxillofac Surg. 2006;64:819–22.
46. Feldmeier J, Carl U, Hartmann K, Sminia P. Hyperbaric oxygen: does it promote growth or recurrence of malignancy? Undersea Hyperb Med. 2003;30:1–18.
47. Sun TB, Chen RL, Hsu YH. The effect of hyperbaric oxygen on human oral cancer cells. Undersea Hyperb Med. 2004;31:251–60.
48. Nerad J, Carter K, LaVelle W, Fyler A, Brånemark PI. The osseointegration technique for the rehabilitation of the exenterated orbit. Arch Ophthalmol. 1991;109:1032–8.
49. Tjellström A, Proops D, Granström G. Chap. 18: Osseointegrated percutaneous titanium implants. In: Maniglia AJ, Stucker FJ, editors. Surgical reconstruction of the face: nose, midface and anterior skull base. Philadelphia: W.B. Saunders Company, (by invitation); 1999. p. 231–43.

Part III
The Anophthalmic Socket

Chapter 11
Maintenance of the Anophthalmic Socket

Erin M. Shriver, Keith Pine, and Elin Bohman

Maintenance of the anophthalmic socket is essential for the long-term health of the socket and the ability of the patient to wear a prosthesis, which is critical to their psychological well-being [1]. A solid grasp of the anatomy and physiology of the anophthalmic socket, the response of the socket to the prosthesis, and the environmental conditions that anophthalmic patients experience is key to understanding the principles behind socket maintenance.

Anophthalmic Socket Anatomy and Physiology

Conjunctiva

The conjunctiva is composed of a deep substantia propria layer and an epithelial layer composed of squamous cells (cylindrical and polyhedral cells), columnar cells, cuboidal cells, and goblet cells [2]. Mucous-producing goblet cells are present in all areas of the conjunctival sac; however the medial third of the fornices has the greatest number, and the superotemporal region has the least [2]. There are no goblet cells in the bulbar conjunctiva near the medial and lateral limbus [2].

E. M. Shriver (✉)
University of Iowa, Department of Ophthalmology and Visual Sciences, Iowa City, IA, USA
e-mail: erin-shriver@uiowa.edu

K. Pine
University of Auckland, School of Optometry and Vision Science, Grafton, Auckland, New Zealand

E. Bohman
St. Erik Eye Hospital, Oculoplastic and Orbital Services, Stockholm, Sweden

T. E. Johnson (ed.), *Anophthalmia*,
https://doi.org/10.1007/978-3-030-29753-4_11

A healthy, comfortable conjunctiva is crucial for prosthesis wear. Conjunctival sensitivity decreases progressively as the distance increases from both the limbus and the lid margin to the fornices [3]. Conjunctival sensation also varies within the menstrual cycle of women, with iris color, and ethnicity. Sensation is known to decrease with age and in those with a history of long-term (poly)methyl methacrylate (PMMA) contact lens wear [3]. This effect of PMMA contact lens wear has led to the theory that prosthesis wear could also be associated with decreased sensation.

Studies have shown that fitting of a prosthesis changes the conjunctiva in other ways. An anophthalmic socket has lower goblet cell density than the companion eye of the same patient. The goblet cells also have greater nucleus-to-cytoplasm ratios especially in the tarsal conjunctiva in anophthalmic sockets compared to companion eyes [4].

Mucous

Throughout the body, mucous is composed of mucins (large, heavily glycosylated proteins) and inorganic salts suspended in water. Lacrimal mucous originates from the lacrimal glands, the epithelial cells, and the goblet cells. Goblet cells are the greatest source of mucous in anophthalmic sockets and typically secrete approximately 2–3 μl of mucous per day per eye. This amount increases when the conjunctiva becomes inflamed [2].

Mucous serves several roles on the ocular surface. The viscosity of mucous limits the spread of microorganisms. It has a lubricating function which aids in eye and eyelid movement and acts as an intermediary layer that enables aqueous tears to remain in contact with the hydrophobic corneal epithelium or prosthesis surface [2]. Mucous also cleans the ocular or prosthetic surface by trapping exfoliated epithelial cells, surface debris, and bacteria [5].

Tears

The normal three layered pre-corneal tear film is composed of a thin superficial lipid layer produced by the meibomian glands of the eyelid, an aqueous center layer, and an inner mucous layer composed of mucoproteins from the conjunctival goblet cells. It typically measures 6–9 μm in thickness immediately after a blink, decreases by 20% after 5 seconds and by over 50% after 30 seconds [6]. In an anophthalmic patient, this three-layer tear film does not form over the anterior surface of a PMMA prosthetic eye but is replaced by a confluent tear film that may form over the prosthesis for a brief period of time. Although glass eyes are not commonly used in the United States, they are preferred in other parts of the world and have been found to have a greater ability to wet and maintain an aqueous tear film than a PMMA prosthesis because of their hydrophilic surface [7].

The height of the tear meniscus also has been found to be lower on the prosthetic eye than in the companion eye [4]. The basal tear volume in the anophthalmic socket is the same as in the companion eye, but overall tear production is less because of absence of reflex tear production [8]. Reflex tearing is decreased in anophthalmic patients because of the lack of the cornea with its increased sensation, likely decreased conjunctival sensation secondary to long-term prosthesis wear, and because the prosthesis shields against external stimulation [7]. Tear volume as measured by Schirmer I and II testing has been reported to be less than the companion eye in 78% of anophthalmic patients [8]. It has been reported that anophthalmic patients who experience socket issues including irritation and discharge have half the basic tear secretion as those without [8]. Another study found that nearly one quarter (23%) of anophthalmic patients required supplemental lubrication [9].

A well-fitting prosthesis is needed for proper tear distribution and drainage in an anophthalmic socket. Tear flow is optimized when the prosthesis is in even contact with all areas of the conjunctival sac and extends into the fornices. Even contact against the orbital and tarsal conjunctiva ensures adequate tear flow and drainage. The anterior surface of the prosthesis should be similar in curvature to the original globe to ensure a proper seal exists between the eyelids and prosthesis surface [7].

Tear Protein Deposits

Tears have both antibacterial and lubricating properties. They also contain proteins that can form deposits that accumulate on the surface of prosthetic eyes. Despite the common perception that the tear protein deposits on the prosthetic eye surface cause inflammation, studies have shown that some deposits are actually associated with less conjunctival inflammation and mucoid discharge [10, 11].

Deposits are distributed on the prosthetic surface in two distinct zones, the retro-palpebral zone where accumulated deposits are in constant contact with the conjunctiva and the inter-palpebral zone where deposits are present but do not accumulate because of the cleansing action of the eyelids during blinking. The inter-palpebral zone deposits experience wetting and drying cycles secondary to the blinking action of the eyelids and cause irritation when they desiccate (Fig. 11.1). As such, the inter-palpebral zone should be kept clear of deposits; however this is not the case with the beneficial retro-palpebral deposits [7].

Surface deposits have been shown to dramatically increase the wettability of prosthetic eyes and therefore may have a useful role in reducing surface hydrophobicity [10, 11]. This finding may explain why frequent cleaning with deposit removal is associated with more severe discharge [10, 11].

Pine et al. evaluated tear deposits on the prosthetic eye surface and found that these deposits build up rapidly during the first 2 weeks of wear and then stabilize until 6 months of continuous wear when they may begin to encroach on the inter-palpebral surface and dry out [10]. This finding serves as the basis for their recommendation that prostheses be cleaned at least every 6 months [7].

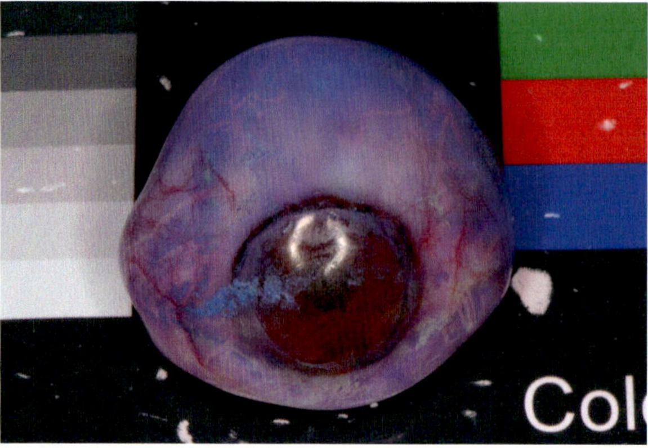

Fig. 11.1 Dried, inter-palpebral zone deposits can lead to irritation, inflammation, and excessive mucous discharge. (Photo courtesy of Pine et al. [28])

The Eyelids

The eyelids play a critical role in the health of the anophthalmic socket. Lagophthalmos is associated with increased mucoid discharge as the prosthesis receives less lubrication, there is more opportunity for increased tear protein deposits, these deposits can desiccate, and there is less clearing of the mucous within the socket.

Eyelids in prosthesis wearers, particularly after 10 years of prosthetic wear, have been found to have significant signs of meibomian gland dysfunction (MGD) and meibomian gland dropout compared to companion eyes [12]. Wearing a prosthesis is associated with hyperkeratinization and associated obstruction of the meibomian glands and lacrimal drainage obstruction [13]. The mechanical rubbing of the lid margins over the prosthesis during blinking, tear meniscus deficiency [14], and tear deposits on the inter-palpebral zone can be contributing factors.

On routine socket evaluations, the eyelids should be evaluated for lagophthalmos, ectropion, entropion, and fornix shortening producing difficulty retaining a prosthesis. The eyelid margins and meibomian glands should be examined as MGD is a significant contributor to prosthetic eye discomfort.

Anophthalmic Socket Phases of Prosthetic Eye Wear

The response of an anophthalmic socket to a prosthesis and the common conditions that affect the socket such as mucoid discharge and papillary conjunctivitis are important in understanding the principles of socket maintenance. A three-phase model has been used to describe the response of the socket to prosthetic eye wear [7].

The *establishment phase* occurs when homeostasis is being established in an anophthalmic socket with a new prosthesis or a newly polished prosthesis. This phase can be as short as a few minutes but can last a month or more as the mucous is distributed over the prosthesis; foreign material is cleared away; and the balance of tear production, evaporation, and drainage is established [15].

The *equilibrium phase* occurs when the mucous is evenly distributed over the prosthesis, surface deposits which aid in wetting of the prosthesis have built up on the prosthesis, and the prosthesis can be comfortably worn. Bacterial homeostasis also occurs during this phase as membrane lipid, iron, and pH all are stabilized [16]. More gram-negative bacteria are typically found in an anophthalmic socket compared to the companion socket, but in the equilibrium phase they do not cause inflammation [17].

The *breakdown phase* occurs when the prosthesis cannot be worn comfortably and inflammation and discharge increase. Deposit buildup occurs and moves toward the inter-palpebral zone which can cause increased mucoid discharge and an allergic response such as giant papillary conjunctivitis (GPC). Although a correlation between contact lens deposits and GPC has been found, the role of prosthesis deposits in GPC has not been well studied [18]. The duration of prosthesis wear has been associated with GPC, however [19]. It is postulated that excessive deposit buildup or inter-palpebral zone deposits drying out and irritating the conjunctiva could be the etiology of GPC and mucoid discharge in some anophthalmic sockets [19].

Care of the Anophthalmic Socket

Lubrication

If the socket has insufficient tears, rapid tear breakup time, and meibomian gland dysfunction or the tears do not flow over the prosthesis evenly, eye movement and blinking may cause irritation to the conjunctiva. Lubricating eye drops, mineral oil, and ointments may be beneficial in improving comfort and eyelid condition. Fett et al. found that 23% of anophthalmic patients required lubrication supplementation [9].

Many ocularists and ophthalmologists recommend mineral oil or lipid-based eye drops which augment the tear film lipid layer and provide a barrier to tear evaporation. Therapies for MGD such as omega III supplementation and warm compresses may also be beneficial for this reason.

Punctal occlusion has also been shown to improve comfort in prosthesis wearers with low tear volume [20].

Removing, Cleaning, and Reinserting the Prosthesis

Many ocularists and ophthalmologists believe that the less a prosthesis is touched the better and advocate for infrequent removal at home. A study of the American Society of Ocularists found that 53% of members recommended that patients remove their prosthesis whenever the socket felt irritated or whenever it was dirty [1].

Removing and reinserting prosthetic eyes disrupts the microenvironment of the socket because of physical forces stressing the socket particularly the lateral canthus, frictional forces of the prosthesis rubbing against the conjunctiva, and disruption of the socket and prosthesis surface environment [7]. The socket environment is altered with manipulation of the prosthesis because it disrupts the conjunctival mucous substrate that both lubricates the prosthesis and enables aqueous tears to remain in contact with the palpebral conjunctival epithelium [2]. Compared to patients who clean their prosthesis less often, patients who clean their prosthesis once a day show significantly less goblet cell density and greater nucleus-to-cytoplasm ratios at the superior tarsal conjunctiva resulting in increased dryness and decreased beneficial mucous [4]. Rapid temperature reduction and evaporative drying of the conjunctiva also can occur with prosthesis removal [7].

Studies have also demonstrated that foreign material and bacteria are introduced into the socket when the prosthesis is manipulated. Patients who frequently handle their prosthesis have a higher proportion of gram-negative bacteria in their socket than their companion eye compared to patients who touch their prosthesis less often [21]. As a result, conjunctival inflammation and excessive mucoid discharge may develop.

When the surface deposits and residual mucous build up on the exposed surface of the prosthesis, irritation can occur, and eyelid closure can be impeded resulting in increased tear evaporation, poor tear distribution, and increased inflammation and discharge. When these deposits are cleaned from the inter-palpebral portion of the prosthesis, eyelid closure in the inter-palpebral region is improved, but there is reduced wettability and rapid tear breakup time on initial reintroduction of the prosthesis [11].

While some advocate not manipulating the prosthesis at home, others recommend establishing a prosthetic eye cleaning regimen which they believe is critical for the management of non-specific mucoid discharge. Pine et al. go as far as to claim that this regimen is likely more important than professional polishing [7]. Their regimen includes the following principles: prosthetic eyes should not be removed and cleaned more than monthly but not less than every 6 months, a paper towel wetted with cold water can be used to wipe all surfaces of the prosthesis clean, and prosthetic eyes should be professionally polished annually to optical quality contact lens standard and be blemish-free with smooth rounded edges [10, 22, 23].

Prosthesis Polishing

Maintenance of the prosthesis with regular professional polishing is critical to minimize excessive mucous discharge and maintain comfortable long-term prosthesis wear. Professional polishing focuses on the inter-palpebral deposits which desiccate, impede the eyelid blink and distribution of tears, and cause conjunctival irritation [7].

The quality of the prosthesis polish and resultant fineness of the surface matrix has been shown to effect surface deposits [10]. PMMA prosthetic surfaces polished with a high "optical quality contact lens standard" accumulated deposits at a slower rate than prosthetic eyes finished with a standard polish [10, 24]. Also, studies have shown that the higher quality the polish, the more wettable the prosthetic eye surface [15].

Although regular polishing is important, it alone is often not sufficient to maintain a healthy socket. Over half (62%) of prosthesis wearers had no improvement in discharge after repolishing or had improvement that lasted less than 1 month [10].

Common Conditions in Anophthalmic Sockets

It is crucial to understand the common issues anophthalmic patients face in order to optimize socket maintenance. The patient should be examined regularly by an ophthalmologist and ocularist to evaluate the socket, eyelids, and prosthesis for common conditions such as excessive mucoid discharge, inflammation, eyelid malposition, and orbital fat atrophy and confirm optimal prosthesis fit. Less common conditions should be excluded as well, including scarring, exposure, or migration of the implant, development of a pyogenic granuloma, and recurrence of a tumor in patients enucleated for a malignancy.

Mucoid discharge is the second most important concern for experienced prosthetic eye wearers after health of their remaining eye and is the most common problem in anophthalmic sockets [1]. A recent study found that prosthetic eye wearers were equally concerned about discharge, visual perception, and appearance both 3 months following loss of the eye and more than 2 years later, although overall their concerns were decreased [25]. Excessive mucoid discharge associated with prosthetic wear has been shown to affect 93% of wearers, over half (60%) on a daily basis [1]. Inflammation is also quite common and is found in 69% of sockets with a prosthesis [11]. It can result in pain, irritation, and increased mucous production.

When mucoid discharge is present, it is important to look for other causes of mucoid discharge such as viral or bacterial infection; nasolacrimal duct obstruction; conditions such as MGD, blepharitis, and ocular rosacea; dry eye; eyelid malposition such as ectropion, giant fornix syndrome, and lagophthalmos; environmental allergens and irritants; conditions that decrease the blink rate such as prolonged computer use; socket conditions such as pyogenic granulomas or implant exposure; and prosthesis-related causes such as chips or scratches on the surface of the prosthesis, significant concavity on the posterior surface of the prosthesis leading to pooling of socket secretions, and rarely an allergy to the prosthetic material itself [7].

Giant papillary conjunctivitis (GPC) is an allergic inflammatory disease of the eye associated with increased numbers of mast cells, eosinophils, and lymphocytes in the conjunctiva [26] (Fig. 11.2). The condition is associated with excess mucous production, itching, and is usually associated with a classic cobblestone appearance

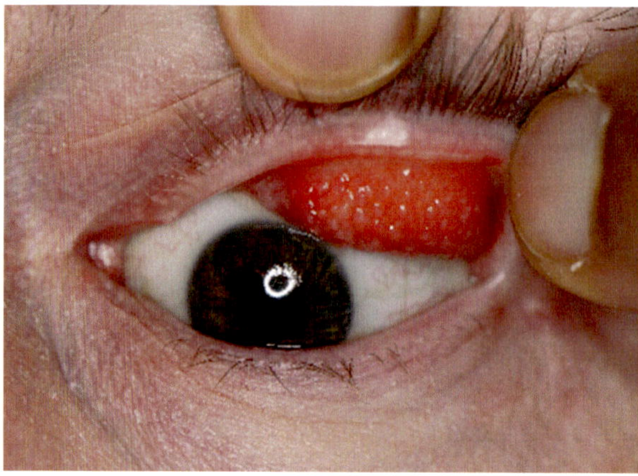

Fig. 11.2 Giant papillary conjunctivitis is an inflammatory condition which causes itching and excess mucoid discharge. (Photo courtesy of Dr. Elin Bohman)

of the upper papillary conjunctiva. Prolonged prosthesis wear has also been shown to be associated with GPC [19].

Monocular Precautions

During socket maintenance checks, it is critical that the health of the remaining eye is evaluated and stressed. This remains the chief concern in anophthalmic patients both at the time of enucleation and after wearing a prosthesis for over 2 years [1].

It is important that patients undergo regular eye examinations at appropriate intervals and that monocular precautions be stressed including the use of protective eyewear comprised of impact-resistant lenses and a large, sturdy frame [27].

It can be extremely rewarding for an ophthalmologist to work closely with an ocularist in caring for anophthalmic patients. Both providers bring their expertise to help the patient maintain a healthy socket and continue with long-term, comfortable prosthesis use.

References

1. Pine K, Sloan B, Stewart J, Jacobs RJ. Concerns of anophthalmic patients wearing artificial eyes. Clin Exp Ophthalmol. 2011;39(1):47–52.
2. Liotet S, Triclot MP, Perderiset M, Warnet VN, Laroche L. The role of conjunctival mucus in contact lens fitting. CLAO J. 1985;11(2):149–54.
3. Ruskell GL, Bergmanson JP. Anatomy and physiology of the cornea and related structures. In: Phillips AJ, Speedwell L, editors. Contact lenses. 5th ed. Edinburgh: Butterworth Heinemann Elsevier; 2007. p. 388–9.

4. Kim JH, Lee MJ, Choung HK, Kim NJ, Hwang SW, Sung MS, et al. Conjunctival cytologic features in anophthalmic patients wearing an ocular prosthesis. Ophthal Plast Reconstr Surg. 2008;24(4):290–5.
5. Adams AD. The morphology of human conjunctival mucus. Arch Ophthalmol (Chicago, Ill: 1960). 1979;97(4):730–4.
6. Guillon JP, Godfrey A. Tears and contact lenses. In: Phillips AJ, Speedwell L, editors. Contact lenses. 5th ed. Edinburgh: Butterworth Heinemann Elsevier; 2007. p. 111–27.
7. Pine KR, Sloan BH, Jacobs RJ. Clinical ocular prosthetics. S.I.: Springer; 2015. p. 364.
8. Allen L, Kolder HE, Bulgarelli EM, Bulgarelli DM. Artificial eyes and tear measurements. Ophthalmology. 1980;87(2):155–7.
9. Fett DR, Scott R, Putterman AM. Evaluation of lubricants for the prosthetic eye wearer. Ophthal Plast Reconstr Surg. 1986;2(1):29–31.
10. Pine KR, Sloan B, Jacobs RJ. Deposit buildup on prosthetic eyes and implications for conjunctival inflammation and mucoid discharge. Clin Ophthalmol (Auckland, NZ). 2012;6:1755–62.
11. Pine KR, Sloan B, Stewart J, Jacobs RJ. The response of the anophthalmic socket to prosthetic eye wear. Clin Exp Optom. 2013;96(4):388–93.
12. Jang SY, Lee SY, Yoon JS. Meibomian gland dysfunction in longstanding prosthetic eye wearers. Br J Ophthalmol. 2013;97(4):398–402.
13. Kashkouli MB, Zolfaghari R, Es'haghi A, Amirsardari A, Abtahi MB, Karimi N, et al. Tear film, lacrimal drainage system, and eyelid findings in subjects with anophthalmic socket discharge. Am J Ophthalmol. 2016;165:33–8.
14. Kim SE, Yoon JS, Lee SY. Tear measurement in prosthetic eye users with Fourier-domain optical coherence tomography. Am J Ophthalmol. 2010;149(4):602–7.e1
15. Pine KR, Sloan B, Han KI, Swift S, Jacobs RJ. Deposit buildup on prosthetic eye material (in vitro) and its effect on surface wettability. Clin Ophthalmol (Auckland, NZ). 2013;7:313–9.
16. Zinni Y. What is bacteria homeostasis? Sciencing; 2017. Available from: https://sciencing.com/bacteria-homeostasis-8706627.html.
17. Christensen JN, Fahmy JA. The bacterial flora of the conjunctival anophthalmic socket in glass prosthesis-carriers. Acta Ophthalmol. 1974;52(6):801–9.
18. Fowler SA, Korb DR, Finnemore VM, Allansmith MR. Surface deposits on worn hard contact lenses. Arch Ophthalmol (Chicago, Ill: 1960). 1984;102(5):757–9.
19. Srinivasan BD, Jakobiec FA, Iwamoto T, DeVoe AG. Giant papillary conjunctivitis with ocular prostheses. Arch Ophthalmol (Chicago, Ill: 1960). 1979;97(5):892–5.
20. Vardizer Y, Lang Y, Mourits MP, Briscoe MD. Favorable effects of lacrimal plugs in patients with an anophthalmic socket. Orbit (Amsterdam, Netherlands). 2007;26(4):263–6.
21. Vasquez RJ, Linberg JV. The anophthalmic socket and the prosthetic eye. A clinical and bacteriologic study. Ophthal Plast Reconstr Surg. 1989;5(4):277–80.
22. Patel V, Allen D, Morley AM, Ercophth RM. Features and management of an acute allergic response to acrylic ocular prostheses. Orbit (Amsterdam, Netherlands). 2009;28(6):339–41.
23. LeGrand J. Chronic exudate: an unnecessary evil. J Ophthalmic Prosthet. 1999;4(1):33–40.
24. Pine KR, Sloan B, Jacobs RJ. Deposit buildup on prosthetic eyes and implications for conjunctival inflammation and mucoid discharge. Clin Ophthalmol. 2012;6(1):1755–62.
25. Pine NS, de Terte I, Pine KR. An investigation into discharge, visual perception, and appearance concerns of prosthetic eye wearers. Orbit (Amsterdam, Netherlands). 2017;36(6):401–6.
26. Bozkurt B, Akyurek N, Irkec M, Erdener U, Memis L. Immunohistochemical findings in prosthesis-associated giant papillary conjunctivitis. Clin Exp Ophthalmol. 2007;35(6):535–40.
27. Vinger PF, Parver L, Alfaro DV 3rd, Woods T, Abrams BS. Shatter resistance of spectacle lenses. JAMA. 1997;277(2):142–4.
28. Pine KR, Sloan BH, Jacobs RJ. Clinical ocular prosthetics. S.I.: Springer International Publishing; 2015. p. 250.

Chapter 12
Anophthalmic Socket Syndrome

Alexandra E. Levitt and Bradford W. Lee

Introduction

Several features characterize the ideal anophthalmic socket. These qualities help to achieve the best possible cosmesis and ocular prosthetic function. First and foremost is the placement of a sufficiently large orbital implant that is well positioned, has appropriate attachment of the rectus muscles, and is covered by native tissue. This restores adequate volume to the orbit and facilitates use of an ocular prosthesis without excessive volume while conferring maximal mobility. The socket should be lined with healthy, native conjunctiva. Fornices should be sufficiently deep to retain the prosthesis. Both upper and lower eyelids should be of normal tone, position, and contour, and the lid crease and superior sulcus should be symmetrical between both sides [1]. In reality, not all of these features may be present due to trauma, disease, or prior surgeries. Moreover, certain pathophysiological changes occur even after the eye removal surgery that can contribute to the development of post-enucleation socket syndrome (PESS) over time.

Pathophysiology of PESS

Various clinical findings and pathophysiological changes are associated with PESS and can lead to suboptimal aesthetic and functional outcomes for the anophthalmic socket (Fig. 12.1).

A. E. Levitt · B. W. Lee (✉)
Bascom Palmer Eye Institute, University of Miami, Miami, FL, USA
e-mail: ALevitt@med.miami.edu; BLee@med.miami.edu

T. E. Johnson (ed.), *Anophthalmia*,
https://doi.org/10.1007/978-3-030-29753-4_12

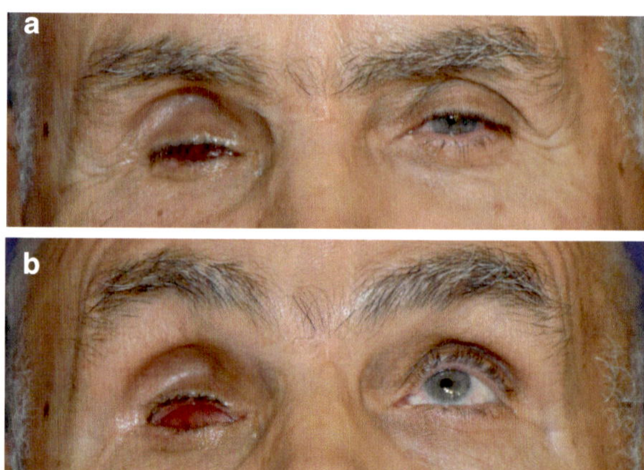

Fig. 12.1 This patient with a history of two penetrating keratoplasties and a glaucoma drainage implant surgery underwent enucleation of the right eye without implant placement due to endophthalmitis and orbital cellulitis. The patient demonstrates classic findings of PESS including enophthalmos, superior sulcus deformity, and ptosis with a conformer in the right socket (Panels **a** and **b**)

Enophthalmos, Superior Sulcus Hollowing, and Orbital Soft Tissue Atrophy

The orbital implant, ocular prosthesis, and orbital soft tissues all contribute to volumizing the socket, so inadequacy of any component can result in enophthalmos or superior sulcus hollowing relative to the contralateral side. The best way to limit enophthalmos and superior sulcus hollowing is via placement of a sufficiently large implant, typically 70–80% of the volume of the native globe, and full-time use of a well-fitted ocular prosthesis [2, 3].

Orbital soft tissue volume is also a function of orbital fat and soft tissue atrophy arising from surgically disrupted vasculature, soft tissue trauma, inflammation associated with globe removal, and any other accidental or surgical trauma to the orbit. For example, if the patient had an orbital fracture and orbital fracture repair with implant or multiple prior socket surgeries, this could cause further vascular disruption and tissue atrophy (Fig. 12.2). All else equal, PESS may be somewhat less severe and less prevalent after evisceration versus enucleation due to less disruption of orbital soft tissue [1, 4].

Finally, computed tomographic analysis of the anophthalmic socket has demonstrated that rotational displacement of orbital soft tissues occurs from superior to posterior and posterior to inferior. This rotation is accompanied by posterior-inferior displacement of the levator/superior rectus complex. These rotational changes result in a backward tilt of the ocular prosthesis and further contribute to hollowing of the superior sulcus [1, 5].

Ptosis, Eyelid Retraction, and Lower Lid Horizontal Laxity

Normal senile and involutional lid changes are accelerated in the anophthalmic socket. Upper lid ptosis frequently occurs as part of PESS and may be caused by enophthalmos due to volume deficiency and the previously described infero-

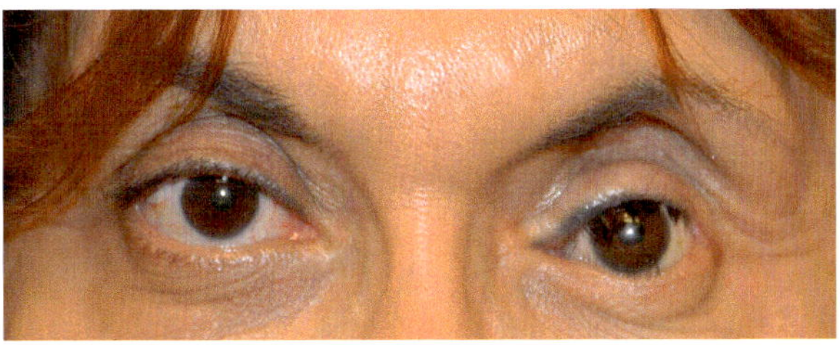

Fig. 12.2 This patient underwent enucleation of the left eye with placement of a pegged implant, which then developed an atypical mycobacteria infection requiring removal of the pegged implant, secondary placement of an 18 mm acrylic implant, and multiple fornix reconstruction surgeries and lower lid-tightening procedures. Prior infection and multiple socket surgeries have contributed to the orbital soft tissue atrophy resulting in enophthalmos, superior sulcus deformity, socket contracture, and lateral canthal tendon disinsertion. The superior sulcus hollowing results in increased superior tarsal platform show

posterior shifting of the levator/superior rectus complex. The posterior rotation of orbital soft tissues also decreases the supporting bulk of the upper lid. An incorrectly sized prosthesis may also cause ptosis and affect the lid position if it does not contribute sufficient volume. Finally, levator damage or injury to the oculomotor nerve during surgery or trauma is another potential contributing factor.

Although ptosis is a common finding in PESS, anophthalmic patients can also have upper lid retraction. This can also occur in the setting of infero-posterior shifting of the levator/superior rectus complex, but other factors can cause this as well such as cicatricial changes of the superior fornix, an oversized prosthesis, or disinsertion of the lateral canthal tendon owing to ongoing manipulation of the prosthesis [4].

The lower eyelid plays a major role in supporting and maintaining the position of an ocular prosthesis, but the weight of the prosthesis and the process of placing and removing the prosthesis can accelerate development of lower lid horizontal laxity, senile ectropion, and lateral canthal tendon disinsertion. When larger volume and thus heavier prostheses are used to restore orbital volume loss, they impose greater gravitational forces that stretch the lower eyelid. If there is significant lower lid laxity due to senile involutional changes and/or years of prosthetic use, a lid-tightening surgery may be necessary to prevent the prosthetic from falling out of the socket (Fig. 12.3). A history of facial trauma, orbito-facial fractures, facial nerve palsy, or cicatricial changes of the lower lid or midface may also affect the orbital and midface structural support, orbicularis tone, and ultimately lid position [1].

Clinical History and Exam

Interventions to address PESS can be aimed toward improved cosmesis or improved function of the ocular prostheses. A thorough history and clinical examination of the anophthalmic socket will help guide treatments that address superior sulcus hollowing,

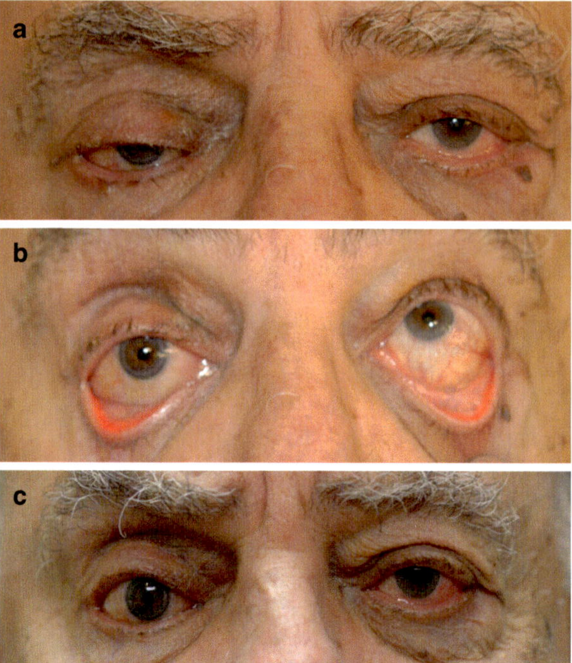

Fig. 12.3 This patient underwent enucleation of the right eye and obtained a custom-fit ocular prosthesis (Panel **a**) but had right upper lid ptosis and difficulty retaining the ocular prosthesis due to lower eyelid laxity (Panel **b**). Following ptosis repair and tightening of the lower lids, the patient was able to retain the ocular prosthetic without problems (Panel **c**)

enophthalmos, and eyelid malpositions and importantly address the patient's specific concerns.

In taking a history, the following information should be elicited:

- Original indication for eye removal and type of procedure performed (e.g., enucleation vs. evisceration, type and size of implant placed if any, whether extraocular muscles were attached to implant)
- History of any subsequent socket complications or surgeries
- History of other ocular, orbital, or eyelid surgeries or procedures
- Ocular prosthetic history and maintenance
- Functional concerns such as pain, discharge, bleeding, or difficulty retaining prosthesis
- Aesthetic concerns such as enophthalmos, superior sulcus hollowing, or eyelid malpositions/asymmetries

The exam with respect to PESS should focus on evaluating:

- Fullness of superior sulcus relative to contralateral side
- Brow position and symmetry insofar as it affects the appearance of the superior sulcus
- Periorbital atrophy involving the lateral canthal, infraorbital, and malar regions

- Upper and lower eyelid position, including measurement of palpebral fissure, levator function, and margin reflex distance (MRD1 and MRD2) measurements
- Lower eyelid horizontal laxity and lateral canthal tendon position
- Facial nerve function including orbicularis oculi tone and function
- Size and thickness of ocular prosthesis
- Depth of fornices, coverage of implant, and health of conjunctiva
- Exophthalmometry with prosthesis in place

If it is unclear whether an implant was placed at the time of eye removal and an implant cannot be palpated in the socket, ultrasound or CT imaging can help determine whether an implant is present, its size, and its placement with respect to the extraocular muscles.

Reconstruction and Management

After listening to the patient's concerns and studying the physical findings, the next challenge is to determine the most effective and least invasive means of addressing these issues. Before undertaking any type of surgery or procedure in the PESS patient, it is important to discuss and collaborate closely with the ocularist. The surgeon should discuss the patient's complaints and determine whether the ocularist can fix some of these by revising the current prosthesis or fashioning a new one. Sometimes, enophthalmos or superior sulcus hollowing can be corrected by creating a thicker prosthesis with more volume. However, this has its limits, since too heavy a prosthesis can put undue strain on the lower lid and accelerate involutional changes of the lower lid. Ptosis or lid retraction can sometimes be addressed by adjusting the height of the prosthesis. If the ocularist and surgeon both agree that a surgery or procedure is necessary, they should discuss the planned procedure, when the patient can be refitted for a new ocular prosthesis, and any procedures anticipated after making the new prosthesis.

When surgery is performed, there is always a risk of scarring and socket contracture, so it is imperative to minimize orbital tissue dissection and cauterization. If there is preexisting socket contracture with no orbital implant, a dermis fat graft can be considered to simultaneously address the contracted socket and the orbital volume deficiency. If the patient has had multiple prior surgeries and there is concern for exuberant cicatrization and socket contracture with any additional surgery, consideration should be given to nonsurgical orbital volume augmentation with injectable fillers or autologous fat transfer to the orbit.

Intraorbital Injection of Filler and Autologous Fat

Minimally invasive options to address enophthalmos and superior sulcus deformity include the intraorbital injection of fillers or autologous fat. While a range of commercially available nonpermanent and permanent fillers are available and could be used off-label for intraorbital injection, an important complication of this procedure is anterior filler migration that causes bulging of the lower lid [6]. For this reason, the authors prefer use of hyaluronic acid gel fillers or calcium hydroxylapatite fillers. Both of these are nonpermanent fillers that are broken down over time, and with hyaluronic acid gel fillers, there is the well-known added advantage of being able to dissolve the filler with hyaluronidase injections in the event of filler migration. It is also important to counsel patients about other potential filler complications including infection, bleeding/orbital hematoma, filler granulomas and granulomatous inflammation, chemosis, filler migration, change in lid position, oculocardiac reflex, and intravascular complications. The patient is advised that the filler will gradually be broken down typically over the course of 1–2 years but that repeat injections can be performed as needed.

This procedure can be performed with intravenous sedation and/or regional local anesthesia. After cleansing the skin, a small amount of local anesthetic can be injected subcutaneously on the lateral lower lid overlying the orbital rim and potentially along the intended tract of filler injection to improve patient comfort. The filler is injected transcutaneously after palpating the orbital rim with the goal of placing the filler into the retrobulbar, extraconal space between the orbital implant and orbital floor. The injection can be performed via a 27-gauge 1.25 inch needle or alternatively via a 25-gauge blunt cannula. Most sockets will require approximately 1–2 cc of filler for correction of enophthalmos, and the volume administered can be titrated during the procedure based on clinical result [7, 8]. If there is concern that there will be residual superior sulcus hollowing even after orbital volume augmentation, the brow fat pad can also be directly injected. To do this, a small amount of local anesthetic is injected below the tail of the brow. The brow is manually lifted above the supraorbital rim, and filler is injected in a pre-periosteal plane to further volumize the superior sulcus. Care should be taken to avoid intravascular injection in the region of the supraorbital neurovascular bundle.

For autologous fat transfer to the orbit, liposuction is performed to harvest the fat typically from the abdominal and flank regions. The lipoaspirate is processed either via centrifugation or a filtration system, and the processed fat is aliquoted into 1 cc syringes and injected on a fine blunt-tipped cannula from the infratemporal orbit. To maximize graft survival, the fat is injected in microaliquots over multiple passes to help avoid large boluses of fat that have a more difficult time engrafting and obtaining an adequate blood supply for survival. With fat, a larger volume must be injected as compared to filler, since not all of the fat transferred will survive. Typically, about 5–10 cc of fat can be injected in a single session. The patient should be monitored for bradycardia throughout the procedure, and if this occurs due to the oculocardiac reflex, the procedure should be paused until the heart rate returns to normal. Postoperatively, patients are given oral analgesics and instructed to place cool towels over the socket. Patients are advised to avoid direct icing of the site since this causes vasoconstriction, reduced tissue perfusion, and

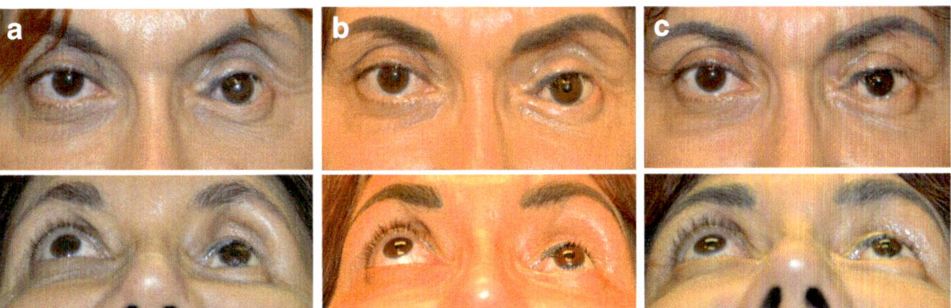

Fig. 12.4 This patient from Fig. 12.2 underwent two sessions of fat transfer from the abdomen to the left inferior orbit, superior sulcus, lateral canthus, and infraorbital hollows. The patient is shown pre-operatively (Panel **a**), after the first session of fat transfer – 12 cc (Panel **b**), and after the second session of fat transfer – 7.5 cc (Panel **c**)

potentially reduced fat graft survival. Patients are instructed that they will be swollen and overcorrected initially and that the final result will be appreciable around 3 months postoperatively, at which time another session of fat grafting can be performed if necessary (Fig. 12.4).

Surgical Orbital Implant Placement

For patients wanting a more definitive and predictable procedure with durable results, various surgical options exist. If no implant was placed at the time of eye removal, a standard and adequately sized orbital implant should be placed secondarily. If an orbital implant was placed previously but there is residual enophthalmos and superior sulcus deformity, a subperiosteal implant can be placed along the orbital floor to further volumize the orbit (Fig. 12.5). This can be performed via a subciliary or transconjunctival approach, and an implant consisting of alloplastic material of the desired volume can be placed. The authors prefer using a porous polyethylene barrier channel sheet implant or an enophthalmos wedge implant. The implant is placed posteriorly in the orbit, and a titanium screw or periosteal closure with suture is performed to prevent anterior implant migration. Placement of a subperiosteal implant, as opposed to performing an implant exchange, avoids the dissection and tissue trauma necessary to remove the existing implant and the potential need to detach the extraocular muscles from the old implant and attach them to a new larger implant. An implant exchange may be necessary or indicated if there is exposure or infection of the existing implant.

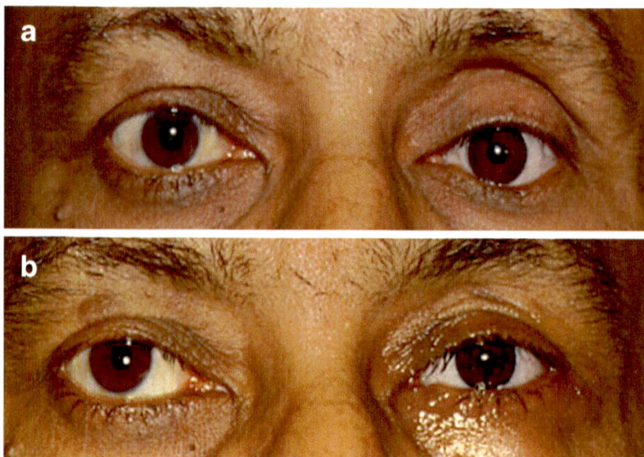

Fig. 12.5 (**a**) Patient with findings of post-enucleation socket syndrome including relative hypoglobus of the left-sided prosthesis and superior sulcus deformity. (**b**) The same patient after subperiosteal wedge implant placement. Note improved position of prosthesis and lid crease symmetry with the additional volume added by the implant. (Photographs courtesy of Dr. Thomas Johnson)

When the anophthalmic socket has a coexisting unrepaired orbital fracture, the orbital fracture can result in volume expansion of the bony orbital confines. In this situation, a standard-sized orbital implant such as a 22 mm spherical implant is often inadequate in preventing postoperative enophthalmos and superior sulcus deformity (Fig. 12.6). If no implant was placed primarily when the eye was removed, a larger-than-normal-sized orbital implant such as a 24 mm spherical implant can be placed to help compensate for mild orbital volume expansion due to a fracture. If an implant was already placed at time of eye removal, or there is significant orbital volume expansion from the fracture, a subperiosteal wedge implant can be placed, or the fracture can be repaired in standard fashion with an alloplastic implant used to recreate the normal anatomical orbital confines and associated orbital volume.

Eyelid Surgery

Once adequate orbital volume has been achieved, a new ocular prosthesis is normally necessary, and the patient meets with the ocularist to get fit for a new prosthesis. It is helpful for the surgeon to again discuss with the ocularist, since the best aesthetic result and prosthesis function are determined jointly by the size and height of the prosthesis and the eyelid position, tension, and function. Once the final prosthetic is made, any ptosis repair or lower lid tightening that is necessary can be performed with the final prosthesis in place.

In conclusion, PESS involves stereotypical findings and pathophysiological changes, and yet every anophthalmic socket must be considered individually based on the patient's history and examination findings. By following a systematic

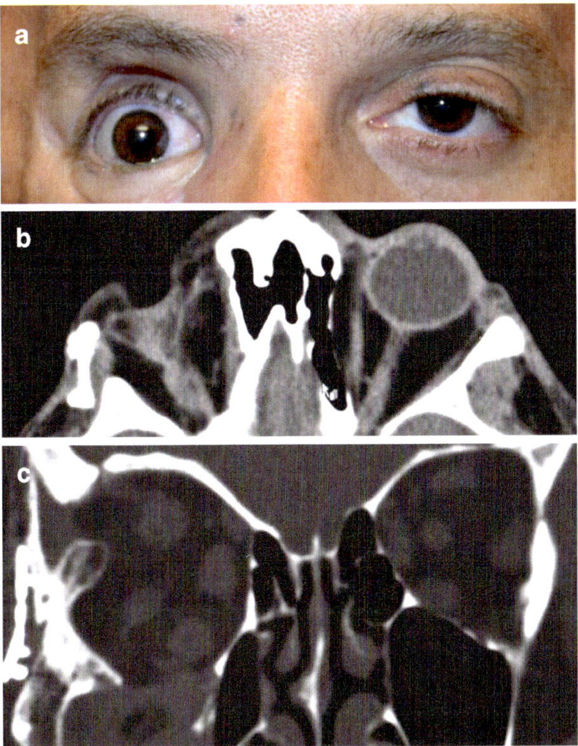

Fig. 12.6 This patient sustained an explosion injury resulting in enucleation of the right eye with no implant, suboptimal reconstruction of orbital and facial fractures with implants, and multiple subsequent reconstructive surgeries. The patient was fit with a large volume ocular prosthesis but demonstrates residual enophthalmos, apparent hypoglobus, superior sulcus deformity, and upper lid retraction (Panel **a**). CT imaging demonstrates lack of a spherical orbital implant (Panel **b**) and the poorly reconstructed orbital floor and zygomaticomaxillary complex fractures that have resulted in bony expansion of the orbit with prolapse of orbital tissues into the maxillary sinus (Panel **c**)

reconstructive process, considering surgical and nonsurgical interventions, and collaborating closely with the ocularist, patients with anophthalmic sockets can achieve excellent symmetry and aesthetic outcomes.

References

1. Jordan DR, Klapper SR. Evaluation and management of the anophthalmic socket and socket reconstruction. In: Black EH, et al., editors. Smith and Nesi's ophthalmic plastic and reconstructive surgery. 3rd ed. New York: Springer; 2012. p. 1131–73.
2. Custer PL, Trinkaus KM. Volumetric determination of enucleation implant size. Am J Ophthalmol. 1999;128(4):489–94.

3. Kaltreider SA, Jacobs JL, Hughes MO. Predicting the ideal implant size before enucleation. Ophthalmic Plast Reconstr Surg. 1999;15(1):37–43.
4. Soll DB. The anophthalmic socket. Ophthalmology. 1982;89(5):407–23.
5. Smit TJ, Koornneef L, Zonneveld FW, Groet E, Otto AJ. Primary and secondary implants in the anophthalmic orbit. Preoperative and postoperative computed tomographic appearance. Ophthalmology. 1991;98(1):106–10.
6. Buchanan AG, Holds JB, Vagefi MR, Bidar M, McCann JD, Anderson RL. Anterior filler displacement following injection of calcium hydroxylapatite gel (Radiesse) for anophthalmic orbital volume augmentation. Ophthalmic Plast Reconstr Surg. 2012;28(5):335–7.
7. Vagefi MR, McMullan TF, Burroughs JR, Georgescu D, McCann JD, Anderson RL. Orbital augmentation with injectable calcium hydroxylapatite for correction of postenucleation/evisceration socket syndrome. Ophthalmic Plast Reconstr Surg. 2011;27(2):90–4.
8. Aletaha M, Salour H, Yadegary S, Fekri Y, Tavakoli M. Orbital volume augmentation with calcium hydroxyapatite filler in anophthalmic enophthalmos. J Ophthalmic Vis Res. 2017;12(4):397–401.

Chapter 13
Socket Inflammation and Infection

Nathan W. Blessing

Introduction

A thorough evaluation of an anophthalmic socket patient includes an overall assessment of the socket's health. Socket inflammation can be multifactorial and can originate from the eyelids, the nasolacrimal system, the conjunctiva, or the prosthesis itself. Each should be assessed individually and treated as necessary. Ensuring the health of the socket allows a patient to wear a prosthesis comfortably. An inflamed or infected socket often presents with copious discharge and possibly socket pain. Treatment of socket issues should be tailored to the individual patient, ideally in concert with their ocularist. Prostheses should be modified and maintained as necessary with regular polishing to reduce associated inflammation and should be customized to fit each individual socket. A poorly fit prosthesis or a "stock" prosthesis can lead to a chronically irritated socket with poor patient satisfaction.

Socket Inflammation

An anophthalmic socket contains all of the tissues necessary to support the health of an eye including the eyelids with their Meibomian glands, the palpebral and forniceal conjunctiva, the conjunctiva overlying the orbital implant, goblet cells, the glands of Krause and Wolfring, the lacrimal gland, and the nasolacrimal drainage

N. W. Blessing (✉)
Dean McGee Eye Institute, University of Oklahoma College of Medicine, Department of Ophthalmology, Oklahoma City, OK, USA
e-mail: nathan-blessing@dmei.org

T. E. Johnson (ed.), *Anophthalmia*,
https://doi.org/10.1007/978-3-030-29753-4_13

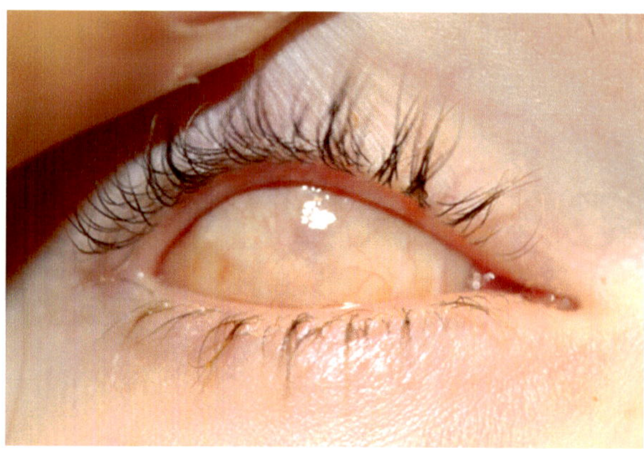

Fig. 13.1 External photo of a right anophthalmic socket. The socket is quiet and healthy as are the eyelids and lashes

system (Fig. 13.1). As in an ophthalmic socket, perturbation of any of these supportive elements may result in the development of local inflammation, e.g., contact lens overwear may result in the development of corneal foreign body sensation and conjunctival injection. Prosthesis-rehabilitated sockets retain a chronic foreign body which requires ongoing maintenance that must be individualized to the patient; there is no definitive standard of care for ocular prostheses, and there are widely variable recommendations in the published literature.

Anatomical Considerations

Although a typical anophthalmic socket contains all of the tissues necessary to support a prosthesis, certain aspects of each socket are both unique to the patient and globally true of all anophthalmic sockets. One prevailing factor is the overall reduction in reflex tear production which renders an anophthalmic socket relatively drier than the companion eye due to loss of the corneal reflex tearing arc [1, 7, 9]. In addition, the presence of a prosthesis alters the normal distribution and transit of socket lubrication such that tears, mucus, and inflammatory debris may become trapped in recesses in and around the ocular prosthesis. Although deposits on the posterior aspect of the prosthesis have not been shown to promote inflammation, interpalpebral deposits on the anterior face of the prosthesis may be proinflammatory either due to mechanical trauma from rubbing or due to the constitution of the deposits themselves. Interpalpebral deposition is promoted by incomplete blinking and lagophthalmos in patients with large prostheses used to correct ptosis or superior sulcus hollowing or to compensate for a relative lack of orbital volume. For unclear reasons, the eyelids of anophthalmic sockets may be more prone to the development of Meibomian gland dysfunction [12]. Tear film debris may obstruct the glands reducing the oily component of the natural tear lubricant, and secondary eyelid inflammation may develop. Large prostheses may also weigh down the lower eyelid creating lid retraction and ectropion with further tear stasis and impaired transit toward the nasolacrimal drainage system. Reduced tear transit through the nasolacrimal system may also explain the presence of at least partial nasolacrimal duct obstructions in some patients, which may further exacerbate the development of socket inflammation.

Patient Symptomatology and Inflammatory Signs

A preponderance of prosthesis-wearing anophthalmic socket patients complain of frequent watering, crusting, and discharge; mucoid discharge can be seen in both quiescent and inflamed or infected sockets, but a progressive increase in socket discharge can signal an increase in overall socket inflammation (Fig. 13.2) [2]. Additionally, some patients may complain of socket soreness although this is less common than complaints of increasing discharge or increasingly viscous discharge. These complaints should prompt the evaluating physician to carefully inspect the socket for tissue signs of inflammation including conjunctival injection, copious mucinous debris, and pyogenic granuloma formation (Fig. 13.3). Pyogenic granuloma formation may also signal the socket's attempt to resolve an occult implant exposure and should be carefully and thoroughly inspected. Pyogenic granulomas can often be treated through a combined approach of prosthesis modification and topical steroid therapy. Refractory lesions may require conservative excision. Although an interval increase in socket discharge may indicate the presence of an infection, mechanical or fundamental socket factors are more likely.

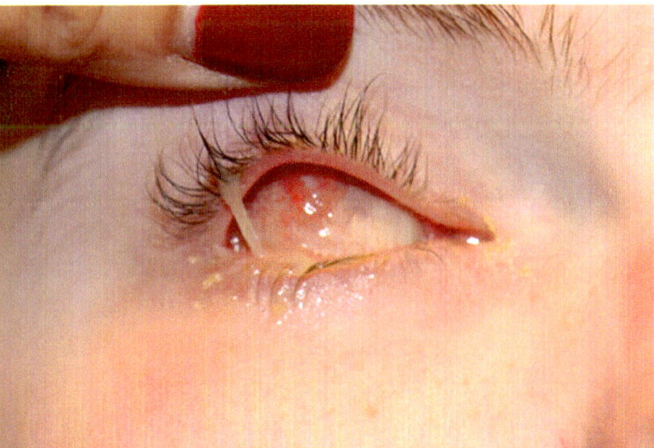

Fig. 13.2 External photo of an inflamed anophthalmic socket showing extensive mucoid discharge and lower eyelash crusting. The patient was successfully treated with a course of topical antibiotic/steroid ointment

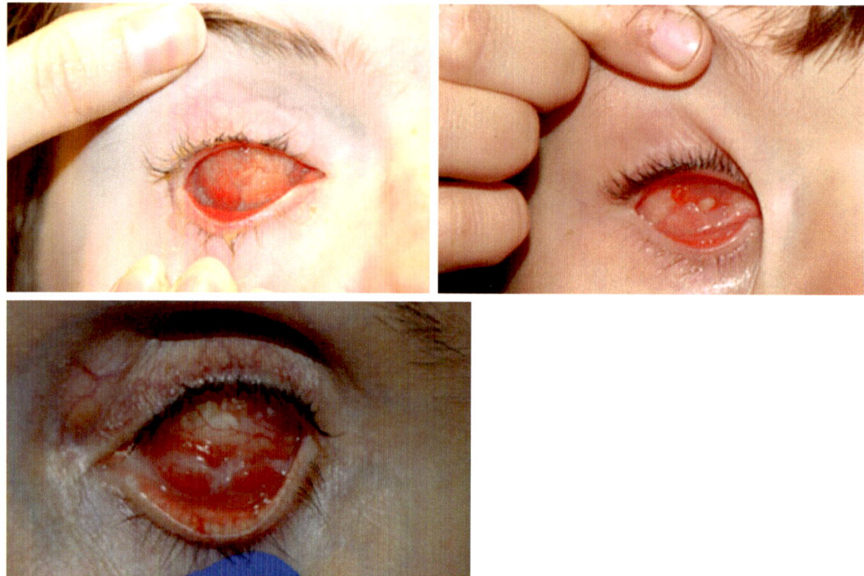

Fig. 13.3 Three different anophthalmic sockets each demonstrating the formation of a conjunctival pyogenic granuloma

Prosthesis Factors

Intrinsic characteristics of a patient's prosthesis may predispose the socket to reactive inflammation [17]. A thorough socket evaluation includes close inspection of the patient's prosthesis including the prosthesis age, material, fit, polish, and surface deposits. It is also important to discuss with the patient their understanding of prosthesis maintenance as some studies have shown that frequent prosthesis manipulation may increase socket inflammation and discharge due to the mechanical trauma associated with removing and replacing the prosthesis, the risk of damaging or scratching the prosthesis when it is manipulated, and the introduction of additional bacterial load when handling the prosthesis in a non-sterile way [3, 8, 14, 20]. Patients who frequently remove their prosthesis for cleaning in response to an increase in socket inflammation or symptomatic discharge may be initiating a reflex cycle whereby increased manipulation leads to persistent or increasing discharge and baseline socket inflammation [10]. Although the best approach to prosthesis and socket hygiene remains controversial, most published or available references have recommended prosthesis removal and cleaning at least every 6 months and not more frequently than monthly [16, 18]. Prostheses should be professionally polished at least once if not twice per year by an experienced ocularist, ideally to an optical quality smooth surface analogous to that of hard contact lenses [11, 13, 19].

Keith Pine's group out of New Zealand has studied the anophthalmic socket and its response to prosthesis wear extensively, and they have proposed a three-phase model of prosthesis and socket homeostasis [15]. First, a clean and freshly polished prosthesis goes through establishment whereby the socket adjusts to the prosthesis. This may include the distribution of mucinous deposits over the prosthesis to improve wettability and lubrication, allowing the posterior portion of the prosthesis to rest comfortably against the socket conjunctiva and the lids to blink smoothly across the anterior portion of the prosthesis face. Additionally, the introduction of the prosthesis may change the socket microbiome requiring the elimination of extraneous or potentially pathogenic bacteria. During this period, there may be an interval increase in mild socket inflammation and discharge which can be ameliorated with topical lubricants such as ophthalmic antibiotic-steroid ointment, mineral oil, or a petroleum-based nighttime eye ointment. The second phase is one of equilibrium whereby the prosthesis has been thoroughly coated with mucin produced by conjunctival goblet cells to improve tear retention and resident bacterial flora are in balance with the antibacterial actions of tear lysozyme. This period should be one of quiescence with minimal baseline socket inflammation and a scant amount of socket mucoid discharge, analogous to a healthy eye in which minimal maintenance is necessary. However, at some point the balance tips toward homeostasis breakdown. The factors predisposing to this disruption of equilibrium may be multiple but presumably begin with the induction of a mild amount of inflammation which cascades into additional inflammation and secondary symptomatology. Inducing events may include the buildup of an excessive amount of mucinous deposits on the prosthesis, an increase in the resident bacterial load, or damages to the finish of the anterior prosthesis due to either protein buildup with secondary drying or finish scratches due to mechanical wiping of the prosthesis by the patient. A rough anterior prosthesis surface may also lead to mechanical damage and reaction of the palpebral conjunctiva in the form of papillary or giant papillary conjunctivitis [5, 6]. It is at this point that the prosthesis requires maintenance cleaning and polishing, and robust socket inflammation can be treated with topical antibiotic-steroid ointment to reduce baseline inflammation and help the patient progress back through the period of re-establishing homeostasis with a clean and smooth prosthesis. If left untreated, these inflamed sockets with poorly maintained prostheses may develop more severe complications including pyogenic granuloma formation, breakdown of socket conjunctiva with underlying implant exposure, socket contracture, giant papillary conjunctivitis (which may be a foreign body allergic reaction to the prosthesis or substantial protein/bacterial deposits on the prosthesis itself), or secondary socket infection.

Pegged Orbital Implants

Some early orbital implants included a buried ring to attach the extraocular muscles and an exposed anterior face with various mechanical interfaces designed to improve motility transmission to the overlying prosthesis. However, these prostheses were often removed due to chronic inflammation or secondary infection. With the advent

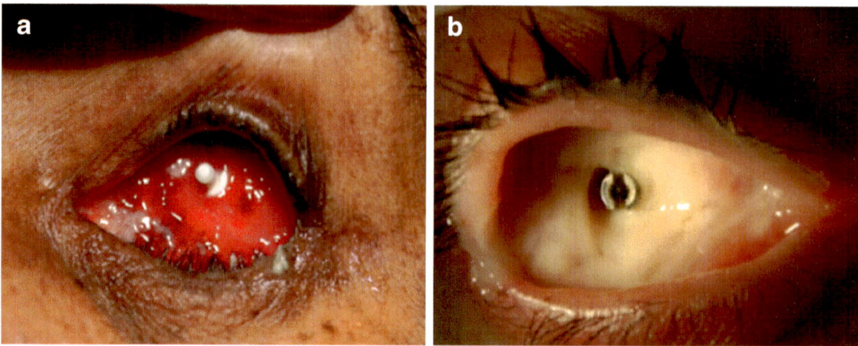

Fig. 13.4 (**a**) Exposed peg with pyogenic granuloma formation. (Photo courtesy of Annie Moreau, M.D.) and (**b**) infected pegged implant with atypical mycobacteria (Photo courtesy of Thomas Johnson, MD)

of the coralline hydroxyapatite implant which permitted fibrovascular integration with the socket, implant pegs were developed in an attempt to again improve implant motility. The assumption was that fibrovascular integration would allow the implant to interface with the peg and prosthesis while retaining a barrier between the buried implant and the outside world. Although peg placement does significantly improve motility, the peg apparatus is susceptible to the same maintenance issues as prostheses in that they may be a nidus for socket inflammation and infection (Fig. 13.4). Although a subset of patients seem to tolerate pegging well, many patients ultimately develop pyogenic granuloma formation, chronic discharge, and possibly implant erosion with secondary infection requiring an implant exchange. As such, many practitioners have abandoned peg placement due to the additional required maintenance and monitoring and the potential complications which may result in significant socket morbidity including contracture. Additionally, it has been the author's experience that exposed porous implants, including porous polyethylene and hydroxyapatite, placed profoundly outside the window of proposed complete fibrovascular ingrowth (years) seem to be surrounded by a superficial fibrovascular capsule as opposed to being completely invested with fibrovascular tissue. This observation undermines the anatomic rationale for peg tolerance over a prolonged period of time, as the peg provides a route for bacteria to colonize the underlying avascular implant.

Socket Infection

An anophthalmic socket is most susceptible to the usual infections seen in ophthalmic sockets. In cases of an acute increase in socket inflammation and discharge, infections are the first etiologies which should be ruled out, especially if a careful examination of the prosthesis reveals no significant abnormalities such as profound

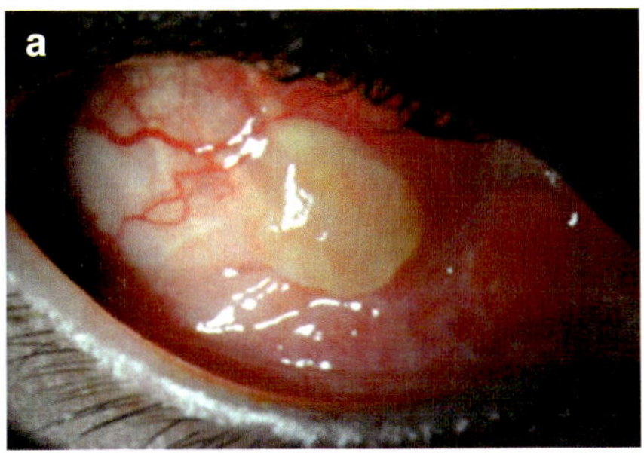

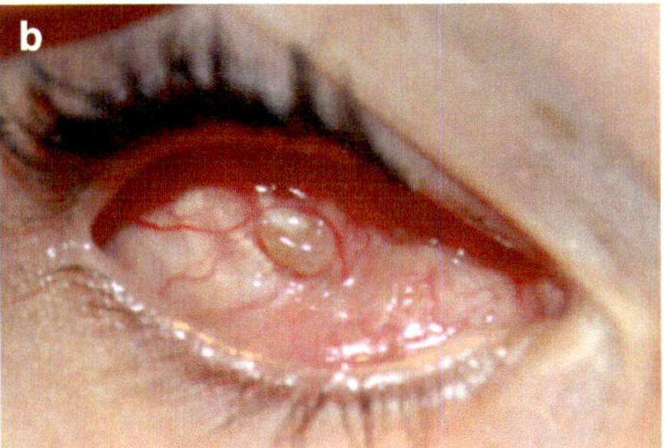

Fig. 13.5 Pyogenic granuloma overlying an exposed HA implant (**a**). Treatment with topical steroids resulted in regression of the pyogenic granuloma revealing the underlying implant exposure (**b**). (Photos courtesy of Annie Moreau, M.D.)

scratches or protein deposition and the prosthesis has been regularly maintained and replaced as needed. Common examples of socket infections include viral conjunctivitis, hordeola, and occasionally bacterial conjunctivitis. An acute increase in socket discharge allows the examining physician to assess the texture and composition of discharged material. Stringy mucoid discharge is most consistent with an inflammatory reaction to an underlying issue, whereas mucopurulent discharge is more suggestive of a bacterial cause, and should be cultured. Routine culture of socket discharge is not recommended because while discharge is common, bacterial superinfection is not and most sockets harbor an array of normal flora which are not pathogenic. Suspected bacterial conjunctivitis should be treated with appropriate empiric topical antibiotics until culture sensitivities are finalized.

In patients who fail to respond adequately to topical antibiotic therapy or whose symptoms recur after antibiotics are stopped and are not otherwise attributable to noninfectious causes of socket inflammation, a careful inspection of the socket should be performed to rule out occult implant exposure with secondary infection. Often these small areas of exposure begin with mechanical trauma from the overlying prosthesis with development of a pyogenic granuloma. The pyogenic granuloma may hide a small area of exposure which tends to enlarge over time without adequate treatment (Fig. 13.5). Suspected superficial infection in the setting of implant exposure may be treated with a course of topical antibiotics and closure of the conjunctival defect. However, a number of these cases may progress to overt implant infection, particularly in the setting of porous implants, necessitating removal of the implant with replacement either at the same time if deeper tissues are deemed healthy or secondary replacement at a later date if the socket itself appears infected [4]. These patients should also be treated with an appropriate course of oral antibiotics, ideally based on culture sensitivities, and their sockets should be thoroughly irrigated with antibiotic solution at the time of surgery. Some patients may present with profound implant exposure (Fig. 13.6) and mucopurulent discharge consistent with bacterial colonization of the implant (most commonly gram-positive organisms such as *Staph* and *Strep* species) and should be treated similarly with oral and topical antibiotics and implant removal. Whereas removal of a smooth (silicone or

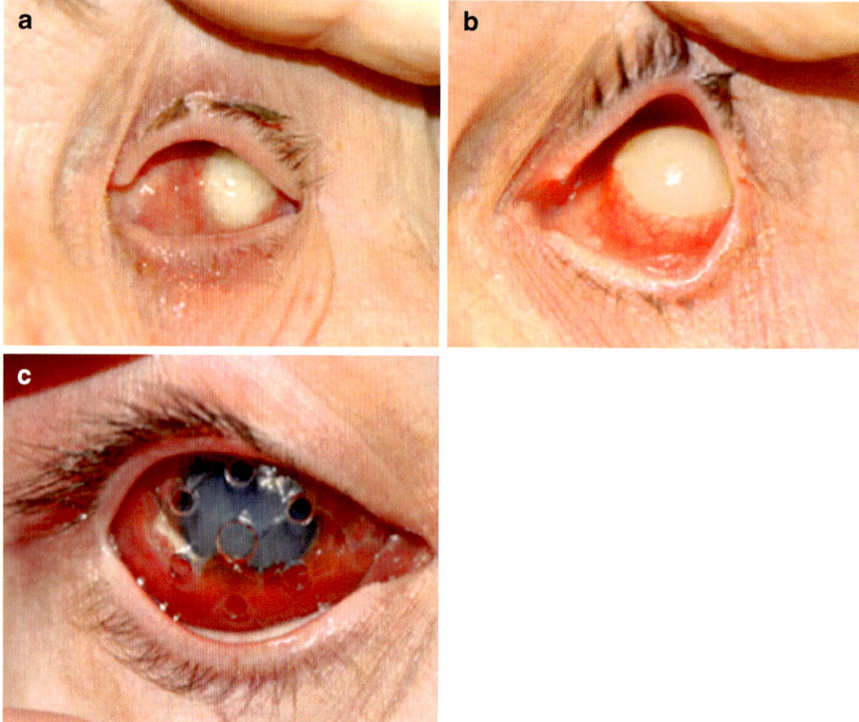

Fig. 13.6 (**a**) Exposed Medpor implant in a patient with poor socket maintenance. (Photo courtesy of Jeremy F. Tan, M.D.). (**b**) Exposed implant in a patient with no socket maintenance for over 20 years. (**c**) Exposed silicone implant in a poorly controlled diabetic patient

PMMA) implant may be easily achieved in the clinic owing to the limited fibrous attachments to the surrounding socket, removal of a porous implant often requires a trip to the operating suite due the extensive superficial fibrovascular capsule that develops around these implants. A subset of patients may develop an infection with atypical mycobacteria which are difficult to culture and difficult to treat even with appropriate antibiotic therapy. Symptomatically, these sockets may more closely resemble a case of benign mild but chronic inflammation, and a high degree of suspicion is necessary in order to arrive at the correct diagnosis.

Finally, there is a subset of anophthalmic patients in which a nasolacrimal duct obstruction develops [17]. Patients whose sockets are otherwise healthy without implant exposure or prosthesis issues but who continue to suffer from recurrent possibly mucopurulent discharge should be assessed for nasolacrimal system patency, as some may harbor an occult underlying chronic dacryocystitis with reflux of retained mucopurulent material from the lacrimal sac. These patients may be treated with dacryocystorhinostomy or simply dacryocystectomy as the socket tends to be relatively dry at baseline. However, dacryocystectomy eliminates the possible transit of excess mucins and proteins through the nasolacrimal system, and these may accumulate in the socket leading to a baseline increase in mucoid discharge.

References

1. Allen L, Kolder HE, Bulgarelli EM, Bulgarelli DM. Artificial eyes and tear measurements. Ophthalmology. 1980;87:155–7.
2. Jones CA, Collin JR. A classification and review the causes of discharging sockets. Trans Ophthalmol Soc U K. 1983;103(Pt 3):351–3.
3. Vasquez RJ, Linberg JV. The anophthalmic socket and the prosthetic eye. A clinical and bacteriologic study. Ophthalmic Plast Reconstr Surg. 1989;5:277–80.
4. Jordan DR, Brownstein S, Faraji H. Clinicopathologic analysis of 15 explanted hydroxyapatite implants. Ophthalmic Plast Reconstr Surg. 2004;20:285–90.
5. Chang WJ, Tse DT, Rosa RH, Huang A, Johnson TE, Schiffman J. Conjunctival cytology features of giant papillary conjunctivitis associated with ocular prostheses. Ophthalmic Plast Reconstr Surg. 2005;21:39–45.
6. Bozkurt B, Akyurek N, Irkec M, Erdener U, Memis L. Immunohistochemical findings in prosthesis-associated giant papillary conjunctivitis. Clin Exp Ophthalmol. 2007;35:535–40.
7. Vardizer Y, Lang Y, Mourits MP, Briscoe MD. Favorable effects of lacrimal plugs in patients with an anophthalmic socket. Orbit. 2007;26:263–6.
8. Kim JH, Lee MJ, Choung HK, et al. Conjunctival cytologic features in anophthalmic patients wearing an ocular prosthesis. Ophthalmic Plast Reconstr Surg. 2008;24:290–5.
9. Kim SE, Yoon JS, Lee SY. Tear measurement in prosthetic eye users with Fourier-domain optical coherence tomography. Am J Ophthalmol. 2010;149:602–7.e1.
10. Pine K, Sloan B, Stewart J, Jacobs RJ. A survey of prosthetic eye wearers to investigate mucoid discharge. Clin Ophthalmol. 2012;6:707–13.
11. Pine KR, Sloan B, Jacobs RJ. Deposit buildup on prosthetic eyes and implications for conjunctival inflammation and mucoid discharge. Clin Ophthalmol. 2012;6:1755–62.
12. Jang SY, Lee SY, Yoon JS. Meibomian gland dysfunction in longstanding prosthetic eye wearers. Br J Ophthalmol. 2013;97:398–402.
13. Pine KR, Sloan B, Han KI, Swift S, Jacobs RJ. Deposit buildup on prosthetic eye material (in vitro) and its effect on surface wettability. Clin Ophthalmol. 2013;7:313–9.
14. Pine KR, Sloan B, Stewart J, Jacobs RJ. The response of the anophthalmic socket to prosthetic eye wear. Clin Exp Optom. 2013;96:388–93.
15. Pine KR, Sloan BH, Jacobs RJ. A proposed model of the response of the anophthalmic socket to prosthetic eye wear and its application to the management of mucoid discharge. Med Hypotheses. 2013;81:300–5.
16. Bonaque-Gonzalez S, Amigo A, Rodriguez-Luna C. Recommendations for post-adaption care of an ocular prosthesis: a review. Cont Lens Anterior Eye. 2015;38:397–401.
17. Kashkouli MB, Zolfaghari R, Es'haghi A, et al. Tear film, lacrimal drainage system, and eyelid findings in subjects with anophthalmic socket discharge. Am J Ophthalmol. 2016;165:33–8.
18. Vargason CW, Mawn LA. Management of inflammation and periocular malignancy in the anophthalmic socket. Int Ophthalmol Clin. 2017;57:103–16.
19. Litwin AS, Worrell E, Roos JCP, Edwards B, Malhotra R. Can we improve the tolerance of an ocular prosthesis by enhancing its surface finish? Ophthalmic Plast Reconstr Surg. 2018;34:130–5.
20. Choi YJ, Oh EK, Lee MJ, Kim N, Choung H, Khwarg SI. Atypical mycobacterial infection in anophthalmic sockets with porous orbital implant exposure. Am J Ophthalmol. 2018;195:131–42.

Chapter 14
Management of Implant Exposure and Extrusion

Benjamin Erickson

Introduction

Porous spheres – whether hydroxyapatite (HA), porous polyethylene (PP), or aluminum oxide (Al_2O_3) – have become the most widely utilized orbital implants following enucleation and evisceration. They confer significant theoretical advantages due to the potential for vascular ingrowth and biointegration, which may reduce the risk of migration or extrusion [1–4]. Their light, porous structure may also slow or reduce the onset of anophthalmic socket syndrome and superior sulcus deformity when compared to heavier solid implants [1, 3, 5]. Drilling with peg placement to improve prosthesis motility has declined in popularity in recent years but remains another potential advantage of porous materials [6].

Nevertheless, the rough outer surface of these implants is thought by some to increase the likelihood of soft tissue erosion and exposure [1, 7]. Many surgeons therefore elect to wrap them with a smooth material, such as donor sclera, which acts as a barrier between the implant and overlying Tenon's fascia but also requires strategic fenestration in order to avoid impeding appropriate vascularization [8, 9]. Alternatively, implants may be engineered with an integrated, smooth anterior barrier with suture tunnels for extraocular muscle attachment (Medpor SST, Stryker [Kalamazoo, MI]) [10].

Despite shifting trends in implant selection, rates of exposure remain between 2% and 10% in most studies, with both technique-dependent and technique-independent factors implicated [11–13]. Significant outliers with very high exposure rates are primarily attributable to use of unwrapped implants for enucleation in the context of pediatric retinoblastoma or to placement by surgeons with limited experience [11, 14]. Nevertheless, orbital implant exposure and extrusion remain significant management challenges, and recognition is often delayed due to the non-

B. Erickson (✉)
Stanford Byers Eye Institute, Department of Ophthalmology, Palo Alto, CA, USA
e-mail: bericksо@stanford.edu

T. E. Johnson (ed.), *Anophthalmia*,
https://doi.org/10.1007/978-3-030-29753-4_14

specific nature of initial symptoms – mild irritation and socket discharge are of course quite common in anophthalmic prosthesis wearers [15].

Small defects (generally those less than 3 mm) may close spontaneously with conservative measures, such as prosthesis removal or vaulting to reduce tension and friction [16]. Larger initial defects or persistent smaller defects, however, require antibiotic treatment and surgical intervention, with undermining and closure, patch grafting, or use of vascularized pedicles [17–19].

When an underlying area of poor implant vascularity is identified in conjunction with the defect, it is typically recommended to burr down and remove it in order to curtail persistent bacterial colonization, which may compromise healing and predispose to recurrent exposure. If the avascular portion of the implant requiring removal is volumetrically significant and/or if there is significant associated conjunctival loss, it may be preferable to employ a technique – such as dermis fat grafting – that can simultaneously address these concerns [12, 20].

Implant exposure not infrequently reaches a point of no return, however, with up to one third of cases ultimately requiring implant removal [11]. When bacteria are able to colonize substantial portions of a porous implant, antibiotic penetration is typically poor due to reduced vascularity and protective biofilm formation [1, 21]. Low-grade infection often persists, resulting in chronic inflammation and intractable exposure or fistula tract formation [1, 21]. Without carefully planned intervention, patients may progress to a state of volume deficiency with contracted fornices, scarred and/or slipped muscles, poor socket vascularity, and poor motility. In severe cases, satisfactory prosthesis retention is ultimately compromised, requiring skin grafting to the anophthalmic socket or other aggressive measures [22].

Factors Related to Exposure

The factors predisposing to implant exposure may be divided into technique-dependent versus technique-independent categories. The former includes such considerations as implant material and size, wrapping material, extraocular muscle anchoring, tissue dragging during implantation (the "cactus syndrome"), and closure technique [11, 23]. The latter includes prosthesis fit and maintenance, as well as host factors that may decrease vascular ingrowth, such as prior trauma, anophthalmic socket surgery, or radiotherapy.

Technique-Dependent Factors

Implant Material Choice

Implant materials do vary slightly with respect to porosity, and there is a theoretical "optimum" pore size, which maximizes fibrovascular ingrowth potential without unduly increasing abrasiveness of the implant exterior [10, 24]. HA implants have been shown to vascularize slightly more rapidly than their PP counterparts in animal studies, but it is not apparent this difference has clinical significance [25].

Clinically, it is difficult to ascertain whether there are meaningful differences in rates of exposure and extrusion when comparing HA, PP, Al_2O_3 (bioceramic), and traditional solid implants due to heterogeneity of patient populations, surgical technique, and follow-up protocols [4]. Custer and colleagues examined pooled data obtained via a English-language PubMed literature search from 1989 to 2004, ultimately reviewing 3777 cases reported in 49 discrete publications [11]. They concluded that a modest observed difference in exposure rates between HA (4.9%) and PP (8.1%) implants was primarily attributable to the controversial practice of inserting unwrapped PP implants, particularly in pediatric retinoblastoma patients [11]. Excluding subjects known to have retinoblastoma resulted in revised exposure rates of 4.2% for PP and 5.1% for HA [11]. Some studies have such low rates or exposure as to render comparisons between implant materials statistically impossible – 1 retrospective analysis of HA and PP implants had only 4 observed exposures across a cohort of 342 patients [26].

Some more recent publications do suggest slightly higher rates of exposure with bioceramic implants, but the level of evidence supporting this conclusion is relatively low [27, 28]. In the absence of compelling outcomes data, choice of implant material is dictated by surgeon preference and comfort.

While biointegration is an oft cited advantage of porous implants, there is some indication that nonporous acrylic spheres may fare as well or better than their porous counterparts with regard to rates of exposure. Custer and colleagues calculated a 3.5% exposure rate for acrylic implants across reported series, but if those wrapped with absorbable mesh are excluded, the rate declined even further to a creditable 1.6% [11]. However, when nonporous implants do become exposed, they are far more likely to spontaneously extrude and are not typically amenable to rescue techniques.

Implant Size

While it is generally agreed that excessive tension on Tenon's fascia due to placement of an oversized implant predisposes to exposure and/or extrusion, this has not been studied in a quantitative fashion [16]. Conversely, routine use of smaller implants may result in the need for a bulky prosthesis with limited motility and excessive tension on the lower eyelid. This may also increase the subsequent need for subperiosteal enophthalmic wedge placement in order to address superior sulcus deformity. It is therefore common practice to use an implant sizing set in order to select the largest implant that permits layered closure of the overlying soft tissues under minimal tension.

Surgeon Experience and Technique

Apart from the choice of whether and how to wrap a porous implant, several other factors appear to influence observed rates of exposure. It is difficult, however, to systematically quantify the impact of slight variations in surgical technique on outcomes data [11].

Reported rates of porous implant exposure were higher in the early 1990s, with surveys of American Society of Ophthalmic Plastic and Reconstructive Surgery membership revealing substantial improvements in recent years – likely indicating an initial community learning curve with biointegrated implants [3, 29]. Nevertheless, noted outliers in rates of exposure do persist, suggesting the presence of individual surgeon and technique-based differences. One particular study identified a tenfold difference in rates of exposure between enucleations performed by an oculoplastic surgeon versus those performed by surgeons lacking subspecialty training [14].

Among other factors, Sagoo and Rose have posited a "cactus syndrome" theory, whereby incorrect sphere implantation is thought to be a major driver of subsequent exposure. When an implant is forced into the orbit with inadequate soft tissue retraction, it can drag superficial fat and fascia, with tissue rebound creating an impetus for postoperative migration [23]. Careful layered closure has also been suggested as an important factor in preventing implant exposure [11].

Some surgeons report an increased rate of exposure with evisceration – presumably due to reduced rate of fibrous ingrowth when a porous sphere is implanted in host sclera and/or avoidance of keratectomy with subsequent reduction of anterior barrier integrity. However, Custer and colleagues did not find statistically significant differences in exposure rates in a comprehensive literature review [11]. Posterior fenestrations are employed by many surgeons both to speed vascular ingrowth and to increase the size of implant that can be placed, particularly with keratectomy, but there remains some concern that these apertures are not routinely made large enough to produce effects comparable to those seen with the rectus muscle windows commonly made in donor sclera for enucleation [30]. However, other advantages of evisceration – such as reduced operative time, faster patient recovery, and potentially slowed progression of anophthalmic socket syndrome – outweigh this theoretical concern in the minds of many surgeons [30].

Certainly, there is an intuitive appeal to attaching extraocular muscles to an implant, not only to promote socket motility but also to speed implant vascularization and promote retention. While this practice is routine with primary enucleations, it is not always possible in cases of ballistic trauma or with secondary orbital implant placement. Notably, exposure and extrusion rates were found to be nearly three times higher for cases in which the rectus muscles were not reattached [31].

Implant Wrapping

The choice of whether to wrap porous implants is still debated, with both proponents and detractors. Creating a barrier between the rough outer surface of an implant and overlying Tenon's fascia and conjunctiva has an intuitive appeal but, without thoughtful execution, could prevent the fibrovascular ingrowth that is the greatest advantage of selecting a porous sphere in the first place [7, 32]. A rabbit model comparing the rate of fibrovascularization of wrapped versus unwrapped HA implants did demonstrate substantial reductions in wrapped spheres, but animals were sacrificed at a 1-week timepoint, and the wrapping technique employed did not closely approximate best surgical practice, casting clinical relevance into doubt [33]. A subsequent rabbit study of HA implants demonstrated that fibrovascularization of all implants occurred by 12 weeks regardless of wrapping material choice [34].

Further studies demonstrate that the most rapid and profound ingrowth originates from windows where the rectus muscles come into direct contact with the implant as well as at the posterior opening facing apical soft tissues [7, 25]. This histological evidence supports the routine practice of fenestrating implant wrappings [1]. Observed rates of exposure approaching 0% with commonly employed wrapping protocols provide further justification for this technique choice, while some of the highest reported rates of exposure are found among patient cohorts with unwrapped implants [11, 13, 26].

Choice of wrapping material also remains a subject of debate. Use of human donor sclera does confer a risk of viral and prion infection, although only one definite case of Creutzfeldt-Jakob disease (CJD) transmission from corneal transplantation has been reported to date and none from the use of donor sclera [35]. At the time of writing, there are no confirmed cases of human immunodeficiency disease (HIV) or hepatitis seroconversion from implantation of donor sclera. On the other hand, pooled evidence suggests excellent clinical results with donor sclera or dura, while wrapping with bovine pericardium or polyglactin mesh may be associated with increased rates of exposure [11, 13, 26]. Some authors assert that use of absorbable wrapping for porous spheres may in fact confer the same exposure risk as use of no wrapping material at all [36]. Autogenous fascia also appears to produce favorable results but at the expense of additional operative time and donor-site morbidity [11].

While wrapping of porous implants is advisable in the majority of circumstances, several important exceptions do exist. Implants that are engineered with an integrated, smooth anterior barrier with suture tunnels for extraocular muscle attachment have favorably low rates of exposure in the absence of wrapping material (Medpor SST, Stryker [Kalamazoo, MI]); Mahoney and colleagues reported a 3.3% exposure rate compared to a calculated 7.1% exposure rate for other porous primary implants in 58 prior studies [10]. Standard porous spheres also may do well unwrapped with careful end-to-end rectus muscle suturing to avoid abrasion of Tenon's fascia and to create a "joint-like" structure over the anterior implant [32].

Implant Pegging

Delayed drilling of porous implants for peg placement is a practice that can substantially improve prosthesis motility but has declined in popularity over time due to potential association with late implant exposure and other complications. While it is agreed by many that peg placement does predispose to late exposure and infection, commonly with latency of up to 6–7 years after pegging, the strength of evidence documenting this is nevertheless relatively weak and circumstantial [6, 37, 38]. Of interest, two thirds of spheres requiring explanation in a histopathological study by

Jordan and colleagues had undergone drilling for peg insertion, and it was suggested that drilling of these implants resulted in bacterial seeding and chronic infection of a poorly vascularized core [11, 15]. It is unclear from this report, however, what the interval was between implant placement and drilling and whether there were other predisposing factors that might have contributed to poor implant biointegration.

Technique-Independent Factors

A number of elements outside of the surgeon's direct control influence the risk of exposure as well. These can broadly be categorized as factors that influence anophthalmic socket health versus factors that impact implant vascularity and/or tissue integrity. Complete implant vascularization normally takes several months, and any factor predisposing to delayed biointegration or tissue contamination can increase the rate of complications [15, 16, 39, 40]. Just as excessively sized and abrasive orbital implants can result in internal erosion, so too can poorly fitting prostheses cause conjunctival abrasion and breakdown with subsequent exposure [16].

Trauma-associated enucleation surgery also appears to be associated with an increased risk of implant exposure, likely due to contamination and/or diminished tissue integrity [11, 30, 36]. Certain surgical histories, with scarring or shortage of conjunctiva and Tenon's fascia, are also anecdotally associated with higher extrusion risk, although systematic data is not currently available to support this clinical impression [11, 30].

Retinoblastoma-associated enucleation is a special case with high rates of reported implant exposure and may have causal factors beyond the controversial practice of using unwrapped porous orbital implants [11, 41]. Double-digit exposure rates have been identified in a number of studies even with wrapped implants [16, 41, 42]. Intravenous chemotherapy consistently arises as a factor potentially predisposing to increased rates of exposure, while the data related to external beam radiotherapy is more mixed [41–43]. Some groups report improved outcomes with nonporous acrylic implants, while others have suggested the importance of frequent prosthesis refitting to prevent tissue breakdown [43, 44].

Implant Exposure Rescue Algorithm

Small defects (generally those less than 3 mm) may close spontaneously with conservative measures [16]. According to a systematic review by Custer et al., 13% of exposures do heal without surgical intervention, although this appears slightly more likely with HA spheres than with their PP counterparts [11]. Use of topical antibiotics and lubricants in combination with tactics to alleviate friction, such as removing or vaulting the prosthesis, may be considered as a preliminary step when there is no clinical evidence of implant infection or compromised vascularity [16].

The majority of exposures, however, do eventually require surgical intervention to promote healing. Larger initial defects or persistent smaller defects may be approached with undermining and closure, patch grafting, or use of vascularized pedicles with as needed burring and removal of any avascular portions of the anterior implant [17–19]. Overall, the literature pertaining to repair is relatively anecdotal, consisting of small cases series with relatively limited follow-up. This makes robust comparison of varying surgical approaches difficult, but some fundamental guiding principles can help to promote successful technique selection. There is also no firm consensus regarding how long it is reasonable to wait prior to surgery, but expert opinion supports repair if a defect has not closed by 8 weeks, with more timely intervention recommended for large or early postoperative exposures [11].

Simple undermining and layered closure is applicable to a limited range of scenarios, as friable tissues surrounding a seemingly small area of exposure may require debridement, and adherence to the principle of closure under minimal tension is of paramount importance to minimize the risk of recurrence. This appears especially true of HA implants [11]. A variety of patch grafts have therefore been utilized and can be classified based on whether the tissue employed is autologous or banked human tissue versus decellularized xenograft. Grafts can also be classified based on which layers they attempt to replace. Some seek to substitute for the conjunctival layer only, while others restore a more robust barrier comparable to fascia/implant wrapping material. With the former, initial healing is rapid, but relatively high rates of melting and re-exposure are reported, particularly when placed on a poorly vascularized implant substrate without an additional blood supply [11, 45]. With the latter, residual conjunctiva and Tenon's fascia are often advanced over the edges of the patch graft to the extent possible without generating undue tension, leaving much of the graft surface to epithelialize secondarily. This results in healing times of up to 3 months, during which time caution with prosthesis fit is especially important, but larger defects may be addressed satisfactorily [46]. The hard palate is relatively unique insofar as it replaces all layers with a single graft, but the keratinized epithelium does still require time to undergo metaplasia [47].

Banked human tissues and processed xenograft materials afford the convenience of avoiding a donor site but may be more susceptible to postoperative inflammation and contraction [48]. As with wrapping materials, they do also confer a small risk of infectious disease transmission [48]. Amniotic membrane has been reported as a conjunctival substitute for small exposures and may be used as an adjunct to promote epithelialization in conjunction with other techniques, while donor sclera, fascia lata, and acellular porcine dermal matrix have been employed with good effect for larger defects [45, 48, 49].

In terms of autologous tissues, buccal mucus membrane grafts may be used for smaller defects as a conjunctival replacement, while posterior auricular muscle, temporalis fascia, pericranium, dermis fat, and hard palate mucosa are typically employed for larger or more challenging defects [29, 48, 50, 51]. Fascia and pericranium may be harvested using approaches familiar and comfortable to oculoplastic surgeons who perform endoscopic brow lifts. Custer and colleagues concluded that placing autologous or donor grafts under conjunctival pedicles is the most successful repair method, based on a comprehensive review of published literature [11].

Vascularized pedicles confer theoretical advantages with regard to healing but may require staged procedures or more extensive extra-orbital dissection and tunneling. Success has been reported with temporoparietal fascia as well as with two-staged tarsoconjunctival flaps with retained Muller's muscle, originating from the ipsilateral upper eyelid [52–54]. Good results have also been reported with local vascularized flaps, such as bulbar conjunctival pedicles combined with oral mucosa, extraocular muscle flaps, and Tenon's fascia/implant capsule flaps [55–58]. It is important to recognize, however, just how considerably the extensive dissection and advancement of these vascularized flaps differ from simple tissue advancement under tension, which is unlikely to succeed.

Each strategy should also seek to address any poorly vascularized portion of the implant, as this typically provides an inadequate substrate for healing of the overlying repaired tissues and may serve as a reservoir for colonizing bacteria, leading to persistent inflammation and recurrent erosion. The highest risk of colonization of a porous implant appears to be in the early postoperative period, before complete fibrovascularization has taken place – when the avascular core can act as an "immune sanctuary" for microorganisms [1]. Studies have demonstrated growth of fibrovascular tissue into the outer two thirds of implants by 3 months, with full vascularization of the core by 7–8 months [59–61]. If implant salvage is deemed feasible, it is generally recommended to burr away any avascular portion of the implant visualized at the time of surgical intervention [12, 16, 62]. The remaining vascularized portion can then serve as a more reliable recipient bed to support placement of grafts or advancement of adjacent flaps [12, 16]. When the area of exposure is large and the portion of the implant excised sizeable, resulting volumetric and forniceal defects can affect subsequent prosthesis fit, and consideration should be given to strategies – such as dermis fat grafting – that replace volume as well as provide coverage of the exposed implant. This can be performed with single or staged surgery, depending on surgeon preference [12, 30, 63]. However, resorption of dermis fat in anophthalmic sockets with resulting suboptimal volume correction is a well-documented problem [30].

Ultimately, implant removal is performed in nearly one third of exposures (Fig. 14.1) [11, 39]. The literature suggests that exposed PP implants are managed more often with primary removal when compared to HA implants, but it is difficult to determine whether this is out of necessity or due to surgeon preference [11]. Regardless, once the center of an implant is colonized, poor vascularization limits antibiotic penetration, and rescue strategies likely become futile [1, 12, 16, 64]. When explanted implants are examined histologically, vascularization is typically limited to the periphery, with presence of chronic inflammatory infiltrate [7, 21]. Gram stain demonstrates frank bacterial colonization in approximately two thirds of implants, with a predominance of gram-positive cocci [1, 21].

When exposure is severe enough to require implant removal, loss of conjunctival tissue and fornix depth is often a significant problem, resulting in difficulty inserting a volumetrically adequate secondary implant and poor prosthesis retention. As with

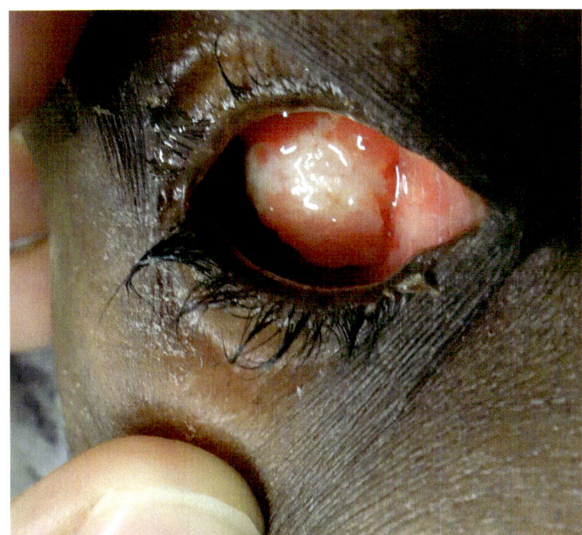

Fig. 14.1 Large exposure of porous polyethylene orbital implant in a right anophthalmic socket, ultimately requiring explanation and replacement. Note the avascular nature of the exposed PP and the thin, friable quality of the overlying mucosa, which required debridement

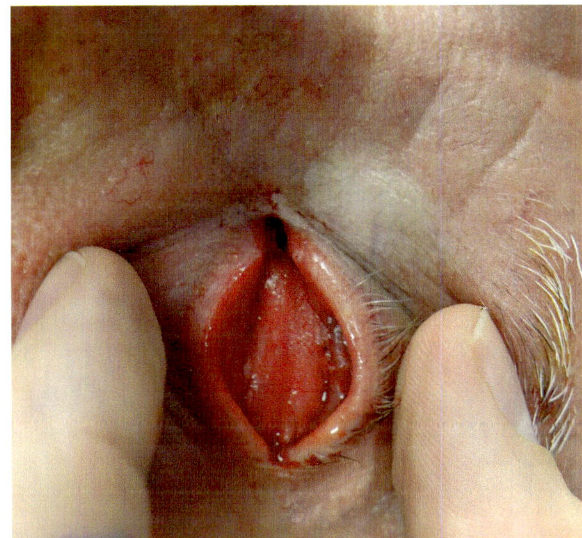

Fig. 14.2 Dermis fat graft *in situ* in a left anophthalmic socket. Note how the de-epithelized dermis serves to compensate for lost conjunctival surface area and promotes reformation of the fornices to permit successful prosthesis wear

cases of extensive burring for implant salvage, dermis fat grafts can be effective for replacing both volume and conjunctival surface area, but may not durably correct the volumetric deficit due to extensive resorption (Fig. 14.2) [12, 21, 65]. An alternative strategy with which the authors have had success is placement of a generously sized scleral-wrapped implant at the expense of forniceal shortening, followed by delayed fornix reconstruction with oral mucus membrane grafting and, when needed, pressure conformers and injection of antimetabolites such as 5-fluorouracil [66].

Conclusion

In spite of advances in orbital implant design, exposure remains a clinically significant and challenging problem to manage. The best approach is to minimize the incidence with careful implant selection, wrapping with fenestration and muscle attachment, and meticulous layered closure. When it does arise, rescue techniques with patch grafts or vascularized flaps are used in conjunction with removal of any visible avascular portion of the implant. Should implant removal be required, thoughtful management of conjunctival and forniceal deficits is essential to maximize the success of future prosthesis wear.

References

1. Chuo JY, Dolman PJ, Ng TL, Buffam FV, White VA. Clinical and histopathologic review of 18 explanted porous polyethylene orbital implants. Ophthalmology. 2009;116(2):349–54.
2. De Potter P, Duprez T, Cosnard G. Postcontrast magnetic resonance imaging assessment of porous polyethylene orbital implant (Medpor). Ophthalmology. 2000;107:1656–60.
3. Su GW, Yen MT. Current trends in managing the anophthalmic socket after primary enucleation and evisceration. Ophthalmic Plast Reconstr Surg. 2004;20(4):274–80.
4. Wladis EJ, Aakalu VK, Sobel RK, Yen MT, Bilyk JR, Mawn LA. Orbital implants in enucleation surgery: a report by the American Academy of Ophthalmology. Ophthalmology. 2018;125(2):311–7.
5. Wang JK, Lai PC, Liao SL. Late exposure of the bioceramic orbital implant. Am J Ophthalmol. 2009;147(1):162–170.e1.
6. Karslıoğlu S, Buttanrı IB, Fazıl K, Serin D, Akbaba M. Long-term outcomes of pegged and unpegged bioceramic orbital implants. Ophthalmic Plast Reconstr Surg. 2012;28(4):264–7.
7. Remulla HD, Rubin PA, Shore JW, Sutula FC, Townsend DJ, Woog JJ, Jahrling KV. Complications of porous spherical orbital implants. Ophthalmology. 1995;102(4):586–93.
8. Inkster CF, Ng SG, Leatherbarrow B. Primary banked scleral patch graft in the prevention of exposure of hydroxyapatite orbital implants. Ophthalmology. 2002;109:389–92.
9. Levine MR. Extruding orbital implant: prevention and treatment. Ann Ophthalmol. 1980;12:1384–6.
10. Mahoney NR, Grant MP, Iliff NT, Merbs SL. Exposure rate of smooth surface tunnel porous polyethylene implants after enucleation. Ophthalmic Plast Reconstr Surg. 2014;30(6):492–8.
11. Custer PL, Trinkaus KM. Porous implant exposure: incidence, management, and morbidity. Ophthal Plast Reconstr Surg. 2007;23:1–7.
12. Lee BJ, Lewis CD, Perry JD. Exposed porous orbital implants treated with simultaneous secondary implant and dermis fat graft. Ophthalmic Plast Reconstr Surg. 2010;26(4):273–6.
13. Oestreicher JH, Liu E, Berkowitz M. Complications of hydroxyapatite orbital implants. A review of 100 consecutive cases and a comparison of Dexon mesh (polyglycolic acid) with scleral wrapping. Ophthalmology. 1997;104(2):324–9.
14. McElnea EM, Ryan A, Fulcher T. Porous orbital implant exposure: the influence of surgical technique. Orbit. 2014;33(2):104–8.
15. Jordan DR, Brownstein S, Dorey M, et al. Fibrovascularisation of porous polyethylene (Medpor) orbital implant in a rabbit model. Ophthal Plast Reconstr Surg. 2004;20:136–43.
16. Kim YD, Goldberg RA, Shorr N, et al. Management of exposed hydroxyapatite orbital implants. Ophthalmology. 1994;101:1709–15.

17. Fountain JA, Helveston EM. A long-term follow-up study of scleral grafting for exposed or extruded orbital implants. Am J Ophthalmol. 1982;93:52–6.
18. Goldberg MF. A simplified scleral graft technique for covering an exposed orbital implant. Ophthalmic Surg. 1988;19:206–11.
19. Schaefer DP. Evaluation and management of the anophthalmic socket and socket reconstruction. In: Nesi FA, Lisman RA, Levine MR, editors. Smith's ophthalmic plastic and reconstructive surgery. 2nd ed. St. Louis: Mosby-Year Book; 1998. p. 1079–124.
20. Lee MJ, Khwarg SI, Choung HK, Kim NJ, Yu YS. Dermis-fat graft for treatment of exposed porous polyethylene implants in pediatric postenucleation retinoblastoma patients. Am J Ophthalmol. 2011;152(2):244–250.e2.
21. Quaranta-Leoni FM, Moretti C, Sposato S, Nardoni S, Lambiase A, Bonini S. Management of porous orbital implants requiring explantation: a clinical and histopathological study. Ophthalmic Plast Reconstr Surg. 2014;30(2):132–6.
22. Hasan SA, Galindo-Ferreiro A, Bigethi C, Meneghim RLSF, Shaikh OA, Schellini SA. Split-skin-graft wrapped conformer to treat severe contracted sockets. J Craniofac Surg. 2018;29:e777–9.
23. Sagoo MS, Rose GE. Mechanisms and treatment of extruding intraconal implants: socket aging and tissue restitution (the "Cactus Syndrome"). Arch Ophthalmol. 2007;125:1616–20.
24. Jung SK, Cho WK, Paik JS, Yang SW. Long-term surgical outcomes of porous polyethylene orbital implants: a review of 314 cases. Br J Ophthalmol. 2012;96(4):494–8.
25. Rubin PA, Popham JK, Bilyk JR, Shore JW. Comparison of fibrovascular ingrowth into hydroxyapatite and porous polyethylene orbital implants. Ophthalmic Plast Reconstr Surg. 1994;10(2):96–103.
26. Christmas NJ, Gordon CD, Murray TG, Tse D, Johnson T, Garonzik S, O'Brien JM. Intraorbital implants after enucleation and their complications: a 10-year review. Arch Ophthalmol. 1998;116(9):1199–203.
27. Jordan DR, Klapper SR, Gilberg SM, Dutton JJ, Wong A, Mawn L. The bioceramic implant: evaluation of implant exposures in 419 implants. Ophthalmic Plast Reconstr Surg. 2010;26(2):80–2.
28. Schellini S, Jorge E, Sousa R, Burroughs J, El-Dib R. Porous and nonporous orbital implants for treating the anophthalmic socket: a meta-analysis of case series studies. Orbit. 2016;35(2):78–86.
29. Yoon KC, Yang Y, Jeong IY, Kook MS. Buccal mucosal graft for hydroxyapatite orbital implant exposure. Jpn J Ophthalmol. 2011;55(3):318–20.
30. Lin CW, Liao SL. Long-term complications of different porous orbital implants: a 21-year review. Br J Ophthalmol. 2017;101(5):681–5.
31. Axmann S, Paridaens D. Anterior surface breakdown and implant extrusion following secondary alloplastic orbital implantation surgery. Acta Ophthalmol. 2018;96(3):310–3.
32. Ye J, Gao Q, He JJ, Gao T, Ning QY, Xie JJ. Exposure rate of unwrapped hydroxyapatite orbital implants in enucleation surgery. Br J Ophthalmol. 2016;100(6):860–5.
33. Gayre GS, Lipham W, Dutton JJ. A comparison of rates of fibrovascular ingrowth in wrapped versus unwrapped hydroxyapatite spheres in a rabbit model. Ophthalmic Plast Reconstr Surg. 2002;18(4):275–80.
34. Klapper SR, Jordan DR, Punja K, Brownstein S, Gilberg SM, Mawn LA, Grahovac SZ. Hydroxyapatite implant wrapping materials: analysis of fibrovascular ingrowth in an animal model. Ophthalmic Plast Reconstr Surg. 2000;16(4):278–85.
35. Tullo AB, Buckley RJ, Kelly T, Head MW, Bennett P, Armitage WJ, Ironside JW. Transplantation of ocular tissue from a donor with sporadic Creutzfeldt-Jakob disease. Clin Exp Ophthalmol. 2006;34(7):645–9.
36. Li T, Shen J, Duffy MT. Exposure rates of wrapped and unwrapped orbital implants following enucleation. Ophthalmic Plast Reconstr Surg. 2001;17(6):431–5.
37. Cheng MS, Liao SL, Lin LL. Late porous polyethylene implant exposure after motility coupling post placement. Am J Ophthalmol. 2004;138(3):420–4.

38. Wang JK, Liao SL, Lai PC, Lin LL. Prevention of exposure of porous orbital implants following enucleation. Am J Ophthalmol. 2007;143(1):61–7.
39. Jordan DR, Brownstein S, Rawlings N, Robinson J. An infected porous polyethylene orbital implant. Ophthalmic Plast Reconstr Surg. 2007;23(5):413–5.
40. Goldberg RE, Dresner SC, Braslow RA. Animal model of porous polyethylene orbital implants. Ophthal Plast Reconstr Surg. 1994;10:104–9.
41. Lee V, Subak-Sharpe I, Hungerford JL, Davies NP, Logani S. Exposure of primary orbital implants in postenucleation retinoblastoma patients. Ophthalmology. 2000;107(5):940–5; discussion 946.
42. Lang P, Kim JW, McGovern K, Reid MW, Subramanian K, Murphree AL, Berry JL. Porous orbital implant after enucleation in retinoblastoma patients: indications and complications. Orbit. 2018;20:1–6.
43. Mourits DL, Moll AC, Bosscha MI, Tan HS, Hartong DT. Orbital implants in retinoblastoma patients: 23 years of experience and a review of the literature. Acta Ophthalmol. 2016;94(2):165–74.
44. Williams BK Jr, Schefler AC, Garonzik SN, Gologorsky D, Shi W, Cavalcante LL, Cavalcante ML, Feuer WJ, Murray TG. Frequent prosthesis refitting to prevent implant exposure in patients with retinoblastoma. J Pediatr Ophthalmol Strabismus. 2011;48(4):238–46.
45. Wu AY, Vagefi MR, Georgescu D, Burroughs JR, Anderson RL. Enduragen patch grafts for exposed orbital implants. Orbit. 2011;30(2):92–5.
46. Ibáñez-Flores N, Abia-Serrano M, Aznar-Peña I, Mascaró-Zamora F, Castellar-Cerpa J, Anaya-Alaminos R, Prieto-Briceño S, Asvat A. Pericranium grafts for exposed orbital implants: an observational case-series study. J Craniomaxillofac Surg. 2015;43(7):1017–20.
47. Choi CJ, Tran AQ, Tse DT. Hard palate-dermis fat composite graft for reconstruction of contracted anophthalmic socket. Orbit. 2018;8:1–6.
48. Sheikh I, Leibovitch I, Selva D, Daya S, Malhotra R. Pericranium grafts for exposed orbital implants. Ophthalmic Plast Reconstr Surg. 2005;21(3):216–9.
49. Lee-Wing MW. Amniotic membrane for repair of exposed hydroxyapatite orbital implant. Ophthalmic Plast Reconstr Surg. 2003;19(5):401–2.
50. Liu CY, Sun MG, Jones S, Setabutr P. Posterior auricular muscle patch graft for exposed orbital implant. Orbit. 2018;13:1–4.
51. Sagoo MS, Olver JM. Autogenous temporalis fascia patch graft for porous polyethylene (Medpor) sphere orbital implant exposure. Br J Ophthalmol. 2004;88(7):942–6.
52. Basterzi Y, Sari A, Sari A. Surgical treatment of an exposed orbital implant with vascularized superficial temporal fascia flap. J Craniofac Surg. 2009;20(2):502–4.
53. Delmas J, Adenis JP, Robert PY. Repair of orbital implant exposure using Müller's muscle flap. J Fr Ophtalmol. 2014;37(8):618–22.
54. Turner LD, Haridas AS, Sullivan TJ. The versatility of the temporoparietal fascial graft (TPFG) in orbital implant exposure. Orbit. 2014;33(5):352–5.
55. Chow K, Satchi K, McNab AA. Combined use of bulbar conjunctival pedicle flap and labial mucous membrane graft for porous orbital implant exposure: long-term outcome. Orbit. 2018;37(4):293–8.
56. Chu HY, Liao YL, Tsai YJ, Chu YC, Wu SY, Ma L. Use of extraocular muscle flaps in the correction of orbital implant exposure. PLoS One. 2013;8(9):e72223.
57. Tawfik HA, Budin H, Dutton JJ. Repair of exposed porous polyethylene implants utilizing flaps from the implant capsule. Ophthalmology. 2005;112(3):516–23.
58. Lu L, Shi W, Luo M, Sun Y, Fan X. Repair of exposed hydroxyapatite orbital implants by subconjunctival tissue flaps. J Craniofac Surg. 2011;22(4):1452–6.
59. Klapper SR, Jordan DR, Brownstein S, Punja K. Incomplete fibrovascularization of a hydroxyapatite orbital implant 3 months after implantation. Arch Ophthalmol. 1999;117(8):1088–9.
60. Nunery WR, Heinz GW, Bonnin JM, et al. Exposure rate of hydroxyapatite spheres in the anophthalmic socket: histopathologic correlation and comparison with silicone sphere implants. Ophthal Plast Reconstr Surg. 1993;9:96–104.

61. Shields CL, Shields JA, De Potter P, Singh AD. Lack of complications of the hydroxyapatite orbital implant in 250 consecutive cases. Trans Am Ophthalmol Soc. 1993;91:177–89; discussion 189–95.
62. Kaltreider SA, Newman SA. Prevention and management of complications associated with the hydroxyapatite implant. Ophthal Plast Reconstr Surg. 1996;12:18–31.
63. Salour H, Owji N, Farahi A. Two-stage procedure for management of large exposure defects of hydroxyapatite orbital implant. Eur J Ophthalmol. 2003;13:789–93.
64. Badilla J, Dolman PJ. Methods of antibiotic instillation in porous orbital implants. Ophthalmic Plast Reconstr Surg. 2008;24(4):287–9.
65. Bosniak SL. Complications of dermis-fat orbital implantation. Adv Ophthalmic Plast Reconstr Surg. 1990;8:170–81.
66. Erickson BP, Johnson TE. An algorithm for staged anophthalmic socket reconstruction. In: 51 Annual Bascom Palmer Resident's Day. Miami, FL; 2015.

Chapter 15
Secondary Orbital Implant Techniques

Andrea Lora Kossler and Ji Kwan Park

Introduction

Most patients undergoing enucleation or evisceration surgery receive the orbital implant at the time of surgery.

The primary orbital implant placement, when adequately sized, facilitates optimal cosmesis and reduces anophthalmic socket complications. Implant placement may be delayed in severe cases of endophthalmitis to allow the infection to resolve or when an implant cannot adequately fit at the time of primary surgery. These patients benefit from secondary implant surgery. Complications from primary orbital implantation, including orbital implant exposure, infection, migration, and enophthalmos, may also require an orbital implant exchange.

Secondary orbital implant surgery requires various surgical techniques and is more complicated than primary enucleation or evisceration. Difficulties arise due to the disruption of anatomic planes, disorganization and rearrangements of orbital tissues, loss of orbital fat, socket contracture, and varying degrees of scar tissue from the previous operation [1]. Secondary implantation requires reestablishing anatomic tissue planes, localization of the rectus muscles, and creating sufficient space for the secondary implant while avoiding additional injury to orbital tissues. Other procedures, such as fornix reconstruction, lower eyelid tightening, ptosis repair, and orbital volume augmentation, may also be required [2]. This chapter describes various surgical techniques to improve success in secondary orbital implantation while minimizing postoperative complications.

A. L. Kossler (✉)
Oculofacial Plastic Surgery & Orbital Oncology, Byers Eye Institute, Stanford University, Stanford, CA, USA
e-mail: akossler@stanford.edu

J. K. Park
Loma Linda University Eye Institute, Department of Ophthalmology, Loma Linda, CA, USA
e-mail: jkpark@llu.edu

T. E. Johnson (ed.), *Anophthalmia*,
https://doi.org/10.1007/978-3-030-29753-4_15

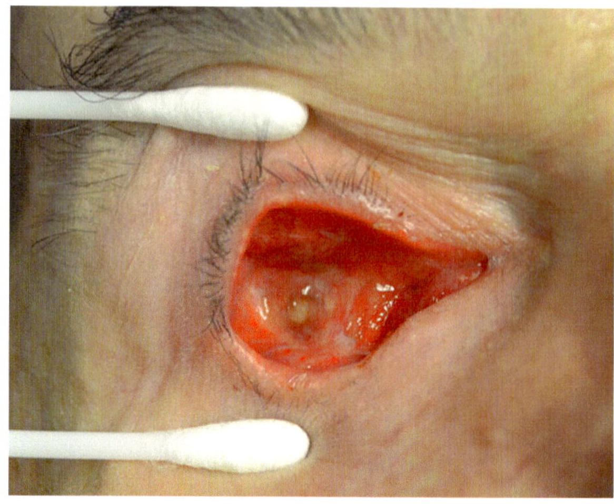

Fig. 15.1 Note the exposed implant at the center of anophthalmic socket with superior and inferior fornix contracture

Indications for Surgery

Secondary orbital implantation is indicated for the following reasons:

1. To insert a new implant into an anophthalmic socket
2. To replace an exposed implant when the exposure, typically greater than 3–4 mm in diameter, cannot be repaired with a patch graft (Fig. 15.1)
3. To replace an infected porous implant or any implant suggestive of chronic infection
4. To replace a migrated implant, particularly when preventing the comfortable wearing of a prosthesis
5. To replace a small implant or augment orbital volume
6. To improve prosthesis motility

Preoperative Surgical Planning

Strategic preoperative planning is crucial to the success of the operation. A complete history and thorough clinical exam are performed to formulate a patient-specific surgical plan. The examination should begin with an assessment of the eyelids and periorbital region, with the best fitting prosthesis positioned correctly in the socket. The medial and lateral canthal tendon attachments as well as eyelid laxity and lid position are assessed. A superior sulcus defect and Hertel exophthalmometry are noted to provide information on orbital volume. The excursion of the prosthesis on vertical and horizontal eye movements is noted. The socket is then assessed with attention to the inferior and superior fornices, the presence of posterior lamellar scarring, the integrity of the conjunctival lining, the position of the orbital implant, and signs of infection or implant exposure [3].

The preoperative evaluation should include the following:

- Etiology of the primary enucleation or evisceration, which may include trauma, cancer, and intraocular causes.
- Time passed since the previous surgery.
- Size, type, and wrapping material of the previous implant.
- Measurement of prosthesis motility.
- Assessment of eyelid position, depth of the sulcus, and lid retraction or laxity.
- Assessment of upper and lower fornices.
- Location of the primary implant to assess for implant migration.
- The diameter of the exposed area, if applicable.
- Any redness, discharge, or pain suggestive of active infection.
- Any evidence of active inflammation or tissue reaction to the primary implant.
- Patient expectations.
- When available, review computed tomography images to identify extraocular muscles, the location of the implant, and possible occult orbital fractures.
- Orbital magnetic resonance imaging may be used to assess implant vascularity.

Surgical Technique

Several techniques exist to address the distortion of anatomical structures, loss of orbital fat, and scarring of orbital tissues that complicate secondary orbital implant placement. Iliff reported a lateral brow incision approach to replace the implant, which he felt avoided further conjunctival scarring and contracture and minimized bacterial implantation [4]. Frueh recommended a transconjunctival approach with the secondary implant wrapped in sclera and attached to the periosteum to improve implant stability [5]. Others recommend the transconjunctival approach with the secondary implant placed behind posterior Tenon's layer with or without tissue wrap [6, 7]. Additionally, the dermis fat graft is described as a secondary implant material [8, 9]. Lee et al. described simultaneous secondary implantation and dermis fat graft placement to address an avascular porous implant exposure with significant conjunctival insufficiency [10]. Similarly, numerous implant materials and wrapping techniques have been introduced [3, 11–13]. Despite these variations, certain core techniques in secondary implant surgery remain unchanged. The surgical steps for orbital implant exchange are outlined below:

Anesthesia

1. Perform the surgery under general anesthesia with a retrobulbar block and intravenous antibiotics. When necessary, surgery can be done under monitored anesthesia care with retrobulbar anesthetic injection and intravenous sedation.
2. Administer a retrobulbar block, consisting of 4–5 mL of a 50:50 mixture of 2% lidocaine with epinephrine (1: 100,000) mixed with 0.5% bupivacaine, into the muscle cone with a 1.25-inch 27-gauge needle for hemostasis, to control the oculocardiac reflex and to mitigate postoperative pain.

Explant Primary Implant After Enucleation

3. Place an eyelid speculum for visualization. Incise the conjunctiva, Tenon's capsule, and scar tissue horizontally. Dissect in a subconjunctival and sub-Tenon's plane to create separate flaps and gain access to the implant. Incise the sclera or wrapping material if present (Fig. 15.2a). Remove the primary orbital implant with blunt and sharp dissection (Fig. 15.2b, c). Of note, some surgeons advocate the removal of the entire pseudocapsule, while others recommend using the pseudocapsule for added volume and implant protection. The authors remove the posterior pseudocapsule, as it may inhibit vascularization of the secondary implant, and leave the anterior pseudocapsule intact. In cases of an implant exchange for a larger implant, if wrapping material from the primary surgery is adequate, take out the implant and insert the implant of choice into the existing wrap. Then,

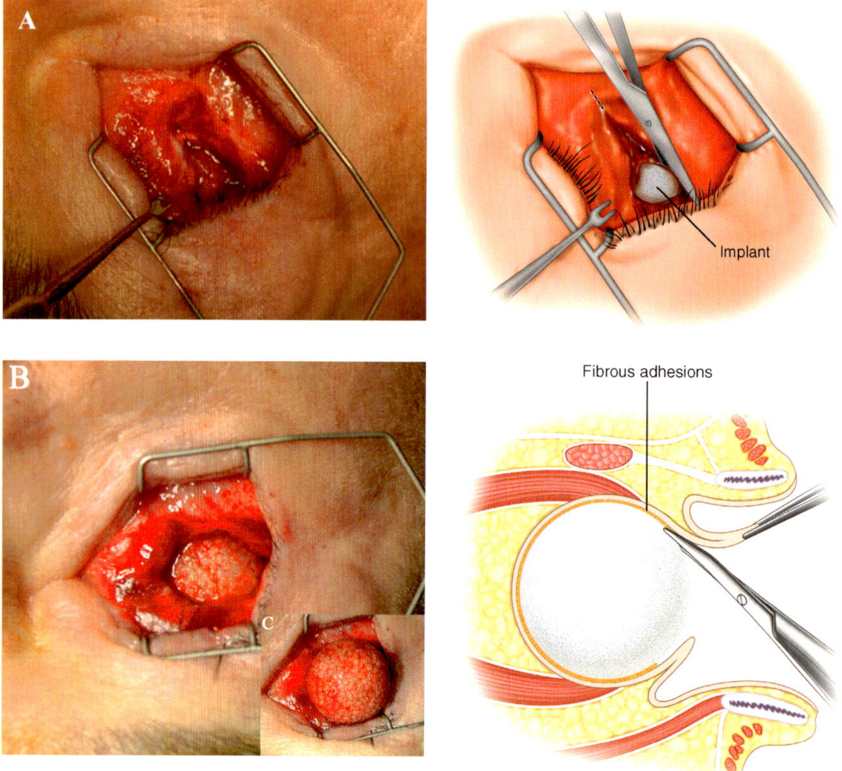

Fig. 15.2 (**a**) Incise through the conjunctiva, Tenon's capsule, and wrapping material to expose the implant. (**b**) Dissect around the implant with blunt and sharp dissection. (**c**) Explant the primary orbital implant

proceed with the closure as described in step #10. If a non-wrapped silicone or acrylic implant is present, the joined ends of the four muscles should be readily identified, separated, and tagged upon incision. In such a case, proceed to step #5. In cases of implant extrusion, excise the infected or epithelialized conjunctival margin, aiming to leave as much conjunctiva and Tenon's as possible to avoid fornix-related complications, and continue onto step #4.

Isolating the Extraocular Muscles

4. If the rectus muscles are attached to the existing implant, isolate and tag each muscle as in an enucleation (Fig. 15.3a). If the rectus muscles are not attached to the primary implant, they can often be found in the fornices after implant removal. Retract the conjunctiva in each quadrant, using the pseudocapsule or scleral remnant as a landmark to place the rectus muscle on stretch, and then dissect into the orbital fat parallel to the muscle belly until the muscle is encountered. Use Stevens scissors and cotton-tipped applicators to bluntly dissect the rectus muscles, isolate them, and reestablish anatomic tissue planes. If no implant is present, the muscles may be found in the fornices, as previously described, or may be found sutured to each other within the orbital fat. Isolate each muscle with a von Graefe or Green muscle hook. Sharply dissect the pseudocapsule, sclera, or surrounding orbital tissues from the anterior muscle tendon to allow for vascular ingrowth to the secondary implant. Tag each muscle with a conventional von Pirquet suture pass using a double-armed 5-0 spatulated polyglactin 910 suture (Ethicon J571, S14 needle). The typical sequence of isolation is medial rectus, lateral rectus, inferior rectus, and then superior rectus. Avoid injury to the superior rectus-levator muscle complex, as well as neural innervation to the rectus muscles during muscle isolation.

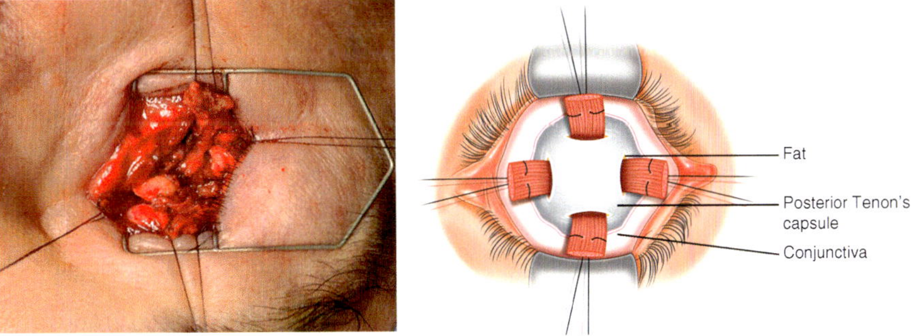

Fig. 15.3 Identify extraocular muscles by exploring the implant, superior and inferior fornices, medial and lateral canthi, and orbital fat. Bluntly dissect the muscle belly within the orbital fat. Hook each muscle, and sharply dissect the surrounding tissues to expose the anterior muscle tendon. Tag each muscle with a von Pirquet suture

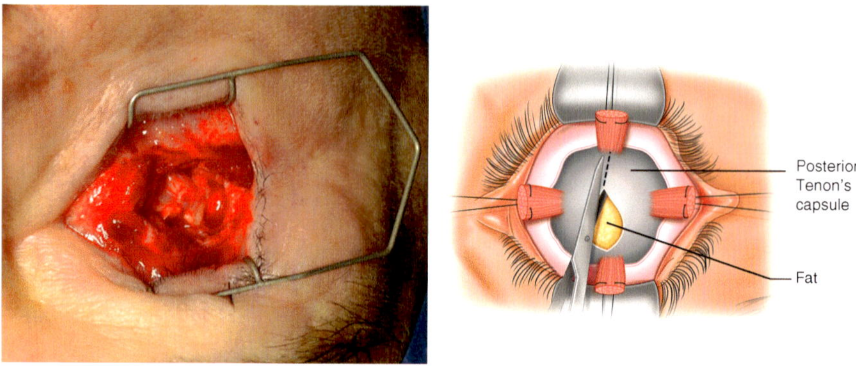

Fig. 15.4 Lyse any posterior orbital scar tissue. Dissect through posterior Tenon's capsule, into the intraconal space until orbital fat is exposed, to make adequate room for the implant

Preparation of the Orbit

5. Evaluate the orbit, and lyse any scar tissue that may prevent proper posterior implant placement (Fig. 15.4). Bluntly and sharply dissect through posterior Tenon's capsule, until the intraconal orbital fat is exposed, to make adequate room for the implant. Avoid excess manipulation of the orbital fat or unnecessary cautery as this may result in postoperative fat atrophy and orbital volume deficiency.

Prepare and Insert the Implant

6. Use an orbital implant sizer to determine the adequate size of the secondary implant (Fig. 15.5a). An 18–20 mm implant is typically placed in adults when possible. Soak the secondary implant in an antibiotic solution for 5 minutes before insertion. An alternative is to place the implant in a 40 cc syringe with antibiotic solution, then pull on the plunger to create a vacuum, and allow the antibiotic solution to saturate the implant completely (Fig. 15.5b).
7. Prepare the wrapping material of choice if used. The authors wrap a high-density porous polyethylene (Medpor®; Porex Surgical Inc., Newnan, GA) implant with whole human donor sclera. Other wrapping options include microporous expanded polytetrafluoroethylene (Gore-Tex, W.L. Gore & Associates, Flagstaff, AZ), polyglactin 910 mesh (Vicryl® mesh, Ethicon, Somerville, NJ, USA), autologous temporalis fascia, or fascia lata. Each of these materials can be sewn over the implant, providing a surface for securing the rectus muscles and an additional tissue barrier to prevent extrusion [3]. When using donor sclera or autologous material, incise four scleral windows at each corresponding muscle site with a No. 15 blade to allow for attachment of the rectus muscles to the implant (Fig. 15.5c). Place the wrapped orbital implant behind posterior Tenon's layer, into the center of the muscle cone, using a sphere introducer (Figs. 15.5d, e). The areas occupied by the implant and the wrapping material should avoid tension when approximating the

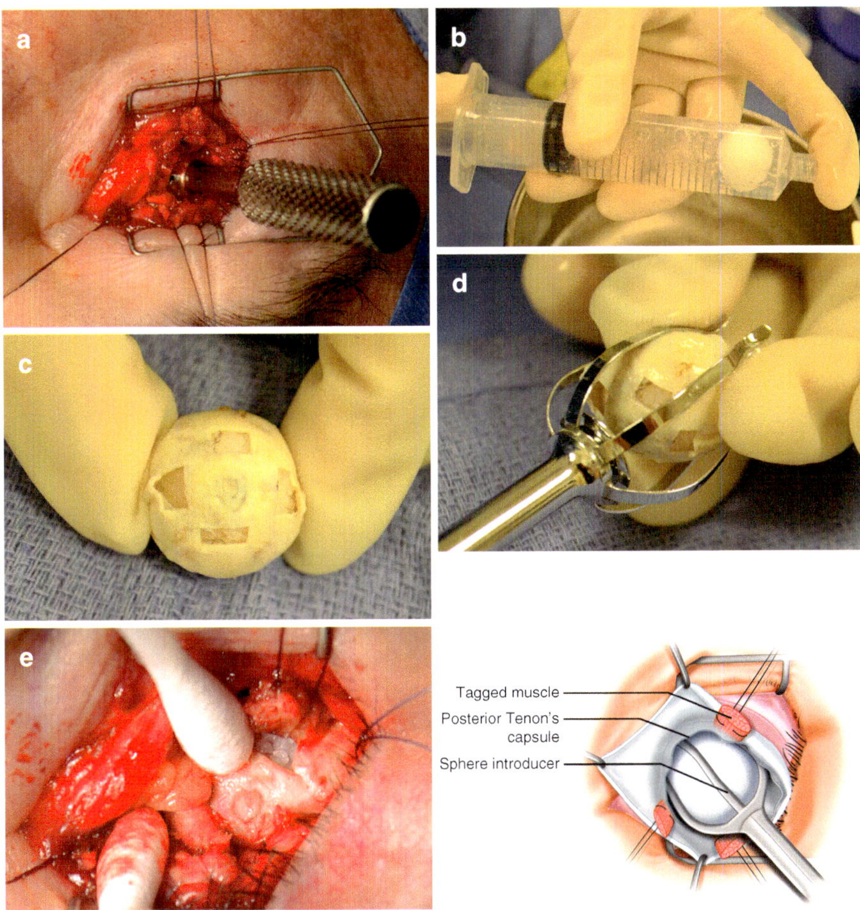

Fig. 15.5 (**a**) Use the orbital implant sizer to determine the adequate size of the secondary implant. (**b**) Place the implant in a 40 cc syringe, and then pull on the plunger to allow the antibiotic solution to saturate the implant. (**c**) Incise four scleral windows at each corresponding muscle site with a No. 15 blade to allow for the attachment of rectus muscles to the porous polyethylene implant. (**d**) Load the wrapped implant into the sphere introducer. (**e**) Place the implant behind posterior Tenon's layer into the center of the muscle cone

anterior soft tissues to ensure adequate space in the conjunctival fornices. Further fornix reconstruction may be needed as discussed in Chap. 17.

Attach the Extraocular Muscles

8. Attach the rectus muscles to the wrapped orbital implant at corresponding anatomical sites using the double-armed 5-0 polyglactin sutures from step # 4. When wrapping with donor sclera, attach the four rectus muscles to the corresponding anterior scleral windows allowing for apposition of the muscle to the implant along the window site (Fig. 15.6). This contact between the

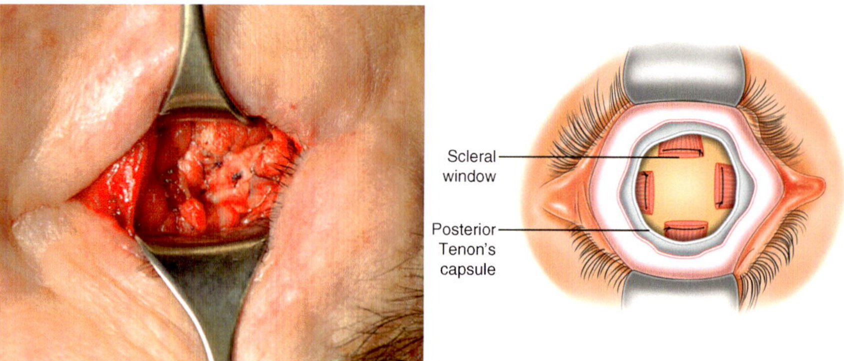

Fig. 15.6 Attach the four rectus muscles to the anterior scleral windows, allowing for the apposition of the muscle to the implant along the window site

porous implant material and the highly vascular muscle tissues ensures good vascularization, retention, and movement of the implant. The muscles can be directly attached to the implant when compatible, such as the smooth surface tunnel porous polyethylene (Medpor® SST™; Porex Surgical Inc., Newnan, GA) implant. If a wrapping material or suture tunneled implant is not used, attach the identified muscles to each other to cover the anterior surfaces of the implant. The inferior oblique muscle can also be attached according to the surgeon's preference. This technique may result in early or late implant migration, particularly when a nonporous implant is used; therefore, the scleral-wrapped porous implant technique is recommended.

Wound Closure

9. If remnant sclera or wrapping material is incised and preserved, then this layer is closed using 5-0 polyglactin sutures. Some surgeons choose to separately close posterior Tenon's layer or the fibrous capsule over the implant in a vertical fashion followed by anterior Tenon's layer in a horizontal fashion (Fig. 15.7c, d), while others close only anterior Tenon's layer. In either option, 5-0 polyglactin buried interrupted sutures are used, and all tails are cut short to minimize exposure, infection risk, and delayed wound healing. A balanced salt solution can be used to delineate the white-appearing Tenon's capsule from the pink-colored conjunctiva (Fig. 15.7a). Approximate the conjunctiva in a running fashion using 6-0 plain gut sutures (Fig. 15.7b).
10. Inject 2–3 ml of 0.5% bupivacaine into the intraconal space at the end of the case for postoperative pain control. Apply antibiotic ointment to the eye socket. Insert a methyl methacrylate conformer of adequate size (small, medium, or large) that will maintain the proper fornix volume. The existing prosthesis can be used if appropriately sized. Proper sizing of the conformer or prosthesis minimizes chemosis, facilitates tissue healing, and prevents

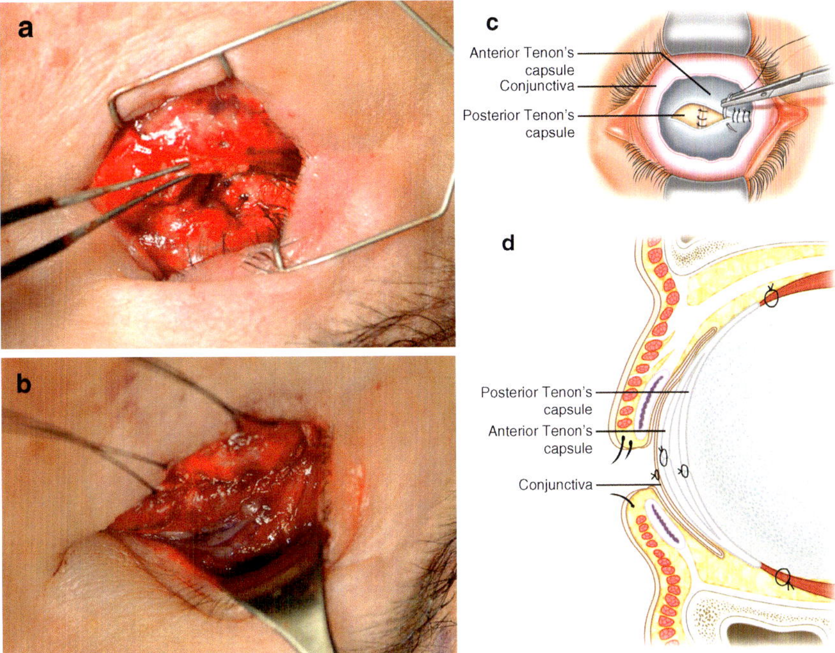

Fig. 15.7 (**a**) Delineate the white-appearing Tenon's capsule from the pink conjunctiva. (**b**) Close the Tenon's capsule with buried interrupted 5-0 polyglactin sutures followed by the conjunctiva with a running 6-0 plain gut suture. This patient also has a mucous membrane graft in the superior (pictured here) and inferior (not shown) fornix. (**c**) A three-layer closure over the implant decreases the risk of recurrent extrusions. Close the posterior Tenon's layer or the fibrous capsule in a vertical fashion, and then close anterior Tenon's layer horizontally. Close the conjunctiva with a running plain gut suture. (**d**) A cross-sectional view of the three-layer closure. Approximate each layer separately. Tie the sutures anterior to the implant

socket contracture. Perform a temporary suture tarsorrhaphy to keep the conformer in place using a 6-0 plain gut suture through the upper and lower lid tarsal margin. An alternative method is to use a double-armed 4-0 silk suture with cotton or rubber bolsters to secure the eyelids.

Dressing and Postoperative Care

11. A firm pressure dressing is maintained for 4–6 days. Oral antibiotics are given for 1 week. Steroids can be prescribed per the surgeon's preference. Oral postoperative pain and anti-nausea medication are also given as needed. The socket is evaluated after the removal of the pressure dressing, and, if the edema has subsided, the tarsorrhaphy suture is removed. A topical antibiotic ointment is applied three times daily for 1 week. The patient is generally ready for fitting of a prosthesis 6–8 weeks postoperatively.

Box 15.1 Implant Exchange

Patient Preparation

- General anesthesia
- Retrobulbar block with 2% lidocaine with epinephrine (1: 100,000) mixed with 0.5% bupivacaine

Primary Implant Removal

- Place an eyelid speculum.
- Incise through the conjunctiva, Tenon's capsule, and wrapping material.
- Bluntly and sharply dissect around the primary implant, and explant the orbital implant.

Isolating the Extraocular Muscles

- Isolate each muscle when rectus muscles are attached to the existing implant.
- If the rectus muscles are not attached to the implant, search the fornices to locate the muscle.
- Retract the conjunctiva in each quadrant, using the pseudocapsule or scleral remnant as a landmark.
- Dissect the orbital fat parallel to the muscle belly using Stevens scissors and cotton-tipped applicators until the muscle belly is encountered.
- Hook the muscle, and sharply dissect the surrounding tissues to expose the anterior muscle tendon.
- Tag the muscle with a von Pirquet suture pass using a double-armed 5-0 spatulated polyglactin 910 suture.
- Repeat the steps until all rectus muscles are isolated and tagged.
- If no implant is present, search within the orbital fat for the joined ends of the muscles. If the muscles were not sutured together during the primary surgery, search for the muscles in the fornices and orbital fat as described.

Preparation of the Orbit

- Lyse any scar tissue in the orbit.
- Bluntly and sharply dissect through posterior Tenon's capsule into the retrobulbar space.

Preparation and Insertion of the Implant

- Use the orbit implant sizer to determine the adequate size of the secondary implant.
- Soak the implant in an antibiotic solution.
- The wrapping material of choice is prepared and secured to the secondary implant.
- Insert the wrapped implant behind posterior Tenon's capsule into the center of the muscle cone.

Extraocular Muscle Attachment

- Suture each rectus muscle to the implant at the corresponding anatomical positions.

Wound Closure

- Close Tenon's layers with interrupted buried 5-0 polyglactin sutures.
- Close the conjunctiva with a running 6-0 plain gut suture.
- Administer a retrobulbar injection of 0.5% bupivacaine.
- Place a methyl methacrylate conformer.
- Suture the upper and lower tarsal margins together using a 6-0 plain gut horizontal mattress suture.

Dressing and Postoperative care

- Place a firm dressing over the operated site for 4–6 days.
- Administer oral and topical antibiotics for 1 week.
- Prescribe oral pain and anti-nausea medications.
- Refer to an ocularist for prosthesis fitting 6–8 weeks after surgery.

Intraoperative Considerations

Secondary Implant Following Evisceration

In patients who underwent evisceration with or without a primary implant, all extraocular muscles are typically left attached at their anatomical positions on the sclera. If the anterior sclera is intact, it is incised, and the implant, if present, is removed. Posterior sclerotomies are performed, if necessary, and the secondary implant is sized and placed as in the standard evisceration procedure. If the sclera is significantly contracted or no implant is present, there are two options: (1) the contracted scleral remnant is enucleated after identifying and tagging the extraocular muscles. A secondary implant is then placed in the intraconal space as previously described. (2) The scleral remnant is incised in a crisscross fashion from the superonasal quadrant to the inferotemporal quadrant and from the superotemporal quadrant to the inferonasal quadrant, to create four scleral petals to allow access to the retrobulbar space. Transect the optic nerve if it is attached to the scleral remnant (Fig. 15.8a). The goal of this dissection is to create a deep intraconal space to seat the new implant. Place the wrapped implant of choice into the muscle cone, posterior to the scleral remnants. Then attach the scleral remnant pieces to the wrapped implant, 4–5 mm anterior to the normal extraocular muscle attachment sites (Fig. 15.8b). In some cases, the scleral remnants can be attached to their counterparts, superior to inferior petal and then nasal to temporal petal, to serve as a double scleral barrier over the implant (Fig. 15.8c, d) [14–16].

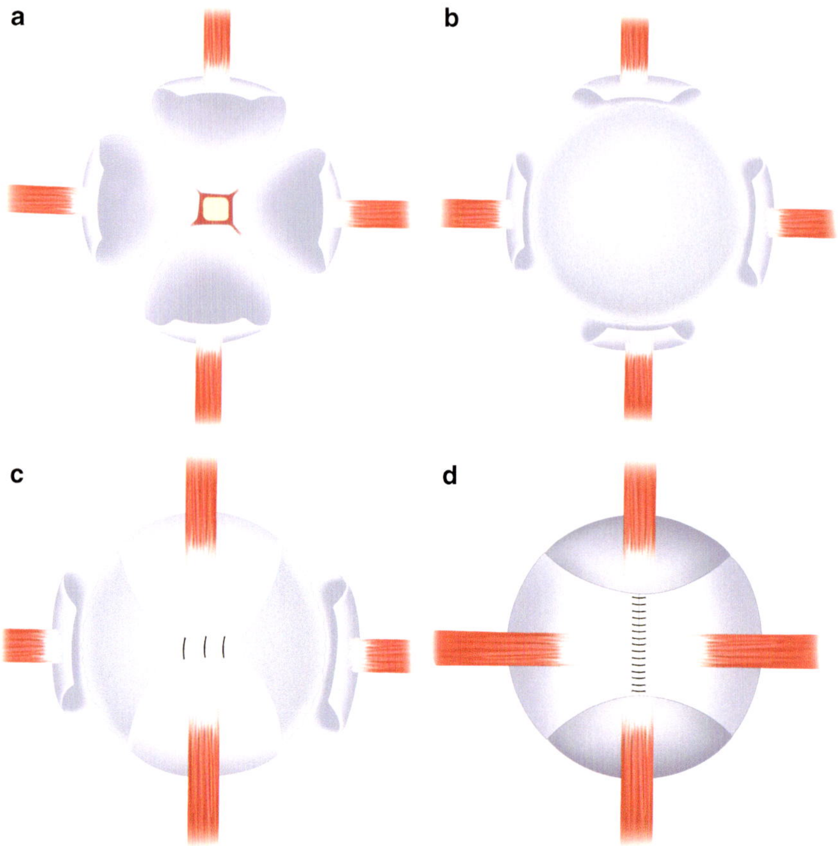

Fig. 15.8 (**a**) Incise the sclera in crisscross fashion and dissect until retrobulbar fat is identified. Transect the optic nerve if it is attached to the scleral remnant. The extraocular muscles stay attached to the scleral remnant. (**b**) Insert the wrapped implant, and attach the anterior scleral remnants over the implant, 4–5 mm anterior to normal extraocular muscle attachment sites. (**c**) Alternatively, the scleral remnants can be attached to its counterparts; superior to inferior petals are sutured first over the implant. (**d**) Then nasal and temporal petals are sutured over the vertical petals, to serve as a double scleral barrier over the implant. (Images reproduced with permission)

Selection of Implant Size

Appropriate implant size selection is vital to minimize subsequent complications. Data from a study showed that patients who received secondary orbital implants had an average of 97% total volume replacement with a mean residual enophthalmos of 1.3 mm and trace to none superior sulcus deformities, which were most noted in children and adults who had primary enucleation in childhood. The size of the bony orbit was smaller in patients who had primary surgery at an early age when compared to the contralateral nonsurgical side. The soft tissue contraction was more severe in the secondary implant group than in the primary implant group. In such patients, the axial length based on the A-scan of the good eye was recommended to estimate the upper limit of the implant diameter, where the implant size = axial length – 2 mm. The size of the primary implant that was removed during the surgery can estimate the lower limit of the new implant size [17]. In most cases, avoid using orbital implants greater than 20 mm to decrease the risk of exposure or fornix shortening while ensuring good projection and symmetric volume. We recommend using implant sizers intraoperatively to ensure adequate coverage of the anterior surface of the implant. The various types of implants and wrapping materials are discussed in Chap. 10.

Identification of Extraocular Muscles

In most secondary orbital implant surgeries, the extraocular muscles are easily identified upon the removal of the existing implant. However, in some cases, the identification of the extraocular muscles can be difficult due to the disruption of normal anatomic planes and the disorganization of orbital tissues. Although some authors reported no postoperative concerns without any attempts to find the extraocular muscles [18], we, and other authors, recommend locating, dissecting, and suturing all extraocular muscles to the implant [2, 11, 12, 14, 19, 20]. Postoperative motility is directly proportional to the number of extraocular muscles attached to the orbital implant [2]. A step-by-step approach to identifying extraocular muscles has been described in the previous section. Despite prior recommendations not to perform fine dissections of tissues in orbit [6], blunt with occasional careful sharp dissection can aid in localizing the extraocular muscles without damaging the surrounding structures [1, 19]. It is crucial to rely on the knowledge of orbital anatomy during these dissections.

If extraocular muscles cannot be identified, tag the corresponding fibrous tissue flaps that contain remains of the medial rectus, lateral rectus, and inferior rectus muscle insertions with the surrounding Tenon's capsule. Attach each flap to the surface of the wrapped implant at its respective muscle insertions, a few millimeters short of the anterior pole, and bring the sutures through Tenon's capsule and conjunctiva. This secures each flap to the respective fornix to allow for movement of the implant while avoiding fornix shortening. The superior rectus muscle and Tenon's capsule are spared to avoid ptosis from traction on the levator muscle [21, 22].

Reconstructive Procedures for Acquired Socket Contracture

When an acquired socket contracture is present on preoperative evaluation, simultaneous secondary implant and fornix reconstruction procedures should be planned. The primary surgical premise in this reconstruction is to select the appropriately

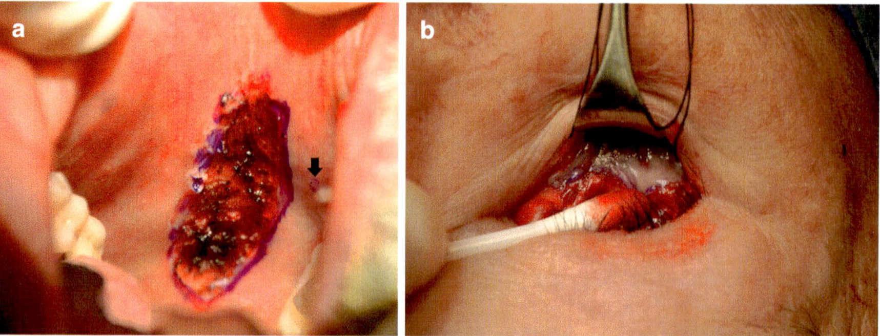

Fig. 15.9 (**a**) Buccal membrane graft defect below Stensen's duct (arrow), which is adjacent to the upper second molar. (**b**) The conjunctival defects are covered with harvested graft to deepen the inferior fornix

sized implant to fill the orbit while ensuring adequate fornix depth for proper prosthesis fit. A variety of techniques have been described to reconstruct the conjunctival fornices and ensure comfortable prosthesis wear and good cosmetic appearance. Oral mucous membrane is the most common tissue used to reconstruct the conjunctiva when treating moderate socket contractions. The graft is usually harvested from the inner lower lip or the buccal mucosa (Fig. 15.9a). A mucous membrane graft has excellent elasticity to cover conjunctival defects after lysis of fornix contraction and to maintain adequate fornix depth for prosthesis fitting (Fig. 15.9b). Another option is amniotic membrane, which promotes natural conjunctival migration and cellular differentiation by providing a new basement membrane [23]. The results of this substrate graft are comparable to mucous membrane grafts [9, 24, 25]. The amniotic membrane graft, however, requires healthy conjunctival tissues, limiting its use in severe contractions [14]. The autologous dermis fat graft can also be harvested from the gluteal region. Studies show good postoperative results in maintaining orbital volume and conserving the conjunctiva [26], without the risk of foreign body reactions, toxic effects from implants, or transfer of pathogens or prions [27]. Lee et al. have described a simultaneous secondary implant and dermis fat graft placement, to address a completely avascular exposed porous orbital implant with conjunctival insufficiency. In this technique, the rectus muscles are drawn over an intraconal polymethyl methacrylate sphere to serve as the host bed for the dermis graft. Following the dissection of conjunctiva from Tenon's layer superiorly and inferiorly, the harvested dermis fat graft is sutured to the surrounding conjunctiva to cover the defect. The authors recommend this technique in patients noted to have an avascular implant after implant drilling [10]. A two-stage procedure that involves primary dermis fat graft and pre-existing implant removal followed by secondary orbital implantation has also been reported [28]. Nonetheless, some authors believe that the dermis fat graft should be reserved for pediatric patients with congenital anophthalmia [29]. In cases of severe socket contractions, multiple autologous grafts may be combined with a mucous membrane graft to reconstruct the conjunctiva and the Tenon's capsule. The management of socket contracture is discussed in greater depth in Chap. 17.

Conjunctival-Sparing Techniques

The anterior transconjunctival approach is most commonly used for secondary implant surgery; however conjunctival-sparing techniques have been described to maximize conjunctiva preservation for adequate closure and to reduce the risk of implant extrusion. A lateral brow approach, as described by Iliff, involves making a 3-cm incision below the lateral brow down to the periosteum. The periorbita is incised in a radial fashion and extended 2.5 cm posterior to the superior orbital rim. The orbital fat is then incised. A pocket is created in the muscle cone sufficient for implant placement. Sharp dissection is performed to remove the central mass of scar tissue, fat, and anterior portions of the scarred extraocular muscles. The conjunctiva is left intact. The implant is inserted through the pocket and into the socket. The soft tissues are closed with plain gut suture [4].

Hart et al. also suggested a conjunctival-sparing technique to avoid further shortening of the fornices in patients who had conjunctival scarring after primary evisceration without implant placement. In this technique, a 10 mm horizontal lateral canthal incision is made followed by blunt dissection to the lateral orbital margin. The lower limb of the lateral canthal tendon and the inferior septum are divided to expose the lateral rectus. The muscle is hooked and divided between two double-armed 6-0 polyglactin sutures and preplaced near its insertion (Fig. 15.10a).

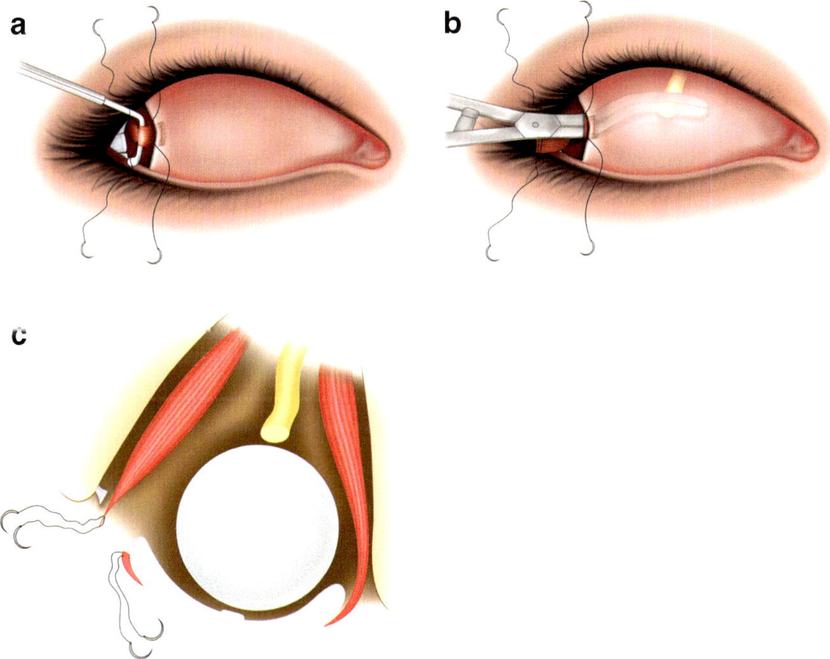

Fig. 15.10 (**a**) A 10 mm lateral canthal incision and inferior cantholysis allows access to the lateral rectus muscle, which is hooked and divided between two double-armed 6-0 polyglactin sutures. (**b**) Dissect the intraconal space to the optic nerve which is then clamped and cut. (**c**) Place the implant through the exposed lateral canthal window into the intraconal space with posterior sclera invaginating the anterior scleral remnant. (Images reproduced with permission)

This procedure allows access to the intraconal space and optic nerve. The optic nerve is clamped and cut (Fig. 15.10b). The posterior sclera can move forward and invaginate the anterior scleral remnant, creating space to accommodate a spherical implant within the muscle cone while forming a double layer scleral cap (Fig. 15.10c). An unwrapped porous implant is placed in the muscle cone. The lateral rectus, lateral canthal tendon, and orbicularis muscles are then repaired [30].

Additional Surgical Techniques and Corrective Procedures

Implant Coverage with the Inferior Oblique Muscle

The inferior oblique muscle can be used for implant coverage, particularly when other rectus muscles cannot be found or when additional vascularization and implant coverage are necessary. The full width of the muscle belly that averages about 7 mm provides robust coverage of the anterior aspect of the implant that is most susceptible to exposure. Once the inferior oblique muscle is tagged in the usual fashion and reflected away from the orbit, spread the muscle over the anterior surface of the implant. Then, attach it to the superior rectus and the lateral rectus muscles or surrounding soft tissues [31, 32]. This technique has been useful in children who have undergone secondary enucleation with subsequent rectus muscle scarring from plaque therapy to treat retinoblastoma [33]. The preserved sclera, pseudocapsule, or retro-orbital fat may also be used to cover the anterior portion of the implant [2].

Secondary Orbital Implant Pegging

Some authors suggest additional pegging of the secondary orbital implants after sufficient time has passed to allow for implant vascularization [2, 5]. Others, including the authors, recommend against the use of pegs for secondary orbital implants due to studies that demonstrate a high, 67.3%, risk of post-drilling complications [10].

Secondary Orbital Implant Wrapping Material

Most experts agree that secondary orbital implantation should be accompanied with a wrapping material [3, 11, 13]. Various wrapping materials and methods are discussed in greater detail in Chap. 10.

Eyelid Malposition

Simultaneous medial and lateral canthoplasty, horizontal tightening procedures, upper and lower blepharoplasty, and ptosis correction may be considered to address residual eyelid malposition following secondary implantation [2]. These procedures are further discussed in Chap. 19.

Complications of Secondary Orbital Implant Surgery

Complication rates are higher in secondary implant surgery when compared to primary enucleation or evisceration [10, 34]. The most concerning complication is implant extrusion. Early exposures are often related to incorrect wound closure techniques, including the closure of wounds under tension, inappropriate implant size and seating, trauma, and infection. Late exposures may be due to friction, pressure points from the prosthesis, inflammation, and infection [35]. The exposure rate in secondary orbital implants ranges from 1 to 15% and is highly variable depending on the study population, surgical techniques, type of implants, use of a peg system, and covering materials [10, 11, 34, 36]. Moreover, up to 83% of the patients who had implant exposures required additional orbital surgeries [11]. An implant larger than 22 mm has been related to high exposure rates due to greater tension on the overlying tissues [37]. Exposure rates are also high when the extraocular muscles are not attached to the secondary implant [36]. As in primary orbital implant exposure, the process is thought to be due to a lack of fibrovascular tissue growth. A "cactus syndrome" may arise when the implant drags the surrounding tissues into the socket as the rough-edged implant is forced into the socket. The process of natural restitution in these tissues results in a gradual return to their original relaxed position along with the anterior migration of the implant, leading to its exposure [38]. Therefore, care should be taken to avoid dragging superficial tissues into the muscle cone during the insertion. The management of exposed implants is discussed in Chap. 15.

Other common postoperative complications include migration of the implant, entropion, blepharoptosis, and deep upper lid sulcus, which may be related to insufficient orbital volume [11, 34]. Patients who received secondary dermis-fat grafts as orbital implants had an average of 2.6 mm enophthalmos compared to 1.6 mm in patients who had primary dermis-fat grafts [39]. Using an adequate implant and conformer of the proper size prevents residual volume deficiencies [29]. A significant number of patients may also develop pyogenic granuloma, transient socket edema, fornix insufficiency, and hypo-ophthalmos [10, 11]. Although the rate of infection in secondary implants may be low at 2–3% [11, 12], all infected implants should be removed.

Conclusion

Secondary orbital implant surgery refers to the placement of a new orbital implant into an anophthalmic socket or the exchange of a previously inserted implant. Surgical techniques to improve outcomes and minimize complications have been described in this chapter. Essential steps include isolation and attachment of the extraocular muscles, the positioning of an appropriately sized implant deeply in the intraconal space, the use of wrapping material, and the simultaneous reconstructive procedures for comfortable prosthesis wear and enhanced cosmetic appearance. The rates of complications are variable depending on the surgical technique, patient factors, type of initial surgery, wrapping materials, quality of ocular prosthesis, socket problems, use of peg systems, and extent of follow-up period. The surgeon should always discuss possible complications with the patients and set outcome expectations before the surgery. All patients should be followed closely for any postoperative concerns.

References

1. Massry GG, Holds JB. Coralline hydroxyapatite spheres as secondary orbital implants in anophthalmos. Ophthalmology. 1995;102(1):161–6.
2. Paik JS, Park HY, Cho WK, Yang SW. Effects of secondary porous orbital implantation in anophthalmic sockets. J Craniofac Surg. 2012;23(6):1677–82.
3. Tse DT. Color atlas of oculoplastic surgery. Philadelphia: Lippeincott Williams & Wilkins; 2011.
4. Iliff CE. The extruded implant. Arch Ophthalmol. 1967;78(6):742–4.
5. Frueh BR, Felker GV. Baseball implant: a method of secondary insertion of an intraorbital implant. Arch Ophthalmol. 1976;94(3):429–30.
6. Soll DB. The anophthalmic socket. Ophthalmology. 1982;89(5):407–23.
7. Soll DB. The anophthalmic socket. In: Management of complications in ophthalmic plastic surgery. Birmingham: Aesculapius; 1976. p. 325–7.
8. Smith B, Petrelli R. Dermis-fat graft as a movable implant within the muscle cone. Am J Ophthalmol. 1978;85(1):62–6.
9. Poonyathalang A, Preechawat P, Pomsathit J, Mahaisaviriya P. Reconstruction of contracted eye socket with amniotic membrane graft. Ophthalmic Plast Reconstr Surg. 2005;21(5):359–62.
10. Lee BJ, Lewis CD, Perry JD. Exposed porous orbital implants treated with simultaneous secondary implant and dermis fat graft. Ophthalmic Plast Reconstr Surg. 2010;26(4):273–6.
11. Shoamanesh A, Pang NK, Oestreicher JH. Complications of orbital implants: a review of 542 patients who have undergone orbital implantation and 275 subsequent PEG placements. Orbit. 2007;26(3):173–82.
12. Sundelin KC, Dafgård Kopp EM. Complications associated with secondary orbital implantations. Acta Ophthalmol. 2015;93(7):679–83.
13. Jordan DR, Klapper SR, Gilberg SM, Dutton JJ, Wong A, Mawn L. The bioceramic implant: evaluation of implant exposures in 419 implants. Ophthalmic Plast Reconstr Surg. 2010;26(2):80–2.
14. Calvano CJ. Smith and Nesi's ophthalmic plastic and reconstructive surgery. New York: Springer Science & Business Media; 2012.
15. Jordan DR, Parisi J. The scleral filet technique for secondary orbital implantation surgery. Can J Ophthalmol (Journal canadien d'ophtalmologie). 1996;31(7):356–61.
16. Sales-Sanz M, Sanz-Lopez A. Four-petal evisceration: a new technique. Ophthalmic Plast Reconstr Surg. 2007;23(5):389–92.
17. Kaltreider SA, Lucarelli MJ. A simple algorithm for selection of implant size for enucleation and evisceration: a prospective study. Ophthalmic Plast Reconstr Surg. 2002;18(5):336–41.
18. Toft PB, Roed Rasmussen ML, Prause JU. One-stage explant–implant procedure of exposed porous orbital implants. Acta Ophthalmol. 2012;90(3):210–4.
19. Jordan DR. Localization of extraocular muscles during secondary orbital implantation surgery: the tunnel technique: experience in 100 patients. Ophthalmology. 2004;111(5):1048–54.
20. Georgiadis NS, Terzidou CD, Dimitriadis AS. Restoration of the anophthalmic socket with secondary implantation of a coralline hydroxyapatite sphere. Ophthalmic Surg Lasers Imaging Retina. 1998;29(10):808–14.

21. Collin JR. A manual of systematic eyelid surgery. 3rd ed. Philadelphia: Elsevier Health Sciences; 2006. p. 212–4.
22. Tyers AG, Collin JR. Baseball orbital implants: a review of 39 patients. Br J Ophthalmol. 1985;69(6):438–42.
23. Koizumi NJ, Inatomi TJ, Sotozona CJ, et al. Growth factor mRNA and protein in preserved human amniotic membrane. Curr Eye Res. 2000;20:173–7.
24. Kumar S, Sugandhi P, Arora R, Pandey PK. Amniotic membrane transplantation versus mucous membrane grafting in anophthalmic contracted socket. Orbit. 2006;25(3):195–203.
25. Bajaj MS, Pushker N, Kumar KS, Chandra M, Ghose S. Evaluation of amniotic membrane grafting in the reconstruction of contracted socket. Ophthal Plast Reconstr Surg. 2006;22(2):116–20.
26. Smith B, Bosniak S, Nesi F, Lisman R. Dermis-fat orbital implantation: 118 cases. Ophthalmic Surg Lasers Imaging Retina. 1983;14(11):941–3.
27. Hintschich C. Dermis-Fett-Transplantat. Ophthalmologe. 2003;100(7):518–24.
28. Kim HK, La TY. Treatment of intractable orbital implant exposure with a large conjunctival defect by secondary insertion of the implant after preceding dermis fat graft. Int J Ophthalmol. 2013;6(2):193.
29. Quaranta-Leoni FM, Sposato S, Lorenzano D. Secondary orbital ball implants after enucleation and evisceration: surgical management, morbidity, and long-term outcome. Ophthalmic Plast Reconstr Surg. 2015;31(2):115–8.
30. Hart RH, Barnes E, Dickinson AJ. Secondary orbital implants after evisceration: a new conjunctiva-sparing technique. Ophthalmic Plast Reconstr Surg. 2005;21(2):129–32.
31. Chu HY, Liao YL, Tsai YJ, Chu YC, Wu SY, Ma L. Use of extraocular muscle flaps in the correction of orbital implant exposure. PLoS One. 2013;8(9):e72223.
32. McInnes AW, Dresner SC. Using the inferior oblique muscle to augment implant coverage in enucleation surgery. Ophthalmic Plast Reconstr Surg. 2011;27(1):52–4.
33. Parulekar MV. Re:"using the inferior oblique muscle to augment implant coverage in enucleation surgery". Ophthalmic Plast Reconstr Surg. 2012;28(4):305.
34. Jung SK, Cho WK, Paik JS, Yang SW. Long-term surgical outcomes of porous polyethylene orbital implants: a review of 314 cases. Br J Ophthalmol. 2011;1:bjophthalmol-2011.
35. Karslioglu S, Buttanri İB, Fazil K, Serin D, Akbaba M. Long-term outcomes of pegged and unpegged bioceramic orbital implants. Ophthalmic Plast Reconstr Surg. 2012;28(4):264–7.
36. Axmann S, Paridaens D. Anterior surface breakdown and implant extrusion following secondary alloplastic orbital implantation surgery. Acta Ophthalmol. 2018;96(3):310–3.
37. Kim YD, Goldberg RA, Shorr N, Steinsapir KD. Management of exposed hydroxyapatite orbital implants. Ophthalmology. 1994;101(10):1709–15.
38. Sagoo MS, Rose GE. Mechanisms and treatment of extruding intraconal implants: socket aging and tissue restitution (the "Cactus Syndrome"). Arch Ophthalmol. 2007;125(12):1616–20.
39. Nentwich MM, Schebitz-Walter K, Hirneiss C, Hintschich C. Dermis fat grafts as primary and secondary orbital implants. Orbit. 2014;33(1):33–8.

Chapter 16
Management of the Contracted Socket

Thomas E. Johnson

Introduction

The ideal anophthalmic socket has the following characteristics: a well-centered orbital implant of adequate volume; a smooth, healthy conjunctival lining; adequate superior and inferior fornices to maintain the prosthesis and permit complete eyelid closure; and functioning upper and lower eyelids to enable complete closure and wetting of the prosthesis [1]. Unfortunately, many patients develop socket issues preventing comfortable and cosmetically pleasing prosthesis wear. These problems have collectively been labelled the "anophthalmic socket syndrome." Inadequate orbital volume results in a sunken appearance with an abnormally deep superior sulcus. Since a larger prosthetic eye is then needed to improve the cosmetic appearance, lower lid sagging occurs due to the increased weight of the prosthesis (Fig. 16.1). Implant migration causes difficulty in maintaining a prosthesis with shallowing of the inferior fornix as well as a deep superior sulcus. Contracture of the conjunctival lining of the socket results in eyelid entropion, inability to close the eyelids over the prosthesis with resultant drying of the artificial eye and loss of luster (Fig. 16.2) and shallowing of the fornices making it difficult to maintain the prosthesis (Fig. 16.3). Patients often note the artificial eye spontaneously extrudes causing embarrassment. The goal of this chapter is to discuss causes of contracture of the socket, preventative measures to combat this problem, and treatment options once contracture has occurred.

T. E. Johnson (✉)
Bascom Palmer Eye Institute, University of Miami Miller School of Medicine, Miami, FL, USA
e-mail: tjohnson@med.miami.edu

T. E. Johnson (ed.), *Anophthalmia*,
https://doi.org/10.1007/978-3-030-29753-4_16

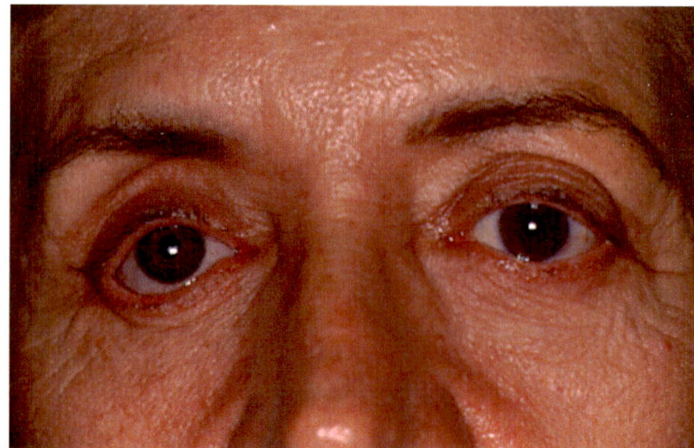

Fig. 16.1 Anophthalmic socket syndrome right side with deep superior sulcus, sunken appearance, inferior displacement of prosthesis, and lower lid sagging due to the weight of the prosthetic eye

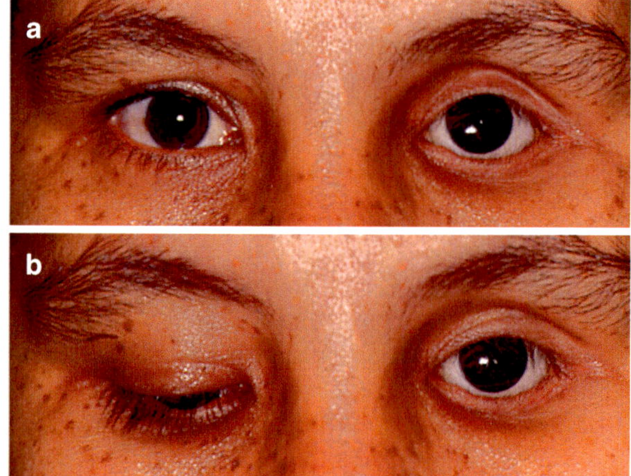

Fig. 16.2 (**a**) Mild socket contracture with entropion of upper and lower eyelids with loss of luster of the prosthesis. (**b**) Mild socket contracture with inability to close eyelids over the ocular prosthesis

Causes of Socket Contracture

Many sockets are predisposed to contracture from the beginning. Trauma-related eye loss often results in significant socket scarring with resultant contracture. Patients enucleated for intraocular malignancies such as retinoblastoma frequently have received radiation therapy, and radiation is a common cause of contracture. Chemical or thermal burns resulting in eye loss can cause significant scarring as

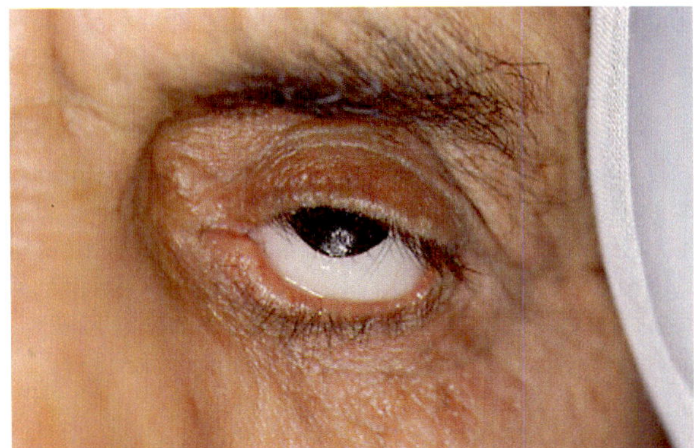

Fig. 16.3 Moderate socket contracture with loss of the inferior fornix and inability to maintain ocular prosthesis

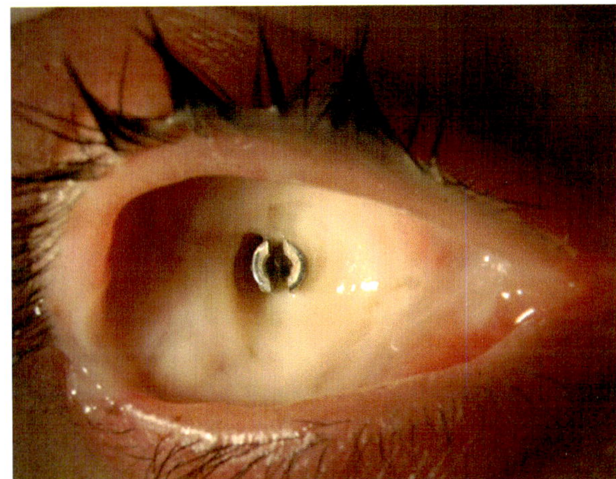

Fig. 16.4 Socket infection with atypical mycobacterial infection in a patient with previous placement titanium motility peg

well. Additionally, multiple socket surgeries induce fibroblast activity, and that in turn causes more aggressive scarring with contracture.

Recurrent infections also result in scarring with forniceal shortening over time. Poor patient hygiene with frequent handling of the prosthesis or failure to keep ocularist and ophthalmologist appointments for prosthesis maintenance causes scarring of the lining tissues. The most common bacterial infections involving the anophthalmic socket are caused by the following bacteria: *Staphylococcus aureus*, pneumococci, pseudomonas, and acinetobacter [2, 3]. Additionally, fungal and atypical mycobacterial infections (Fig. 16.4) can affect the conjunctival lining of the socket. When infection is suspected, cultures of the socket discharge should be taken and patients treated with appropriate topical as well as systemic antibiotics.

Recurrent noninfectious inflammations are common in anophthalmic sockets. This syndrome is referred to as giant papillary conjunctivitis (GPC) and is more common in younger individuals with robust immune systems [4]. The cause is unknown but may be due to mechanical irritation of the tissues due to irregularities or protein deposits on the prosthesis [5]. Prevention includes frequent prosthesis cleaning and polishing (at least every 6 months) and treatment with topical steroid solutions or ointments when present. Old or cracked prostheses should be changed, as they may cause more inflammation and more GPC.

Prevention

The key to maintain an ideal, healthy socket is preventive medicine. Once a patient has an artificial eye, he or she has embarked on a lifelong relationship with his or her ophthalmologist and ocularist. It is important that these two health professionals work together to ensure optimal socket health. Of course, monocular precautions with wearing of polycarbonate safety glasses are imperative for all affected patients to protect their remaining good eye. The ocularist needs to clean and polish the prosthetic eye usually about every 6 months and even more frequently in those predisposed to develop GPC. The ophthalmologist needs to carefully examine the socket every 6 months to detect infections and GPC and treat appropriately when present. This exam includes eversion of the upper lid to closely examine the tarsal conjunctiva, the most frequent area of GPC involvement. Prosthetic eyes don't last forever even when well-maintained, as the acrylic breaks down over time. Therefore, a new prosthesis is needed about every 5 years to ensure the health of the lining tissues. An adequately sized orbital implant should be placed during the initial eye removal to prevent the need for future surgeries including implant exchanges.

Stages of Socket Contracture

Socket contracture can be classified as mild, moderate, or severe. In mild contracture, upper and lower eyelid entropion results in the eyelashes rubbing against the ocular prosthesis. There is incomplete eyelid closure resulting in drying and crusting of the anterior surface of the artificial eye. Patients note discomfort and poor cosmesis. Moderate contracture results in shortening of the inferior and superior fornices. Initially, the ocularist compensates for this by making a smaller prosthesis. Patients later may note the inability to maintain the prosthesis due to inadequate fornices, and the artificial eye extrudes easily. Severe socket contracture results in complete loss of the fornices as well as horizontal shortening of the socket, and prosthesis wear is not possible (Fig. 16.5).

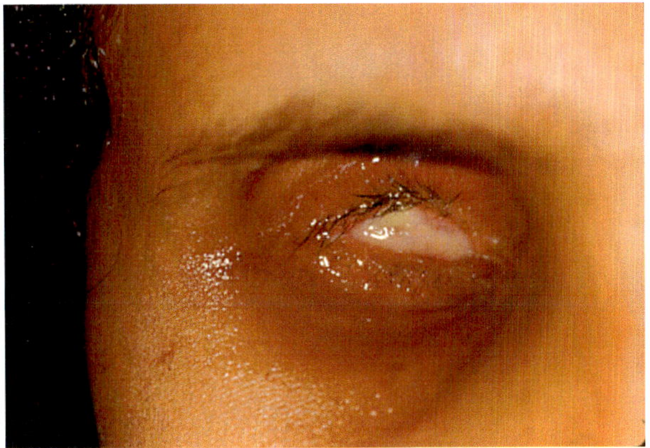

Fig. 16.5 Severe socket contracture with complete loss of both superior and inferior fornices as well as horizontal shortening of the palpebral fissure. Prosthesis wear is not possible

Entropion

Early socket contracture can manifest as upper or lower eyelid entropion. If the upper eyelid turns in, the lashes can touch the ocular prosthesis and cause dulling of the luster of the artificial eye. This problem can be treated with entropion repair surgery. One useful method is the upper eyelid tarsotomy or tarsal fracture procedure. The surgery can be performed under local or general anesthesia. The upper eyelid is injected from both the skin surface and the conjunctival surface with 2% lidocaine with epinephrine. Three 4-0 silk sutures are passed through the gray line of the upper eyelid, and the lid is everted over a chalazion clamp. An incision is made through the conjunctiva and tarsal plate approximately 2 mm from the lid margin the entire length of the tarsal plate. Blunt dissection is carried out between the tarsal plate and the lid margin and in the plane between tarsal plate and overlying muscle. A groove is therefore formed at the lid margin. Three double-armed sutures of 5-0 polyglactin 910 are passed in a lamellar fashion through the tarsal plate and then brought into the groove and out through the eyelid skin just above the eyelash margin (Fig. 16.6a). The silk sutures are removed. The double-armed polyglactin 910 sutures are tied over foam bolsters or brought through the foam material found in the 4-0 silk suture pack (Fig. 16.6b). These bolsters are left in place for 2 weeks. In a similar fashion, entropion repair can be performed on the lower eyelid using a Weis procedure. However, one must be careful not to shallow the inferior fornix. Oftentimes, a mucous membrane graft is a better procedure to treat lower lid entropion in the setting of socket contracture.

Mucous Membrane Grafting with Fornix-Deepening Sutures

The mainstay of treatment of contracted anatomic sockets is mucous membrane grafting. Oftentimes the inferior fornix becomes shallow resulting in incomplete closure of the eyelids and the inability to maintain the ocular prosthesis. Patients

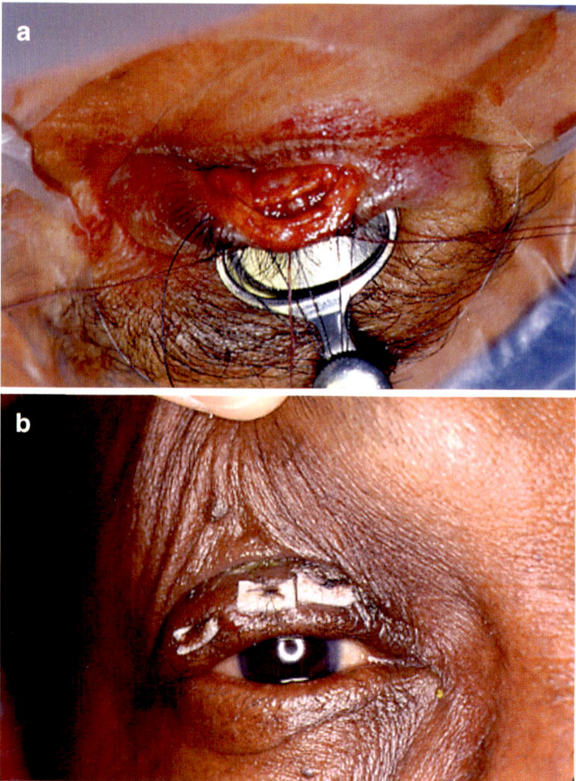

Fig. 16.6 (**a**) Surgeons' view, posterior tarsotomy for upper lid entropion repair. Lid has been everted over a large chalazion clamp after placement of three 4-0 silk sutures through the gray line. Incision has been made through conjunctiva and tarsal plate approximately 2 mm from the lid margin. A groove has been fashioned at the lid margin, and three 5-0 Vicryl™ sutures have been placed in a lamellar fashion through the superior segment of tarsal plate. The sutures have been passed through the groove to exit the skin just above the eyelash line. (**b**) Posterior tarsotomy completed with good upper lid eversion and presence of three 5-0 Vicryl™ sutures exiting the skin just above the eyelashes and tied over foam bolsters fashioned from a 4-0 silk suture pack

often complain that the prosthesis falls out spontaneously, and this causes embarrassment. The cosmetic appearance is also affected. Harvesting mucous membrane from the inside of the lower lip is a useful technique to address this problem. This surgery can be performed under either local or general anesthesia. Initially, the inferior fornix is injected with 2% lidocaine with epinephrine. A 4-0 silk suture is placed through the gray line of the lower eyelid margin to enable eversion of the lid and good exposure of the inferior fornix. An incision is made in the inferior fornix several millimeters below the inferior border of the tarsal plate. Blunt and sharp dissection is carried down to the level of the inferior orbital rim which is easily palpable. A conformer is placed in the socket to ensure that the dissection is adequate. After that, the conformer is removed, and attention is directed to the lower lip which is everted and injected with 2% lidocaine with epinephrine. A large

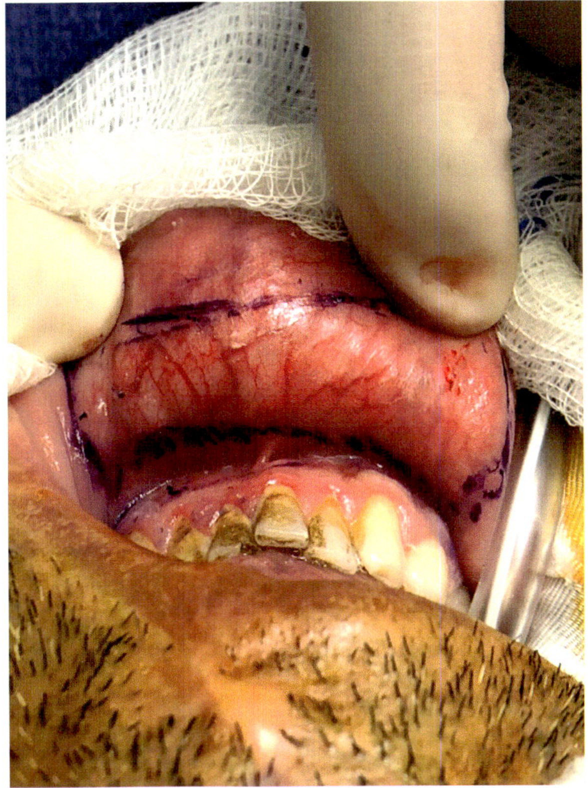

Fig. 16.7 Harvesting large full-thickness mucous membrane graft from inside of the lower lip. The entire length of the lip is used, and the width of the graft extends from just in front of the frenulum posteriorly to the wet-dry junction of the lip anteriorly

mucous membrane graft is outlined with a marking pen (Fig. 16.7). Full-thickness grafts are preferable to partial thickness grafts as there is less contracture of the tissue postoperatively [6]. The rectangle marked is incised with a number 15 Bard-Parker blade, and the graft is dissected using blunt Westcott scissors and forceps. Care is taken to avoid cautery to this area, as this can result in postoperative discomfort. Good hemostasis can usually be obtained by placing oxidized cellulose polymer (Surgicel™) gauze on the donor bed and applying gentle pressure. The mucous membrane is thinned of submucosal tissue. The authors usually harvest a graft sized approximately 30 mm by 10 mm. When implanted, the narrow sides of the rectangle are sutured horizontally, as the graft can usually be stretched from the medial to the lateral canthus. The long limbs of the rectangle are needed to extend the mucous membrane deep into the fornices and back (Fig. 16.8). The harvested graft is sutured into position using four cardinal interrupted sutures of 7-0 Vicryl™, one in each corner, and the mucous membrane is gently draped into the inferior fornix with a muscle hook (Fig. 16.9). Next, running 7-0 Vicryl™ sutures on the superior and inferior aspects of the wound are used to secure the tissue in position. After the graft has been successfully fixated in place, fornix-deepening sutures are added. Two double-armed sutures of 5-0 polyglactin 910 are brought through either a small piece of a vein or nerve retractor or a retinal encircling element cut into a

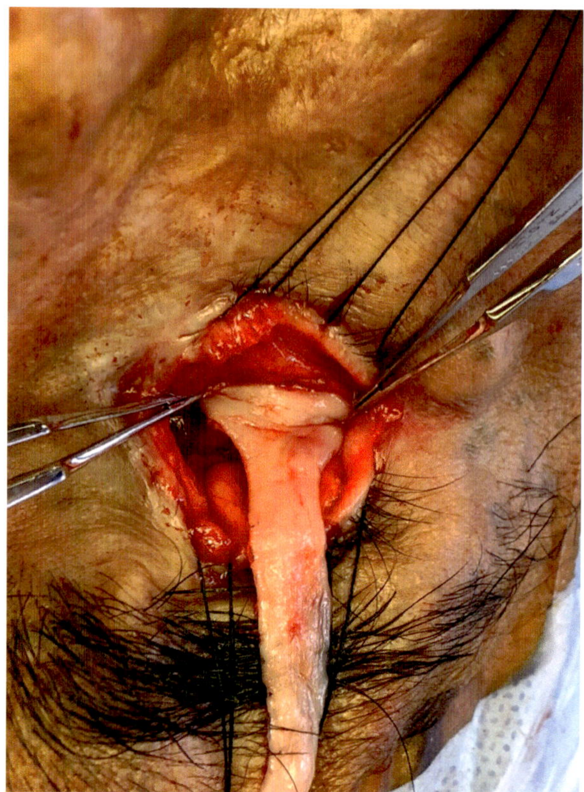

Fig. 16.8 Mucous membrane graft is sutured into the newly dissected inferior fornix. An incision has been made several centimeters beneath the tarsal plate the entire length of the lid. Dissection has been carried out down to the inferior orbital rim. The graft is being sutured into position using absorbable sutures. Note the short end of the rectangular graft is oriented horizontally and stretched from the medial to the lateral canthus

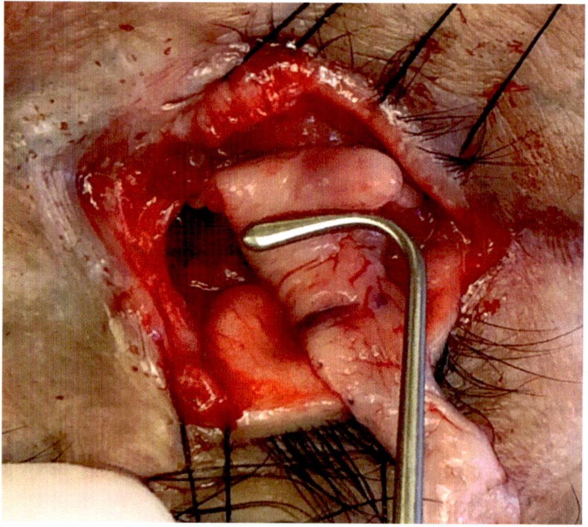

Fig. 16.9 A muscle hook is used to gently advance the mucous membrane graft into the newly constructed fornix down to the level of the inferior orbital rim

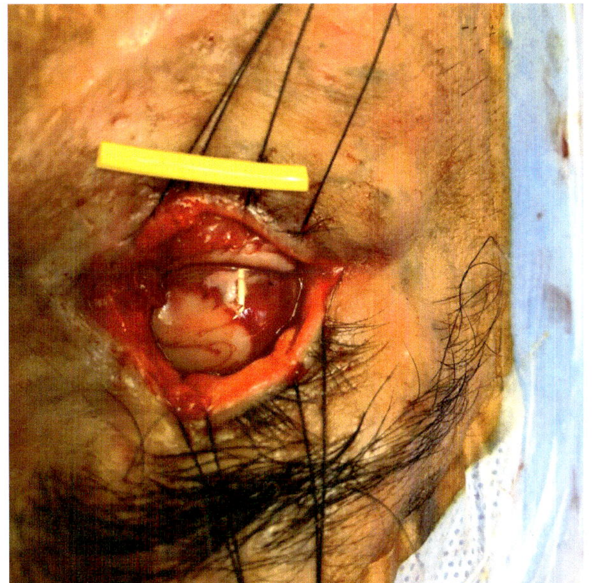

Fig. 16.10 The mucous membrane graft has been sutured into position and a large conformer placed. A small segment of a nerve retractor approximately 15 mm in length has been cut to size for placement of fornix-deepening sutures

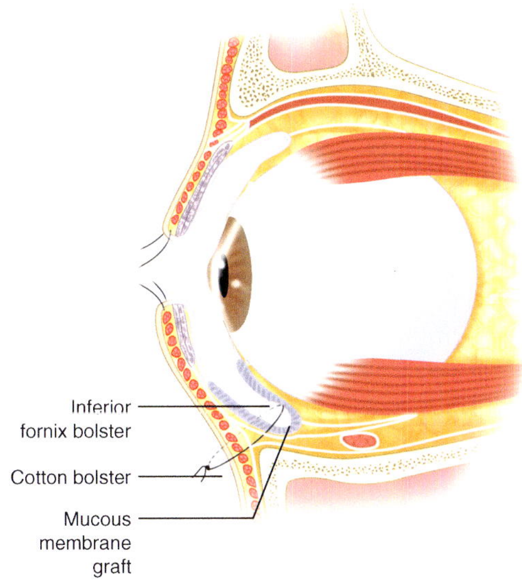

Fig. 16.11 Cross-sectional diagram showing mucous membrane graft sutured into position in the inferior conjunctival fornix with fornix-deepening sutures passing through an inferior fornix bolster. The sutures scrape the periosteum at the inferior orbital rim and exit the skin approximately 12–15 mm below the lower eyelid margin. They are then tied over a cotton bolster made from the end of a cotton-tip applicator. (Illustration by Alison Bozung)

size of about 15 mm in length (Fig. 16.10). The needles are removed from the 5-0 polyglactin 910 sutures, and a larger free needle is selected. The free needle is used to pass the suture through the mucous membrane graft into the inferior fornix scraping the periosteum at the inferior orbital rim and exiting through the skin approximately 12–15 mm below the eyelid margin. The two double-armed sutures are tied over cotton bolsters made by removing the cotton tips from cotton-tip applicators (Figs. 16.11 and 16.12). This technique creates a deep inferior fornix,

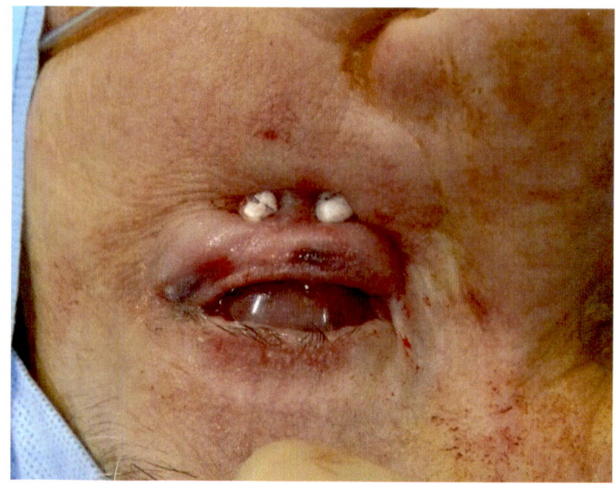

Fig. 16.12 Two double-armed sutures of 5-0 Vicryl™ have been passed through the nerve retractor and their needles removed. A large free needle has been used to pass the sutures through the mucous membrane graft at the depth of the inferior fornix scrapping the periosteum at the inferior orbital rim and exiting the skin. The sutures have been tied over cotton bolsters and will stay in position for about 2 weeks

and sutures are left in place for approximately 2–3 weeks. They are removed in the clinic along with the inferior fornix bolster. Mucous membrane grafting can be combined with a lateral canthal tightening when needed for lateral canthal laxity. Rarely some patients with adequate conjunctiva lose their inferior fornix due to loss of adhesions between the inferior fornix and inferior orbital rim. These patients have anterior migration of orbital fat and shallowing of the fornix, making it difficult to maintain their prosthesis. They can also benefit from fornix-deepening sutures, suturing the inferior conjunctival tissues to the periosteum just inside the inferior orbital rim [7]. It takes approximately 1 month for mucous membrane grafts to become fully vascularized, and functional success rates have been reported to be over 80% [8].

Superior Fornix Shortening

The superior fornix can also contract causing difficulty closing the eyelids and drying of the prosthesis. This conjunctival shortage is addressed using a superior mucous membrane graft. If more mucous membrane is needed than can be obtained on the inside of the lower lip, one can also harvest mucous membrane from the inside of the cheek. Care must be taken to avoid damage to Stenson's duct adjacent to the upper second molar. A superior fornix incision is made with Westcott scissors, and blunt and sharp dissection is carried out to the superior orbital rim. The mucous membrane graft is sutured into position in this area using 6-0 plain or 7-0 Vicryl™ sutures, and fornix-deepening sutures can be used in a similar fashion to those used in the lower eyelid. However, they are often not needed. If both the inferior and superior fornices are reconstructed using mucous membrane grafts, a temporary tarsorrhaphy is performed after a conformer is placed to hold the grafts in proper position.

The eyelids are split at the gray line into anterior and posterior lamellae. The mucocutaneous junction is removed using sharp Westcott scissors. The anterior surface of the tarsal plate is exposed using Westcott scissors, and several interrupted sutures of 5-0 polyglactin 910 are placed in a lamellar fashion from the tarsus of the lower lid to the tarsus of the upper lid, connecting the two tarsal plates. The skin is closed to skin using a running suture of 7-0 polyglactin 910. After 1–2 months, the tarsorrhaphy can be opened using blunt Westcott scissors.

Complete Socket Contracture

Severe scarring due to trauma, chemical burns, thermal burns, or chronic infections can result in complete socket contracture. The upper and lower eyelids are adherent, and there is little discernible socket tissue. These cases are challenging, and extensive dissection and mucous membrane grafting are needed. One surgical technique involves completely wrapping a conformer with a large mucous membrane graft. The smooth side of the mucous membrane is directed inward toward the conformer, and the submucosal tissues are directed into the graft bed. This procedure can be performed under either local or general anesthesia. The scarred tissues are injected with 2% lidocaine with epinephrine. An incision was made between the upper and lower eyelids with a 15 Bard-Parker blade or sharp Westcott scissors. Dissection is carried out superiorly to create a superior fornix, aiming for the superior orbital rim, and inferiorly to the inferior orbital rim. When a large pocket has been created, a conformer is placed into the socket to confirm that adequate dissection has been performed. A large mucous membrane graft is harvested from the inside of the cheek and is used to completely wrap the conformer. The mucous membrane graft is sutured over the conformer using absorbable sutures. This wrapped conformer is placed into the socket, and a permanent tarsorrhaphy is placed. The tarsorrhaphy remains closed for approximately 6 months to ensure that the conformer will not extrude during the postop period. After the tarsorrhaphy is opened, a custom-made pressure conformer is fitted with the ocularist's help to maintain pressure in the newly formed socket and help prevent re-contracture. It is recommended that the patient use a pressure conformer at night for several months after opening the tarsorrhaphy to prevent re-contracture, a common complication after surgery on severely contracted sockets (Fig. 16.13a, b). Other surgical options for severely contracted sockets include using hard palate mucosal grafts with temporary tarsorrhaphies [9]. Yet another technique includes a deep socket reconstruction using a special conformer with pre-drilled holes for placement of wires or sutures that are attached to the superior and inferior orbital rims [6].

In a severely contracted dry socket without viable wet mucosal tissue, mucous membrane grafts often shrink and fail. In those cases, skin grafts can be used to reestablish fornices [10]. One technique involves wrapping a conformer with a split-thickness supraclavicular graft [11] or split-thickness postauricular graft [12]. However, skin grafts have the disadvantage of not lubricating the surface of the

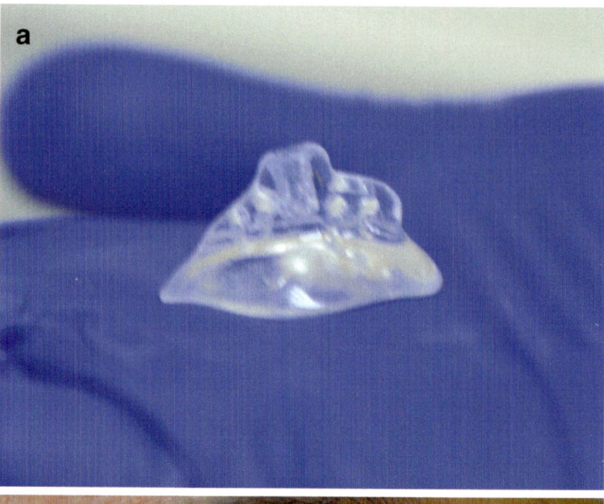

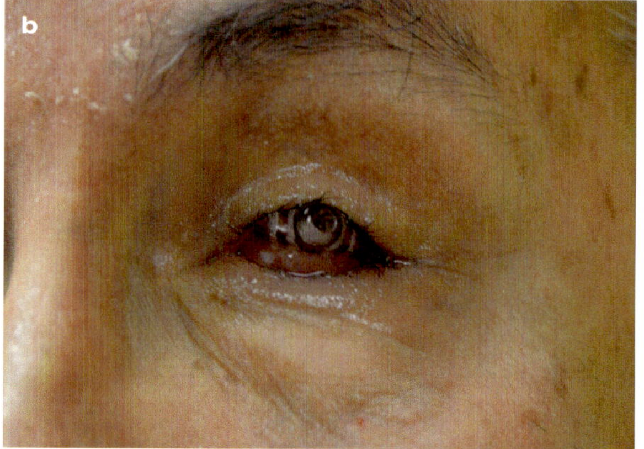

Fig. 16.13 (**a**) A custom-made pressure conformer has been made by the ocularist. Note it has an opening to accommodate a disk-shaped outer component to apply continuous pressure to the healing mucous membrane graft to prevent contracture of the tissues. (Courtesy of Yasser Bataineh B.C.O.). (**b**) Custom-made pressure conformer in place. (Courtesy Yasser Bataineh B.C.O)

artificial eye, resulting in a dull and unrealistic appearance. Also, skin continually desquamates, resulting in chronic odor and hygiene issues related to buildup of keratin in the socket [10].

Amniotic Membrane in Socket Contracture Surgery

Amniotic membrane grafting is also used in the reconstruction of contracted anatomic sockets. This material is mainly beneficial in the management of mild to moderate socket contracture [13]. Its main advantage is that it avoids the necessity of harvesting autologous grafts from the inside of the lip and cheek, therefore resulting in less patient morbidity and discomfort [14–16]. Some authors have described success rates using amniotic membrane similar to those of mucous membrane grafts [15]. The disadvantage of using this material is that it can result in more re-contracture later, especially in severely contracted sockets, and the increased cost of using this material. Mucous membrane is the gold standard and, if harvested in a full-thickness fashion, usually will not re-contract easily. The surgical technique for implantation of amniotic membrane is like that of mucous membrane grafting. Dissection is carried out in the superior and inferior fornices. The amniotic membrane is hydrated and placed into the socket bed and sutured into position with absorbable sutures. A conformer is placed, and one may place a temporary tarsorrhaphy. Fornix-deepening sutures can be placed, but care must be taken to avoid damage to the more fragile amniotic membrane.

Hard Palate Grafts and Auricular Cartilage Grafts

Hard palate graft mucosa and auricular cartilage grafts have also been successfully used in the treatment of contracted anophthalmic sockets. Holck and coauthors reported ten patients who underwent hard palate mucosal grafts with forniceal sutures. 8/10 patients were able to comfortably wear an ocular prosthesis afterward, but 2 developed socket recurrent contracture and were unable to wear a prosthesis [9]. Smith and coworkers used postauricular cartilage grafts in 54 patients with lower conjunctival fornix contraction and reported a 92.6% success rate [17].

Dermis-Fat Autografts

Dermis-fat grafting is another option in the rehabilitation of the contracted anophthalmic socket and was described in 1978 by Smith and Petrelli [18]. These grafts are sometimes used for primary enucleations in place of implanting a spherical alloplastic orbital implant. Either the left lower abdominal flank or buttocks are usually selected as the donor site. A circular graft of the skin and fat is harvested, and the epidermis is removed. Care is taken to harvest the graft perpendicularly through the fat to obtain an ample cylinder of fat (Fig. 16.14). Dissection is then carried out

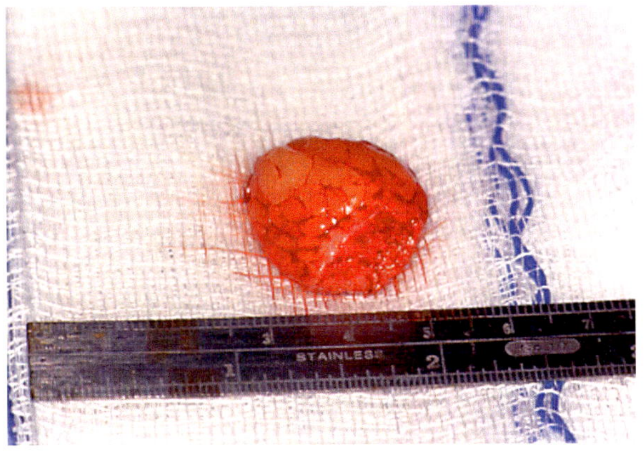

Fig. 16.14 Harvested dermis-fat graft with epidermis removed. Note that a cylinder and a cone of fat has been harvested

through the scarred conjunctival tissues, and a space is created to gently insert the graft. The conjunctiva is sutured to the edges of the dermis with 7-0 Vicryl™ sutures, and a conformer with antibiotic ointment is placed. The socket is pressure-patched for 1 week. This technique has unique benefits including increasing the surface area of the socket and supplying volume as well. However, complications can occur. Atrophy of the graft, infection, and shrinkage can result in failure. Minor complications include granulomas, keratinization, conjunctival cyst, and graft hirsutism [15–19]. Shore and coworkers reported 66 patients who underwent socket reconstruction with dermis-fat grafts and noted 24 complications, the most common being failure of conjunctival resurfacing of the graft. Complications most commonly occurred in severely traumatized sockets, those patients with a history of extensive earlier ocular surgery, and those with systemic diseases causing defective wound healing [20].

Composite Hard Palate-Dermis-Fat Grafts

Choi and coauthors described the use of a composite hard palate and dermis-fat graft for reconstruction of severely contracted anophthalmic sockets. In their four patients, they used this composite grafting technique for reconstruction of both inferior and superior fornices. Adjunctive 5-FU injections were added, and they reported good functional and cosmetic results [21].

Other Non-autologous Grafts

Porcine acellular dermis grafts have been used as spacer grafts in contracted anophthalmic socket reconstruction. However, they take longer to vascularize and undergo more shrinkage with time compared to autologous buccal mucosal grafts [22].

Antimetabolites in Socket Contracture Surgery

Anophthalmic socket surgery is often complicated by re-contracture due to increased fibroblastic activity within the conjunctiva. Patients that have had multiple surgeries on their anophthalmic sockets are prone to this complication. Therefore, one tries to minimize the number of procedures performed. With time, the socket can become completely scarred with loss of the fornices and inability to wear an ocular prosthesis. Treatment with injections of antimetabolite medications can often help prevent re-scarring of the tissues. One such medication, 5-fluorouracil (5-FU), is a pyrimidine analogue that inhibits fibroblast growth and interferes with collagen lattice contraction [23]. It has been used extensively in glaucoma surgery, conjunctival neoplasia, and in the treatment of cutaneous skin cancers. Studies have shown that it can reduce the incidence of re-contraction after socket repair. Kamal and coworkers found that weekly subconjunctival injections of 10 mg of 5-FU starting about 4 weeks after surgery resulted in better outcomes compared with controls. Their patients received weekly subconjunctival injections of 10 mg of 5-FU in the superior and inferior fornices weekly for 4 weeks [23]. Mitomycin C has also been used both at the time of surgery and in the postoperative period. Priel and coworkers reported a nonrandomized retrospective review of five patients with complex anophthalmic socket scarring in which the patients had multiple previous unsuccessful surgeries. The authors injected either 5-FU (three patients) or mitomycin C (two patients) intraoperatively and gave their three patients who had initially received 5-FU postoperative 5-FU injections. All patients had tarsorrhaphies for 3 months, and all were then able to retain an ocular prosthesis [24].

Other Methods

Free radial forearm flaps have been described in the reconstruction of "malignant contracture" in patients who had undergone exenteration of the orbit followed by radiation therapy during infancy [25].

Conclusions

The loss of an eye can result in psychological distress and loss of self-esteem. Healthcare professionals can do a lot to alleviate anxiety and help return patients to a normal, healthy life with confidence in their cosmetic appearance. Excellent initial surgical eye removal technique, meticulous postoperative care and maintenance, and a thoughtful graded approach to socket reconstructive procedures enable us to achieve these goals.

References

1. Bosniak SL. Reconstruction of the anophthalmic socket: state of the art. Adv Ophthalmic Plast Reconstr Surg. 1987;7:313–48.
2. Vasquez RJ, Linberg JV. The anophthalmic socket and the prosthetic eye. A clinical and bacteriologic study. Ophthalmic Plast Reconstr Surg. 1989;5(4):277–80.
3. Mahajan VM. Acute bacterial infections of the eye: their aetiology and treatment. Br J Ophthalmol. 1983;67(3):191–4.
4. Srinivasan BD, et al. Giant papillary conjunctivitis with ocular prostheses. Arch Ophthalmol. 1979;97(5):892–5.
5. Chang WJ, et al. Conjunctival cytology features of giant papillary conjunctivitis associated with ocular prostheses. Ophthalmic Plast Reconstr Surg. 2005;21(1):39–45.

6. Putterman AM, Scott R. Deep ocular socket reconstruction. Arch Ophthalmol. 1977;95(7):1221–8.
7. Neuhaus RW, Hawes MJ. Inadequate inferior cul-de-sac in the anophthalmic socket. Ophthalmology. 1992;99(1):153–7.
8. Kim CY, et al. Postoperative outcomes of anophthalmic socket reconstruction using an autologous buccal mucosa graft. J Craniofac Surg. 2014;25(4):1171–4.
9. Holck DE, et al. Hard palate mucosal grafts in the treatment of the contracted socket. Ophthal Plast Reconstr Surg. 1999;15(3):202.
10. Vistnes LM, Iverson RE. Surgical treatment of the contracted socket. Plast Reconstr Surg. 1974;53(5):563–7.
11. Hasan SA, et al. Split-skin-graft wrapped conformer to treat severe contracted sockets. J Craniofac Surg. 2018;29:e777–9.
12. AlHassan S, et al. Deepening fornix technique using central split-medium thickness skin graft to treat contracted anophthalmic sockets. J Craniofac Surg. 2018;29:1607–11.
13. Tawfik HA, Raslan AO, Talib N. Surgical management of acquired socket contracture. Curr Opin Ophthalmol. 2009;20(5):406–11.
14. Kumar S, et al. Amniotic membrane transplantation versus mucous membrane grafting in anophthalmic contracted socket. Orbit. 2006;25(3):195–203.
15. Bajaj MS, et al. Evaluation of amniotic membrane grafting in the reconstruction of contracted socket. Ophthalmic Plast Reconstr Surg. 2006;22(2):116–20.
16. Poonyathalang A, et al. Reconstruction of contracted eye socket with amniotic membrane graft. Ophthalmic Plast Reconstr Surg. 2005;21(5):359–62.
17. Smith RJ, Malet T. Auricular cartilage grafting to correct lower conjunctival fornix retraction and eyelid malposition in anophthalmic patients. Ophthalmic Plast Reconstr Surg. 2008;24(1):13–8.
18. Smith B, Petrelli R. Dermis-fat graft as a movable implant within the muscle cone. Am J Ophthalmol. 1978;85(1):62–6.
19. Starks V, Freitag SK. Postoperative complications of dermis-fat autografts in the anophthalmic socket. Semin Ophthalmol. 2018;33(1):112–5.
20. Shore JW, et al. Management of complications following dermis-fat grafting for anophthalmic socket reconstruction. Ophthalmology. 1985;92(10):1342–50.
21. Choi CJ, Tran AQ, Tse DT. Hard palate-dermis fat composite graft for reconstruction of contracted anophthalmic socket. Orbit. 2018;38:1–6.
22. Teo L, et al. Surgical outcomes of porcine acellular dermis graft in anophthalmic socket: comparison with oral mucosa graft. Korean J Ophthalmol. 2017;31(1):9–15.
23. Kamal S, et al. Serial sub-conjunctival 5-Fluorouracil for early recurrent anophthalmic contracted socket. Graefes Arch Clin Exp Ophthalmol. 2013;251(12):2797–802.
24. Priel A, et al. Use of antimetabolites in the reconstruction of severe anophthalmic socket contraction. Ophthalmic Plast Reconstr Surg. 2012;28(6):409–12.
25. Tahara S, Susuki T. Eye socket reconstruction with free radial forearm flap. Ann Plast Surg. 1989;23(2):112–6.

Chapter 17
Socket Malignancy

Apostolos G. Anagnostopoulos and Thomas E. Johnson

Introduction

The anophthalmic socket can often be associated with postoperative complications. Usually patients present with the following post-enucleation socket syndromes: enophthalmos with deepening of the superior sulcus, upper eyelid ptosis, and lower eyelid laxity associated with ill-fitting of the ocular prosthesis and resulting poor cosmesis [1–3]. Also, a common concern of anophthalmic patients is change in the amount of discharge produced by the socket itself [4]. The development of a malignant tumor in an anophthalmic socket is considered a rare entity. Although most anophthalmic patients are closely followed up with frequent visits with ophthalmologists, oculoplastic surgeons, and their ocularists, such entities can be overlooked for long periods of time [5]. Only a handful of cases of malignant tumors originating in the anophthalmic socket, such as ocular surface squamous neoplasia (OSSN) and conjunctival malignant melanoma (MM), have been reported in the literature.

Pathophysiology

Different mechanisms have been considered responsible for carcinogenesis in the anophthalmic socket. Environmental conditions including ultraviolet light exposure, radiation, smoking, viral infections (HPV types 16, 18 or HIV), and genetic

A. G. Anagnostopoulos (✉)
University of Miami, Bascom Palmer Eye Institute, Ophthalmic Plastic and Reconstructive Surgery, Miami, FL, USA
e-mail: axa1753@miami.edu

T. E. Johnson
Bascom Palmer Eye Institute, University of Miami Miller School of Medicine, Miami, FL, USA

T. E. Johnson (ed.), *Anophthalmia*,
https://doi.org/10.1007/978-3-030-29753-4_17

mutations contribute to carcinogenesis, but are not specific for the anophthalmic socket. One of the main suspected mechanisms is chronic inflammation created as the conjunctiva is in constant contact with an ocular prosthesis. Giant papillary conjunctivitis (GPC), a type 1 hypersensitivity reaction, is a common finding in anophthalmic sockets. Immunologically a B-cell-driven IgE response and immunohistochemically an IL-4 and eotaxin process, GPC could be related to carcinogenesis. High levels of IgE have been positively but also negatively correlated with breast cancer [6]. IL-4 has been shown to decrease the antitumor activity of CD8 T cells while eotaxin (a chemokine which attracts eosinophils) has a positive correlation with prostate and ovarian cancers [7–9]. Although these findings could suggest a positive correlation between GPC and anophthalmic socket malignancy, there is currently no data to back up this hypothesis.

Ocular Surface Squamous Neoplasia (OSSN)

OSSN consists of a wide variety of premalignant and malignant diseases which involve the abnormal growth of squamous epithelial cells of the ocular surface. These include conjunctival intraepithelial neoplasia (CIN), squamous cell carcinoma (SCC), and mucoepidermoid carcinoma (entities which include corneal involvement will not be discussed here). The prevalence of OSSN ranges from <0.2 cases/million/year to 35 cases/million/year depending on the geographic region [10, 11]. CIN is by definition noninvasive, while SCC is malignant with a metastatic potential. Mucoepidermoid carcinoma is a very rare aggressive variant of SCC [12, 13].

Generally, OSSN is considered the third most common ocular surface tumor (following melanoma and lymphoma) while being the most common malignant conjunctival tumor [14, 15]. Although a relatively common ocular tumor, only a few cases of OSSN in the anophthalmic socket have been reported. All cases had one thing in common: the occurrence of the malignancy presented a long time after enucleation, with a median time of wearing of the ocular prosthesis of 44.3 years [16]. Patients often presented with an ill-fitting prosthesis; a serous, mucoid, purulent or sanguineous discharge; and a conjunctival mass which resembled a papilloma or granuloma [17–21].

Treatment of OSSN depends on the pathology of the underlying tumor. Noninvasive small lesions whose size does not create problems with prosthesis fitting can be treated medically with topical and/or intralesional IFN-a_{2b}, mitomycin C (MMC), or 5-fluorouracil (5-FU), therapies that have been gaining in popularity over the past years [22, 23]. Surgical excision combined with cryotherapy (double freeze–thaw technique) combined with this topical therapy is preferred. Wide excision (4 mm margins) combined with adjuvant therapy to kill any remaining tumor cells provides a low recurrence rate up to 33% when surgical margins are negative [24]. Positive margins increase the recurrence rate to 50% [25]. In refractive cases or cases not responding to topical chemotherapy, extensive surgery including exenteration or high doses of radiation with proton beam therapy (PBT) or iodine-125 brachytherapy can be delivered [26].

As noninvasive and aggressive tumors cannot be distinguished clinically, suspicious lesions should be considered and treated as if invasive in order to decrease the chance of recurrence.

Conjunctival Malignant Melanoma (MM)

Conjunctival MM is considered a rare ocular tumor. The incidence is up to 0.08 cases per 100.000. An important factor is that 50% of the cases arise from preexisting melanocytic intraepithelial neoplasia [27]. To date, only two cases have been described in the literature of conjunctival MM in the anophthalmic socket. One presented with MM after enucleation for a blind painful eye with no obvious risk for malignancy [28]. The second case occurred in a young patient with bilateral retinoblastoma (treated with excision, chemotherapy, and radiation); the malignant tumor and the history of radiation can increase the risk for further malignancies [29]. In contrary to OSSN which seems to occur many years after enucleation, both of the melanoma cases presented 3 years after the primary operation.

Treatment of such cases includes surgical excision combined with topical MMC, brachytherapy, or PBT. Each case should be treated individually, as no current guidelines exist for their treatment due to the rarity of this lesion (Fig. 17.1).

Tumor Recurrence

Primary orbital tumors that are aggressive in nature or other tumors that metastasize to the orbit may require orbital exenteration in conjunction with chemotherapy or radiation therapy. Such therapy will increase the chance of total tumor removal, eliminate the risk of metastasis, and increase life expectancy.

Tumor recurrence after orbital exenteration is common and ranges from 24% to 50% [30–32]. As recurrence is difficult to be determined on clinical examination, it

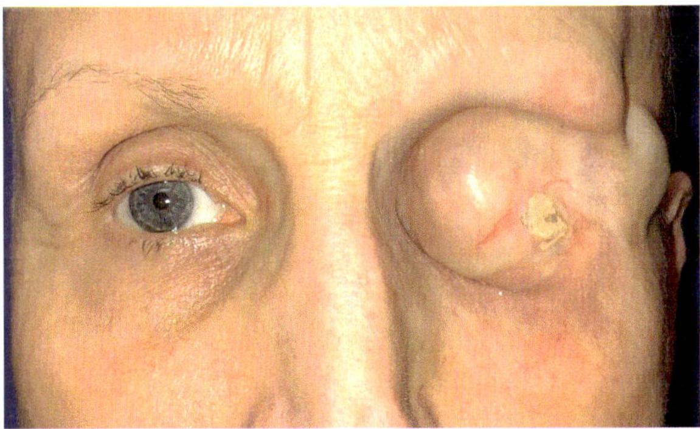

Fig. 17.1 Recurrent malignant melanoma in exenterated socket

is essential to obtain imaging studies at regular intervals after the initial treatment for early detection and possible re-treatment. Although MRI and CT imaging are mostly used for the detection of tumor recurrence, it is often difficult to differentiate between scar tissue (post-surgical or post-radiation) and tumor recurrence. The imaging characteristics of any recurrence may be similar to that of the original excised tumor; also, they are often different from any soft tissue flaps used for socket reconstruction during post-exenteration. PET/CT imaging can be helpful in certain circumstances in those cases in which conventional CT or MRI techniques are unable to detect recurrences [33]. In order to prevent delay in detection, regular clinical examinations together with imaging studies every 3–4 months should be carried out for the first 2 years after exenteration [32].

Conclusions

The anophthalmic socket is a constantly changing environment. Mucoid discharge is one of the most common reasons why anophthalmic patients seek care. Most often this symptom is a result of the microenvironment of the socket itself or conjunctival reaction to the continuous contact with the ocular prosthesis appearing as GPC. Less often the presence of a conjunctival lesion can increase the amount of mucoid discharge. Anophthalmic sockets should be examined on a regular basis and more frequently when there is a change in discharge amount or discomfort in prosthesis wearing. The presence of deep fornices with healthy pink conjunctiva without injection, edema, erosion, purulent discharge, or GPC are signs of a healthy socket. As chronic inflammation has been related to cancer, changes or increase in GPC should be promptly treated by ophthalmologists.

The exenterated socket should also be thoroughly examined. Any lesions should be excised and sent to pathology for further investigation. Imaging studies should be considered where there is any suspicion of orbital involvement or recurrence.

References

1. Tyers AG, Collin JR. Orbital implants and post enucleation socket syndrome. Trans Ophthalmol Soc U K. 1982;102(Pt 1):90–2.
2. Murchinson AP, Robert Bernardino C. Evaluation of the anophthalmic socket. Rev Ophthalmol. 2006. www.reviewofophthalmology.com/content/d/plastic_pointers/i/1301/c/25050/. Accessed 12 Oct 2018.
3. Nerad J. Techniques in ophthalmic plastic surgery. 1st ed. Elsevier; 2010. p. 463–486.
4. Pine K, Sloan B, Stewart J, Jacobs RJ. Concerns of anophthalmic patients wearing artificial eyes. Clin Exp Ophthalmol. 2011;39(1):47–52.
5. American Society of Ocularists. When should you see an ocularist. www.ocularist.org/resources_see_ocularist.asp. Accessed 12 Oct 2018.
6. Bozkurt B, Akyurek N, Irkec M, Erdener U, Memis L. Immunohistochemical findings in prosthesis-associated giant papillary conjunctivitis. Clin Exp Ophthalmol. 2007;35(6):535–40.

7. Li Z, Chen L, Qin Z. Paradoxical roles of IL-4 in tumor immunity. Cell Mol Immunol. 2009;6(6):415–22.
8. Heidegger I, Hofer J, Luger M, Pichler R, Klocker H, Horninger W, Steiner E, Jochberger S, Culig Z. Is Eotaxin-1 a serum and urinary biomarker for prostate cancer detection and recurrence? Prostate. 2015;75(16):1904–9.
9. Nolen BM, Lokshin AE. Targeting CCL11 in the treatment of ovarian cancer. Expert Opin Ther Targets. 2010;14(2):157–67.
10. Newton R, Ziegler J, Ateenyi-Agaba C, Bousarghin L, Casabonne D, Beral V, Mbidde E, Carpenter L, Reeves G, Parkin DM, Wabinga H, Mbulaiteye S, Jaffe H, Bourboulia D, Boshoff C, Touze A, Coursaget P, Uganda Kaposi's Sarcoma Study Group. The epidemiology of conjunctival squamous cell carcinoma in Uganda. Br J Cancer. 2002;87(3):301–8.
11. Newton R, Ferlay J, Reeves G, Beral V, Parkin DM. Effect of ambient solar ultraviolet radiation on incidence of squamous-cell carcinoma of the eye. Lancet. 1996;347(9013):1450–1.
12. Hwang IP, Jordan DR, Brownstein S, Gilberg SM, McEachren TM, Prokopetz R. Mucoepidermoid carcinoma of the conjunctiva: a series of three cases. Ophthalmology. 2000;107(4):801–5.
13. Yadav R, Battoo AJ, Mir AW, Haji AG. Bulbar conjunctival metastasis from mucoepidermoid carcinoma of parotid-a case report and review of literature. World J Surg Oncol. 2017;15(1):10.
14. Hamam R, Bhat P, Foster CS. Conjunctival/corneal intraepithelial neoplasia. Int Ophthalmol Clin. 2009;49(1):63–70.
15. Pe'er J. Ocular surface squamous neoplasia. Ophthalmol Clin North Am. 2005;18(1):1–13, vii.
16. Vargason CW, Mawn LA. Management of inflammation and periocular malignancy in the anophthalmic socket. Int Ophthalmol Clin. 2017;57(1):103–16.
17. Campanella PC, Goldberg SH, Erlichman K, Abendroth C. Squamous cell tumors and ocular prostheses. Ophthalmic Plast Reconstr Surg. 1998;14(1):45–9.
18. Whittaker KW, Trivedi D, Bridger J, Sandramouli S. Ocular surface squamous neoplasia: report of an unusual case and review of the literature. Orbit. 2002;21(3):209–15.
19. Nguyen J, Ivan D, Esmaeli B. Conjunctival squamous cell carcinoma in the anophthalmic socket. Ophthalmic Plast Reconstr Surg. 2008;24(2):98–101.
20. Espana EM, Levine M, Schoenfield L, Singh AD. Ocular surface squamous neoplasia in an anophthalmic socket 60 years after enucleation. Surv Ophthalmol. 2011;56(6):539–43.
21. Barrett RV, Meyer DR, Carlson JA. Conjunctival squamous cell carcinoma in situ in the anophthalmic socket. Ophthalmic Plast Reconstr Surg. 2010;26(1):52–3.
22. Venkateswaran N, Mercado C, Galor A, Karp CL. Comparison of topical 5-fluorouracil and interferon Alfa-2b as primary treatment modalities for ocular surface squamous neoplasia. Am J Ophthalmol. 2019;199:216–22.
23. Blasi MA, Maceroni M, Sammarco MG, Pagliara MM. Mitomycin C or interferon as adjuvant therapy to surgery for ocular surface squamous neoplasia: comparative study. Eur J Ophthalmol. 2018;28(2):204–9.
24. Giaconi JA, Karp CL. Current treatment options for conjunctival and corneal intraepithelial neoplasia. Ocul Surf. 2003;1(2):66–73.
25. Tabin G, Levin S, Snibson G, Loughnan M, Taylor H. Late recurrences and the necessity for long-term follow-up in corneal and conjunctival intraepithelial neoplasia. Ophthalmology. 1997;104(3):485–92.
26. Stannard C, Sauerwein W, Maree G, Lecuona K. Radiotherapy for ocular tumours. Eye (Lond). 2013;27(2):119–27.
27. Kenawy N, Lake SL, Coupland SE, Damato BE. Conjunctival melanoma and melanocytic intra-epithelial neoplasia. Eye (Lond). 2013;27(2):142–52.
28. Scuderi G, Balestrazzi E. Conjunctival melanoma in an anophthalmic orbit. Ophthalmologica. 1973;166(3):172–4.
29. Mahajan A, Shields CL, Eagle RC Jr, Mashayekhi A, Freire JE, Shields JA. Conjunctival melanoma 3 years after radiation and chemotherapy for retinoblastoma. J Pediatr Ophthalmol Strabismus. 2007;44(5):300–2.

30. Kuo CH, Gao K, Clifford A, Shannon K, Clark J. Orbital exenterations: an 18-year experience from a single head and neck unit. ANZ J Surg. 2011;81(5):326–30.
31. Nemet AY, Martin P, Benger R, Kourt G, Sharma V, Ghabrial R, Danks J. Orbital exenteration: a 15-year study of 38 cases. Ophthalmic Plast Reconstr Surg. 2007;23(6):468–72.
32. Lee PS, Sedrak P, Guha-Thakurta N, Chang EI, Ginsberg LE, Esmaeli B, Debnam JM. Imaging findings of recurrent tumors after orbital exenteration and free flap reconstruction. Ophthalmic Plast Reconstr Surg. 2014;30(4):315–21.
33. Lane KA, Bilyk JR. Preliminary study of positron emission tomography in the detection and management of orbital malignancy. Ophthalmic Plast Reconstr Surg. 2006;22(5):361–5.

Chapter 18
Cosmetic Interventions in Anophthalmia

Michelle W. Latting, Ann Q. Tran, and Wendy W. Lee

Introduction

Following enucleation or evisceration, a primary goal of the surgeon is to construct a socket capable of maintaining an ocular prosthesis that together with the surrounding adnexal structures has a natural appearance and is symmetric with that of the contralateral eye and adnexa. In the management of the anophthalmic socket, the distinction between functional and aesthetic indications for surgery is often indistinct. At one end of the continuum lie patients who experience contraction of the socket with obliteration of the conjunctival fornices and complete inability to maintain an ocular prosthesis. Management of socket contracture is discussed elsewhere within the text. At the other end of the continuum lie patients who are able to maintain an ocular prosthesis but who are bothered by asymmetries between the anophthalmic socket and the healthy contralateral eye and adnexa.

Following enucleation or evisceration, many patients develop what is called post-enucleation/evisceration socket syndrome (PESS) characterized by enophthalmos, a deep superior sulcus, blepharoptosis, and laxity of the lower eyelid. Laxity of the lower eyelid and subsequent inferior displacement of the ocular prosthesis together give rise to the "dropped socket" appearance of the anophthalmic orbit (Fig. 18.1).

While the purpose of many surgical interventions for the anophthalmic socket is to improve the ability to maintain an ocular prosthesis or to enhance comfort associated with ocular prosthesis wear, other surgeries will have both functional and cosmetic implications. For example, tightening the lower eyelid to correct lower eyelid laxity may improve ability to maintain an ocular prosthesis while also placing the ocular prosthesis in a position that improves the appearance of a sunken superior

M. W. Latting · A. Q. Tran · W. W. Lee (✉)
Bascom Palmer Eye Institute, University of Miami Miller School of Medicine, Miami, FL, USA
e-mail: WLee@med.miami.edu

T. E. Johnson (ed.), *Anophthalmia*,
https://doi.org/10.1007/978-3-030-29753-4_18

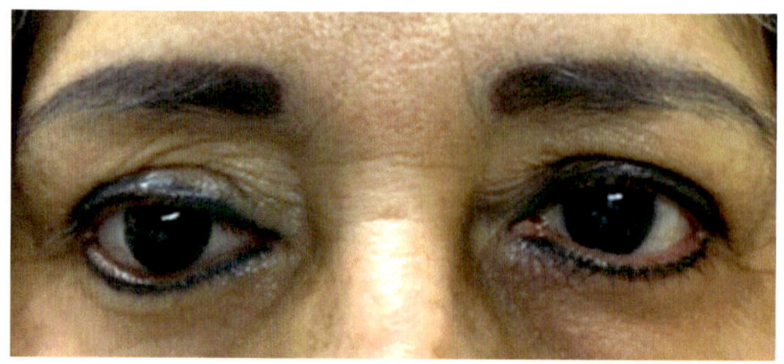

Fig. 18.1 Right anophthalmic socket with inferior displacement of the right upper eyelid, right lower eyelid, and right ocular prosthesis giving rise to a "dropped socket" appearance

sulcus. Similarly, interventions principally driven by the patient's desire to achieve greater symmetry and a more natural appearance may have additional functional benefits. For example, volume augmentation procedures to address anophthalmic enophthalmos may improve both facial symmetry as well as the fit and motility of an ocular prosthesis. As with strabismus surgery in densely amblyopic or non-seeing eyes, there are psychosocial benefits to restoring a natural, and symmetric appearance for the patient with an anophthalmic socket, even in the absence of functional complaints.

Aesthetic concerns in patients with anophthalmia largely fall into two general categories: those secondary to orbital volume deficiency and others related to eyelid malpositions. Considerable overlap exists between categories as orbital volume deficiency may contribute directly or indirectly to eyelid malposition.

In addition to aesthetic concerns related to orbital volume deficiency and eyelid malposition, additional cosmetic concerns may arise related to adjacent facial contour abnormalities, for example, in the setting of facial fractures, following soft tissue lacerations or in the setting of prior radiation therapy. Addressing these concerns may require the use of custom facial implants, autologous fat grafts, facial fillers, or cosmetic lasers and chemotherapeutic agents for the purpose of scar revision. Discussion of these interventions is beyond the scope of this chapter. Cosmetic concerns related to the appearance of the ocular prosthesis itself are addressed elsewhere in the text.

Orbital Volume Deficiency: Etiologies and Clinical Findings

Much of the asymmetry seen with an anophthalmic socket is due to the relative deficit in the soft tissue volume of the anophthalmic orbit. At the time of enucleation or evisceration surgery, a primary orbital implant is typically placed that together with the ocular prosthesis will replace the majority of the volume lost with removal of the eye or intraocular contents. The average volume of the adult globe is 8 cm^3. According to Smit et al., at the time of enucleation, an additional 4 cm^3 of soft tissue loss occurs [1]. Placement of a 20-mm spherical implant replaces approximately 4 cm^3. Placement of an ocular prosthesis replaces an additional 1.5–4 cm^3 [1]. This results in a residual volume deficit of 6.5–4 cm^3. In the presence of unrepaired

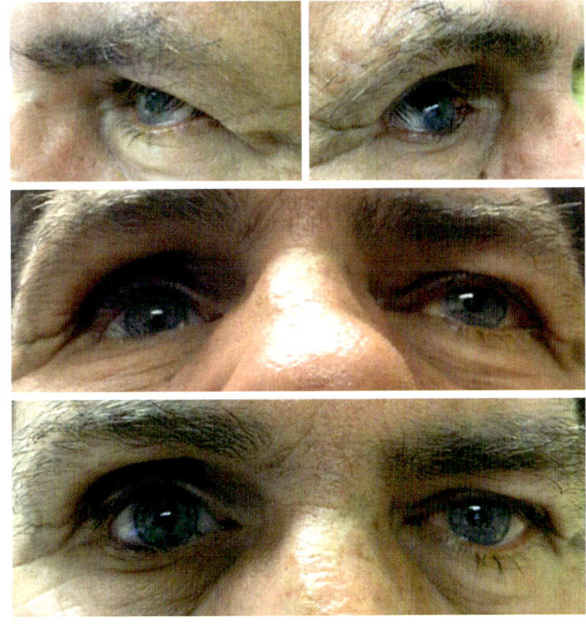

Fig. 18.2 Right anophthalmic socket with severe volume deficiency in a patient with a remote history of trauma. The superior sulcus above the right upper eyelid is deep and has a sunken appearance. A CT scan is obtained to confirm the absence of orbital wall fractures given the history of trauma

orbital fractures, orbital radiation, or other causes of soft tissue fibrosis, the soft tissue volume deficit may be even greater.

In some cases, such as in the setting of infection, the surgeon may defer placement of a primary orbital implant in favor of placement of a secondary orbital implant at a later time. In the absence of orbital volume replacement, significant enophthalmos may result.

Signs of volume deficiency on exam include relative enophthalmos as measured by Hertel exophthalmometry (comparing the anterior projection of the surface of the ocular prosthesis with anterior surface of the cornea of the contralateral eye), and a deepened superior sulcus which is referred to as the superior sulcus deformity (Fig. 18.2).

Etiologies for orbital soft tissue volume deficiency in anophthalmic enophthalmos are diverse, and include absence of a primary implant, implant of insufficient volume, fat atrophy (for example, in the setting of trauma or prior radiation), tissue fibrosis or contraction, and relative volume deficiency due to orbital fractures resulting in bony orbital volume expansion.

Compounding the loss of volume are the effects of gravity and destabilization of the orbital suspensory ligaments either from trauma or secondary to the enucleation or evisceration surgery. These factors result in inferior displacement of orbital contents, giving rise to a relative lack of volume within the superior orbit. Together, these factors contribute to the sunken in appearance of the superior sulcus that characterizes the superior sulcus deformity.

Prior to any non-surgical or surgical intervention to address orbital volume deficiency in an anophthalmic patient, a thorough history and physical exam should be performed. The patient history should include the indication for removal of the globe, the type of surgery performed (enucleation or evisceration), history of orbital trauma and associated fractures, prior periocular or orbital malignancy, and history of radiation therapy.

Additionally, the surgeon should obtain the prior operative report detailing the initial enucleation or evisceration surgery. On reviewing the prior operative report, the surgeon should ascertain if an orbital implant was placed, the type and size of the implant, and whether the extraocular muscles were secured to the implant or wrapping material. If this information is unavailable, a non-contrast CT scan of the orbit may be obtained to determine the presence or absence of an orbital implant and its location within the orbit. In the patient with a history of prior trauma, a CT scan should be obtained to rule out orbital fractures and subsequent orbital volume expansion as this information may alter the surgeon's choice of procedure for volume restoration.

Orbital Volume Deficiency: Options for Management

Numerous non-surgical and surgical options exist for the patient with cosmetic concerns related to orbital volume deficiency. If the volume deficiency is mild, satisfactory outcomes may be achieved by revision of the ocular prosthesis alone. If revision of the ocular prosthesis alone is unable or unlikely to produce adequate results, then a procedure to increase the apparent soft tissue volume within the orbit may be indicated.

In patients for whom a primary implant was not placed at the time of the initial evisceration or enucleation procedure, volume augmentation may be achieved by placement of a secondary orbital implant, most commonly an alloplastic spherical implant or dermis fat graft. Patients with anophthalmic enophthalmos despite the presence of an orbital implant may benefit from implant exchange with placement of an implant of larger volume. Techniques for secondary orbital implant placement and implant exchange are addressed elsewhere in the text.

Revision of Ocular Prosthesis

In patients with mild volume deficiency, revision of the ocular prosthesis alone may be sufficient to minimize the appearance of enophthalmos. Anophthalmic patients should therefore be referred to the ocularist for ocular prosthesis revision prior to proceeding with any non-incisional procedure or incisional surgery to address their concern of asymmetry. In addition to improving the appearance of enophthalmos, replacing the ocular prosthesis with a thicker ocular prosthesis or one with a more prominent projection into the superior orbit may also help to augment the sunken appearance of the superior sulcus and improve blepharoptosis. The vast majority of the weight of the ocular prosthesis is born by the lower eyelid. Consequently, increasing the size or thickness of the ocular prosthesis may, with time, worsen lower eyelid laxity and contribute to the dropped socket appearance.

For many patients, revision of the ocular prosthesis alone is unable to produce adequate reduction in the appearance of enophthalmos and achieve the patient's goal of improved symmetry. For patients unable to achieve satisfactory cosmesis by a revision of the prosthesis, a number of non-incisional procedures and surgical options are available to improve symmetry and enhance cosmesis.

Volume Augmentation with Supplemental Implant Material: Non-surgical/Non-incisional Options for Volume Augmentation

Increasingly, patients are seeking non-surgical/non-incisional options to address their cosmetic and functional concerns. Non-incisional options for addressing orbital soft tissue volume deficiency in the anophthalmic socket largely involve injection of various biocompatible substances into the orbit to restore volume. Injectable silicone, non-cross-linked collagen, cross-linked collagen, hyaluronic acid gel, calcium hydroxylapatite, and autogenous fat have all been used as injectable materials for the purpose of achieving orbital volume restoration.

Non-surgical alternatives for volume restoration have several advantages compared to traditional surgeries. The procedures involve minimal to no surgical morbidity and consequently, little to no surgical downtime. Furthermore, these procedures can be performed in patients with medical comorbidities that make them poor surgical candidates. Many providers chose to perform injections in the office or minor OR setting negating operating room costs and the risks of general anesthesia. Additionally, injections can be done in a graded, stepwise fashion to achieve the desired results.

Similar to surgically implanted materials designed to remedy orbital volume loss, injectable products have a risk of infection, migration, extrusion, and localized inflammation. Additional risks of intraorbital injection include orbital ache, vasovagal response/oculocardiac reflex bradycardia, foreign body reactions, allergic reactions, eyelid swelling, orbital cellulitis, peribulbar hemorrhage, intravascular injection, and globe perforation. Some injectable substances partially or completely resorb with time. The lack of permanent effect and need for subsequent volume augmentation will lead some patients to favor more permanent surgical options over injections.

In general, injections are made transconjunctivally or transcutaneously, most commonly with the point of entry for transcutaneous injections occurring at the lateral third of the lower eyelid at the level of the inferior orbital rim. The material injected may be injected into the subperiosteal, supraperiosteal, extraconal, or intraconal space or into the preaponeurotic fat. Injection into the preaponeurotic fat

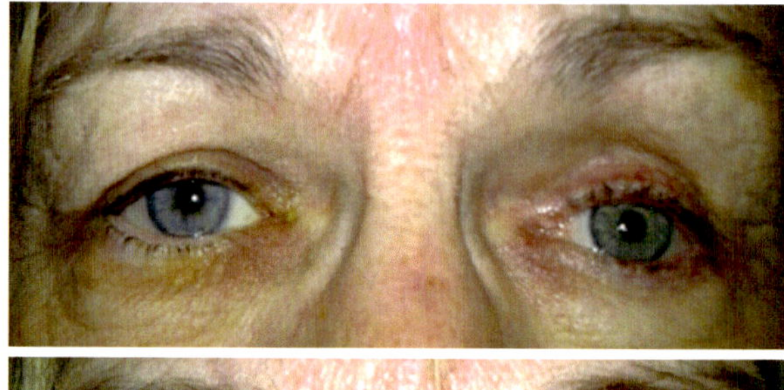
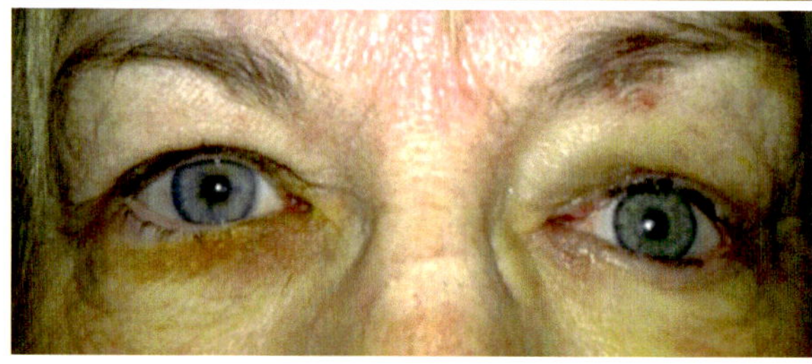

Fig. 18.3 Hyaluronic acid filler was injected into the left superior sulcus to correct a superior sulcus deformity in a patient with an anophthalmic left socket. Before (top image) and after (bottom image) injection of hyaluronic acid filler

of the upper eyelid carries the risk of causing or exacerbating upper eyelid blepharoptosis due to local effects on the levator palpebrae superioris muscle and its aponeurosis. A trial injection of saline may be used prior to injection of the volume-enhancing substance in order to confirm the absence of ptosis following injection. To fill a superior sulcus deformity injections may be given just beneath or anterior to the superior orbital rim directly into the sulcus in a supraperiosteal plane (Fig. 18.3). Care should be taken to inject conservative volumes, as material can be easily evident as lumps, bumps, or Tyndall effect under the thin upper eyelid skin. As well, care must be taken to avoid intravascular injection which can lead to soft tissue necrosis.

Patients with a history of multiple prior orbital surgeries, severe trauma, prior radiation therapy, or other causes of extensive orbital soft tissue fibrosis may be less likely to respond to volume augmentation procedures due to orbital fibrosis and subsequent immobility of the orbital implant. Patients with extensive fibrosis and immobility of the orbital implant may be more likely to have anterior migration of filler and should be specifically advised of this increased risk. Some clinicians recommend a trial injection of local anesthetic or normal saline to confirm implant mobility and the potential for treatment benefit with volume augmentation. Although some clinicians aim for intraconal injection, others avoid injecting within the intraconal space due to concern that resistance from the extraocular muscles will limit the desired anterior displacement of the implant and that stretch of the extraocular muscles may cause patient discomfort. Injection at the orbital apex is avoided to prevent inadvertent intravascular injection within the larger vessels that travel within the superior and inferior orbital fissure. Additionally, intravascular injection may be avoided by using a large bore, blunt-tipped cannula and injecting small aliquots while withdrawing the needle or injection cannula.

Injection of Hyaluronic Acid Gel

Hyaluronic acid is a cross-linked, naturally occurring polysaccharide commonly used for facial soft tissue augmentation. Intraorbital injection of the hyaluronic acid gel, Restylane Sub-Q (Restylane Sub-Q; Q-med, Uppsala, Sweden), has been described by several authors for the purpose of addressing volume deficits in anophthalmic sockets, although this product is not FDA approved for use in the United States [2–4]. Injection of hyaluronic acid gel into the orbit can be performed transconjunctivally or transcutaneously. If a transconjunctival approach is employed, topical anesthetic may be applied to the conjunctiva followed by betadine or other antibacterial solution. A 23-gauge 25-mm needle or 19 G blunt-tipped cannula is inserted into the inferotemporal conjunctival fornix and directed posteriorly. If a transcutaneous injection is employed, a peribulbar injection of local anesthetic may be delivered prior to injection of the hyaluronic acid gel. Peribulbar injection of local anesthetic may make it difficult to determine the quantity of hyaluronic gel necessary to achieve the desired effect. Some clinicians avoid peribulbar injection of local anesthesia for this reason.

Hyaluronic acid gel may be injected into the intraconal or extraconal space, posterior to the equator of the implant if present. 2–4 ml of hyaluronic acid gel is typically injected. Multiple authors have advocated injection as a single bolus to create a "lake" of hyaluronic acid gel to minimize the surface area to volume ratio and decrease the rate of resorption [2].

Hyaluronic acid can be dissolved with hyaluronidase resulting in a reversible effect if side effects or undesired outcomes result. Hyaluronic acid products resorb naturally with time, and repeat injections may be necessary to maintain adequate orbital volume. Zamani et al. found a shorter duration of effect with injection of hyaluronic acid gel in the orbit compared with injection in the dermis [2]. The reason for the shorter duration of affect is unknown.

Injection of Calcium Hydroxylapatite

Like hyaluronic acid products, calcium hydroxylapatite (CaHA) is most commonly injected into facial soft tissues but can be used off label for orbital volume augmentation. Several authors have described intraorbital injection of Radiesse (Merz Aesthetics., Raleigh, NC, U.S.A.) for orbital volume augmentation in anophthalmic sockets. Radiesse is composed of 30% CaHA microspheres in an aqueous gel carrier. Similar to the injection of hyaluronic acid gel, calcium hydroxylapatite filler can be injected transconjunctivally or transcutaneously.

Kotlus et al. describe transconjunctival intraorbital injection of calcium hydroxylapatite filler [5]. After instillation of a topical anesthetic, the calcium hydroxylapatite filler is injected transconjunctivally into the subperiosteal space of the orbital floor using a 25-gauge 1.5-inch needle. The calcium hydroxylapatite filler is injected beneath the periosteum, posterior to the orbital implant.

Vagefi et al. describe transcutaneous intraorbital injection of calcium hydroxylapatite filler [6]. Local anesthesia is achieved by injection of lidocaine into the lateral aspect of the lower eyelid and along the orbital floor prior to injection of filler. Alternatively, 0.2 ml of 2% lidocaine hydrochloride can be mixed with each syringe of filler. Vagefi et al. switched from the former approach to the latter approach due to peribulbar hemorrhage in one patient following injection of local anesthetic as well as difficulty judging the volume of filler needed after injection of local anesthetic [6]. A 27-gauge 1.25-inch retrobulbar needle can be passed transcutaneously through the lower eyelid into the medial, inferior, and lateral extraconal space. Vagefi et al. reported a 2.4-mm mean improvement in enophthalmos for each syringe of filler used [6]. Buchanan et al. advise against injecting while withdrawing the needle through the eyelid to avoid anterior displacement of the filler [7].

Unlike hyaluronic acid products, calcium hydroxylapatite filler cannot be dissolved by hyaluronidase, and the effect cannot easily be reversed if the patient is dissatisfied with the cosmetic result. A longer duration of effect has been reported with injection of calcium hydroxylapatite filler in the orbit compared with injection into the facial soft tissues, presumably due to decreased movement within the orbit. Other postulated reasons for the longer duration of effect with intraorbital injection include decreased vascularity and absence of lymphatic drainage [6].

Injection of Autologous Fat

Injection of autologous fat has less risk of rejection or sensitivity reaction when compared with injection of fillers. Fat can be harvested from the abdomen or thigh using an aspiration cannula and microsuction technique. A feathered approach may be employed to prevent contour irregularities in the area of fat removal. The processed fat may be injected transconjunctivally or transcutaneously into the intraconal and extraconal space using a 14-gauge needle or 16-gauge blunt-tipped cannula. Injecting while withdrawing the needle or cannula helps to prevent inadvertent intravascular injection.

Avoid significant extraconal injection as this may cause shallowing of the conjunctival fornices and inability to retain an ocular prosthesis. Hardy et al. advise injecting in 0.1–0.2-ml aliquots in different locations to reduce graft volume to surface ratio and consequently enhance vascularization and survival of the graft [8]. Injection of 1 ml of fat yields approximately 1-mm reduction in relative enophthalmos as measured by Hertel [9]. Compared with block fat grafts, injection of autologous fat is associated with minimal donor site morbidity and may have less secondary volume loss due to resorption.

Volume Augmentation with Supplemental Implant Material: Surgical Options for Volume Augmentation

Patients with profound enophthalmos, coexisting orbital wall fractures, or prior sub-optimal response to non-incisional volume-enhancing procedures may benefit from surgical volume augmentation. Surgical options for orbital volume restoration involve the placement of alloplastic implants or autologous grafts within the orbit or periorbital space. Alloplastic implants include bone cement, PMMA, silicone and porous polyethylene wedge-shaped implants, blocks, or sheets, room temperature vulcanizing silicone, cadaver costal cartilage, glass beads, and Proplast (synthetic porous composite of Teflon polymer and alumina). Autogenous grafts used in orbital volume restoration include dermis, fat (block transplants), bone (ex. split calvarial bone grafts), and cartilage.

With the exception of block fat transplants, alloplastic materials and autogenous grafts placed surgically to restore orbital volume generally do not resorb. Consequently, a surgically placed implant may be preferred by the patient seeking a more permanent solution to orbital volume deficiency. Risks of surgery include migration or extrusion of the implant, infection, and foreign body reaction.

Following orbital injection of filler or fat, patients are typically able to resume wear of their ocular prosthesis or be fitted for a new ocular prosthesis without a significant delay to allow for healing. By contrast, most surgical procedures to restore orbital volume require a period of rehabilitation during which time the patient is unable to wear their ocular prosthesis or be fitted for a new prosthesis. Anticipated recovery time and limitations during surgical rehabilitation should be discussed with the patient prior to surgery.

To augment orbital volume, surgical implants are most commonly placed in the subperiosteal space along the orbital floor accessed via a transcutaneous subciliary incision or a transconjunctival incision through the inferior fornix. The secondary implant is placed with the greatest volume immediately posterior to the equator of the spherical implant to push the spherical implant anteriorly and superiorly. After placement of the implant, many surgeons will close the periosteum over the implant to prevent implant extrusion. A frost suture is commonly left in place for several days to prevent the development of lower eyelid retraction.

Although less commonly utilized, the subperiosteal space along the superolateral orbital wall may be accessed via an incision over the lateral canthus. Positioning the implant within the subperiosteal space of the superior orbit provides general volume augmentation and also has a direct effect on the appearance of a sunken superior sulcus.

Direct augmentation of the superior sulcus can be achieved by placement of an implant within the retroseptal space of the superior orbit anterior to the preaponeurotic fat. This region can be accessed via an upper eyelid crease incision with little to no visible scar after the healing process is complete. Materials that may be surgically implanted in this space include free fat, a dermis-fat graft, Alloderm, and temporoparietal fascia. The placement of an implant within the preaponeurotic space may reduce the appearance of a sunken superior sulcus but does not improve enophthalmos and may worsen blepharoptosis due to its effect on the levator palpebrae superioris and its aponeurosis.

Eyelid Malposition

Upper Eyelid Blepharoptosis

In general, blepharoptosis in the patient with anophthalmia can be thought of as caused by one of three factors: primary issues with the levator superioris muscle or its aponeurosis (ex. dehiscence, lack of innervation), inadequate support of the levator muscle complex (ex. orbital soft tissue deficiency, orbital floor fracture with depressed intraorbital contents, small or displaced orbital implant), and issues related to the prosthesis itself (ex. small prosthesis, prosthesis with protein deposits causing secondary conjunctival inflammation).

Trauma to the levator muscle or aponeurosis may occur at the time of initial globe injury, at the time of enucleation or evisceration, or over time with repeated removal and insertion of an ocular prosthesis. Orbital fractures, particularly orbital floor fractures, may be associated with herniation and inferior displacement of orbital contents and subsequent alterations in the suspensory system that supports the levator muscle complex. Additionally, disruption of the suspensory ligaments within the orbit at the time of enucleation may alter the points of support that allow the levator muscle to exercise its maximal effect. Similarly, loss of soft tissue volume within the orbit due to orbital fat atrophy of any cause may affect the ability of the levator muscle to function optimally. With both enucleation and evisceration surgeries, excessive advancement of the conjunctiva over an orbital implant may result in secondary advancement of the superior rectus-levator complex and subsequent blepharoptosis.

On exam, upper eyelid ptosis may be masked by concurrent lower eyelid laxity and inferior displacement of the ocular prosthesis. An increase in the distance between the upper eyelid margin and upper eyelid crease may provide quantitative evidence of blepharoptosis as a contributing factor to the patient's asymmetry. Prosthetic surface irregularities, giant papillary conjunctivitis, and conjunctival pyogenic granulomas should be ruled out as a cause of blepharoptosis.

Non-surgical options for addressing mild blepharoptosis include modification of the ocular prosthesis. Adding a superior projection to the ocular prosthesis may provide support for the levator aponeurosis providing modest elevation of the upper eyelid. Similarly, adding volume to the corneal apex of the prosthesis may provide support for the upper eyelid preventing downward descent. Adding volume to the ocular prosthesis, however, increases the weight of the prosthesis and may exacerbate lower eyelid laxity. A particularly bulky prosthesis may also give the appearance of a bulging eye. Prior to any surgical intervention, the patient should be referred to an ocularist for optimization of the ocular prosthesis. For the patient who wishes to avoid surgical intervention, custom eyewear may aid in disguising facial asymmetry. Glasses in which the superior rim of the spectacle frame bisects the upper eyelid may provide a visual distraction from the upper eyelid height.

Many patients with anophthalmic sockets will have both blepharoptosis and evidence of loss of orbital soft tissue volume. In some cases, restoring orbital soft tissue volume alone may be sufficient to correct mild ptosis by reestablishing structural support to the levator superioris muscle and its aponeurosis. Kaltreider et al. found that orbital volume augmentation with an intraconal or extraconal implant lead to improvement in blepharoptosis in 30% of anophthalmic patients [10]. Thus, one should consider volume augmentation, prior to blepharoptosis surgery in the anophthalmic patient with both enophthalmos and blepharoptosis.

When blepharoptosis surgery is indicated, levator resection or advancement is often preferred to Müller's muscle conjunctival resection as external blepharoptosis repair avoids loss of conjunctiva and minimizes the risk of socket contracture. Care should be taken to avoid the removal of large amounts of preaponeurotic fat as fat removal can exacerbate the appearance of a sunken superior sulcus.

Although preservation of conjunctiva is a top priority in patients with anophthalmic sockets, many surgeons will consider Müller's muscle conjunctival resection (MMCR) for the correction of blepharoptosis in select patients, particularly those with an enlarged superior conjunctival fornix. 10% phenylephrine testing performed with the patient's prosthesis in place may be used to assess the likely response to surgery. Putterman and Urist were the first to describe the MMCR procedure [11]. Since their initial report, several authors have described conjunctival sparing Müller's muscle resection procedures that may be of particular value in patients with anophthalmic sockets for whom preservation of healthy conjunctiva is desired [12, 13].

Upper Eyelid Retraction

Upper eyelid retraction has been reported rarely in patients with anophthalmic sockets [14, 15]. It is thought to be a late complication of anophthalmia with the postulated mechanism being contracture of the levator palpebrae superioris muscle due to its role as an antagonist to an underused orbicularis oculi muscle [15]. Upper eyelid retraction is thought to occur most commonly many years after the initial enucleation or evisceration surgery. Upper eyelid retraction may be corrected by recession of the levator palpebrae superioris or Müller's muscle.

Lower Eyelid Laxity

In many instances, anophthalmic enophthalmos and blepharoptosis may be improved by revision of the ocular prosthesis. However, the weight of the ocular prosthesis is borne by the lower eyelid and increasing the weight of the prosthesis may cause or exacerbate lower eyelid laxity. Lower eyelid laxity is most often corrected by horizontally shortening the lower eyelid using the lateral tarsal strip procedure. Although uncommonly utilized, a fascia lata sling may be used to provide additional structural support [16, 17]. As well, dermal filler can be injected into the middle lamella for structural support. Lower eyelid laxity should be addressed prior to surgical correction of upper eyelid blepharoptosis as correction of lower eyelid laxity may alter the position of the ocular prosthesis and consequently the position of the upper eyelid.

Lower Eyelid Retraction

Lower eyelid retraction may occur in the anophthalmic patient due to contraction of the posterior lamellae. If the retraction is 2 mm or less, a simple release of the lower eyelid retractors may suffice. If more than 2 mm of retraction exists, a spacer graft may be necessary. A hard palate mucosa graft can serve as a spacer between the inferior border of the tarsus and the lower eyelid retractors increasing the vertical height of the lower eyelid. Other alternatives for spacer grafts include dermis, auricular cartilage, a free tarsal graft from the upper eyelid, and non-autologous implants including cross-linked porcine collagen (ENDURAGen), and acellular cadaveric dermis (AlloDerm) [18].

Conclusion

Rehabilitation of the patient with an anophthalmic socket includes interventions to reduce cosmetic deformities associated with loss of the globe. A variety of non-surgical and surgical options are available to decrease disfigurement and restore a natural appearance. Optimization of the ocular prosthesis should be achieved prior to any surgical intervention as mild deformities may be improved with revision of the prosthesis alone. As a general rule, orbital volume replacement should precede eyelid surgery as the appearance, motility, and overall function of the eyelids may be improved by restoring normal orbital soft tissue volume. When surgery is indicated to address eyelid malpositions, tightening of the lower eyelid should proceed surgical correction of upper eyelid blepharoptosis as laxity of the lower eyelid will alter the position of the ocular prosthesis and confuse the assessment of upper eyelid blepharoptosis. After any surgical procedure, the patient should be referred back to the ocularist to reassess the fit of the ocular prosthesis. Close collaboration between the surgeon and a skilled ocularist is key to achieving optimal results.

References

1. Smit TJ, Koornneef L, Zonneveld FW, et al. Computed tomography in the assessment of the postenucleation socket syndrome. Ophthalmology. 1990;97(10):1347–51.
2. Zamani M, Thyagarajan S, Olver JM. Adjunctive use of hyaluronic acid gel (Restylane Sub-Q) in anophthalmic volume deficient sockets and phthisical eyes. Ophthalmic Plast Reconstr Surg. 2010;26(4):250–3.
3. Tay E, Olver J. Intraorbital hyaluronic acid for enophthalmos. Ophthalmology. 2008;115(6):1101–1101.e2.
4. Malhotra R. Deep orbital Sub-Q restylane (nonanimal stabilized hyaluronic acid) for orbital volume enhancement in sighted and anophthalmic orbits. Arch Ophthalmol. 2007;125(12):1623–9.
5. Kotlus BS, Dryden RM. Correction of anophthalmic enophthalmos with injectable calcium hydroxylapatite (Radiesse). Ophthalmic Plast Reconstr Surg. 2007;23(4):313–4.
6. Vagefi MR, McMullan TF, Burroughs JR, Georgescu D, McCann JD, Anderson RL. Orbital augmentation with injectable calcium hydroxylapatite for correction of postenucleation/evisceration socket syndrome. Ophthalmic Plast Reconstr Surg. 2011;27(2):90–4.
7. Buchanan AG, Holds JB, Vagefi MR, Bidar M, et al. Anterior filler displacement following injection of calcium hydroxylapatite gel (Radiesse) for anophthalmic orbital volume augmentation. Ophthalmic Plast Reconstr Surg. 2012;28(5):335–7.
8. Hardy TG, Joshi N, Kelly MH. Orbital volume augmentation with autologous micro-fat grafts. Ophthalmic Plast Reconstr Surg. 2007;23(6):445–9.
9. Hunter PD, Baker SS. The treatment of enophthalmos by orbital injection of fat autograft. Arch Otolaryngol Head Neck Surg. 1994;120(8):835–9.
10. Kaltreider SA, Shields MD, Hippeard SC, et al. Anophthalmic ptosis: investigation of the mechanisms and statistical analysis. Ophthalmic Plast Reconstr Surg. 2003;19(6):421–8.
11. Putterman AM, Urist MJ. Müller muscle-conjunctiva resection. Technique for treatment of blepharoptosis. Arch Ophthalmol. 1975;93(8):619–23.
12. Saha K, Leatherbarrow B. Conjunctival sparing Müller's muscle resection for the management of blepharoptosis in the anophthalmic patient. Clin Exp Ophthalmol. 2011;39(5):478–9.
13. Vreck I, Hogan RN, Rossen J, Mancini R. Conjunctiva-sparing posterior ptosis surgery: a novel approach. Ophthalmic Plast Reconstr Surg. 2016;32(5):366–70.
14. Shams PN, Selva D, ANZSOPS Eyelid Retraction in Anophthalmia Survey Group. Upper eyelid retraction in the anophthalmic socket: review and survey of the Australian and New Zealand Society of Ophthalmic Plastic Surgeons (ANZSOPS). Ophthalmic Plast Reconstr Surg. 2014;30(4):309–12.
15. Zolli CI. Upper eyelid retraction in long-standing anophthalmic sockets. Ann Ophthalmol. 1983;15:621–4.
16. Nolan WB 3rd, Vistnes LM. Correction of lower eyelid ptosis in the anophthalmic orbit: a long-term follow up. Plast Reconstr Surg. 1983;72(3):289–93.
17. Vistnes LM, Iverson RE, Laub DR. The anophthalmic orbit. Surgical correction of lower eyelid ptosis. Plast Reconstr Surg. 1973;52(4):346–51.
18. Massry GG, Hornblass A, Rubin P, et al. Tarsal switch procedure for the surgical rehabilitation of the eyelid and socket deficiencies of the anophthalmic socket. Ophthalmic Plast Reconstr Surg. 1999;15(5):333–40.

References Not Directly Quoted

Cahill KV, Burns JA. Volume augmentation of the anophthalmic orbit with cross-linked collagen (Zyplast). Arch Ophthalmol. 1989;107(11):1684–6.

Coleman SR. Avoidance of arterial occlusion from injection of soft tissue fillers. Aesthet Surg J. 2002;22(6):555–7.

Ding J, Ma X, Xin Y, et al. Correction of lower eyelid retraction with hard palate graft in the anophthalmic socket. Can J Ophthalmol. 2018;53(5):458–61.

Jones DF, Lyle CE, Fleming JC. Superior conjunctivoplasty-mullerectomy for correction of chronic discharge and concurrent ptosis in the anophthalmic socket with enlarged superior fornix. Ophthalmic Plast Reconstr Surg. 2010;26(3):172–5.

Karesh JW, Putterman AM, Fett DR. Conjunctiva-Müller's muscle excision to correct anophthalmic ptosis. Ophthalmology. 1986;93(8):1068–71.

Mombaerts I, Groet E. Upper eyelid ptosis surgery using a preparatory ocular prosthesis. Ophthalmic Plast Reconstr Surg. 2009;25(2):90–3.

Nerad JA. Techniques in ophthalmic plastic surgery: a personal tutorial. 1st ed. New York: Elsevier; 2010.

Quaranta-Leoni FM. Treatment of the anophthalmic socket. Curr Opin Ophthalmol. 2008;19(5):422–7.

Smith RJ, Malet T. Auricular cartilage grafting to correct lower conjunctival fornix retraction and eyelid malposition in anophthalmic patients. Ophthalmic Plast Reconstr Surg. 2008;24(1):13–8.

Tse D. Color atlas of oculoplastic surgery. 2nd ed. Philadelphia: Lippincott Williams & Wilkins; 2012.

Part IV
Pediatrics and Oncology

Chapter 19
Conservative Treatment of Congenital Clinical Anophthalmia

Chad Zatezalo, Yasser Bataineh, and Thomas E. Johnson

Introduction

Congenital anophthalmos (CA) is defined as the complete failure of outgrowth of the primary optic vesicle. This failure results from the arrest of ocular and orbital organogenesis during the fourth to seventh weeks of gestation. In cases of partial outgrowth failure, an underdeveloped globe and orbit occurs leading to a condition termed congenital microphthalmia (CM). The incidences of CA and CM have been estimated at 0.18–0.4/10,000 and 1.5–1.9/10,000, respectively [1–3]. Congenital anophthalmos and CM are often clinically indistinguishable and require similar management. In more severe cases of CM, the term clinical anophthalmos is often used. Both CA and CM may be unilateral or bilateral and associated with other systemic abnormalities, especially in bilateral cases [4]. In unilateral cases, there may also be anomalies of the contralateral eye including coloboma, lens irregularities, and optic nerve abnormalities [5]. The etiology of CA and CM is usually sporadic in nature, but environmental, toxic, and genetic factors have been cited. These factors include intrauterine infections such as rubella and cytomegalovirus, exposure to chemicals such as thalidomide, vitamin A deficiency, and radiation. Autosomal-dominant, autosomal-recessive, and X-linked anophthalmia have all been reported. A mutation in the SOX2 gene has been postulated to result in bilateral anophthalmia [6].

C. Zatezalo (✉)
The Zatezalo Group, Oculoplastics Private Practice, North Bethesda, MD, USA

Y. Bataineh
International Ocular Center, Inc, Miami and Palm Beach Gardens, FL, USA

T. E. Johnson
Bascom Palmer Eye Institute, University of Miami Miller School of Medicine, Miami, FL, USA

T. E. Johnson (ed.), *Anophthalmia*,
https://doi.org/10.1007/978-3-030-29753-4_19

Clinical Findings

Patients with CA present with a constellation of findings: no visible ocular remnant, hypoplastic bony orbit, deficient socket mucous membrane, phimotic eyelid fissure, small hypoplastic eyelids, decreased distance from the eyelashes to brow cilia, and facial asymmetry in unilateral cases.

Timing and Goals of Treatment

In the setting of CA, the bony orbit has no stimulus for growth, resulting in a greatly reduced orbital volume compared to age-matched orbits. The goals in the management of CA and CM are to replace the absent orbital volume, stimulate bony growth, enlarge the surface area of the socket mucous membrane, and lengthen and promote the growth of the eyelids. Early socket expansion and orbital volume replacement reduces facial deformity and should be started soon after birth. The normal-sized eye in a child at birth is approximately 70% that of an adult eye. By contrast, the normal-sized face at birth is only 40% that of an adult face. During the first 2 years of life, there is rapid growth of the face, and by the age of two, the face is 70% that of an adult face and reaches 90% by age 5.5 years. The rapid growth of the facial bones during the first years of life illustrates the importance of early orbital volume replacement to promote bone and soft tissue facial development [7].

Treatment Options

The treatment options for socket expansion and volume replacement include a variety of techniques: pressure conformers, serial expansion conformers, orbital tissue expanders, balloon expansion therapy, hydrophilic expanders, and surgical expansion of the orbit [8–14]. Early surgery and overly aggressive expansion using tissue expanders and expandable orbital implants can result in conjunctival scarring and socket deformity. Additionally, surgically altering the lateral canthus (i.e., canthotomy) often compromises the integrity of the canthal structures and leads to poor prosthetic retention with an undesirable cosmetic outcome [15].

The authors prefer initially treating CA with a conservative nonsurgical strategy using a sequence of gradually enlarging acrylic conformers. The expansion phase is followed by a single surgical intervention at around the age of 4–5 years. This approach requires an experienced ocularist using serial expansion conformers to accomplish the following: expand the socket soft tissue, stimulate bony orbital growth, and lengthen the eyelid fissures. Optimal results rely on close collaboration between the ocularist and the ophthalmologist.

Other treatments, including early surgery, osmotic implants, and tissue expanders, have several possible pitfalls including the need for multiple surgical interventions, high rates of complications and failures, and lack of long-term results. Overly aggressive surgical approaches can lead to the destruction of key orbital and socket anatomy [13, 16–18].

In our conservative method, patients with CA are seen as soon as possible after birth and most definitely before 1 year of age. On initial evaluation, a complete ophthalmic evaluation including ultrasound is performed, and patients are referred to a pediatrician for a systemic evaluation. Successful expansion of the socket demands patience from all members of the team.

On clinical examination, the congenital anophthalmic orbit usually has a depression or "pit" at the apex of the socket and an "acorn shape" [19]. This pit plays a crucial role in the successful expansion of the socket, and the shape of the expansion conformer should reflect the posterior pit (Fig. 19.1) [19].

Initially small acrylic conformers are used to expand the phimotic socket. As the socket tissue has a rapid initial expansion, the conformers may be changed weekly. However, the time interval between changing the expanders is gradually lengthened as the process advances. The conservative expansion process should imitate natural orbital and eyelid growth. The ocularist takes an impression and fabricates a conformer that is sequentially 1–2 mm larger each treatment session, depending on the severity of contraction found in each patient. In the early stages, that requires increasing the size and shape both horizontally and vertically. Initially, the thickness and shape of the conformer is changed approximately weekly as the socket can tolerate a larger conformer at each phase. Slowly a "balanced expansion zone" is

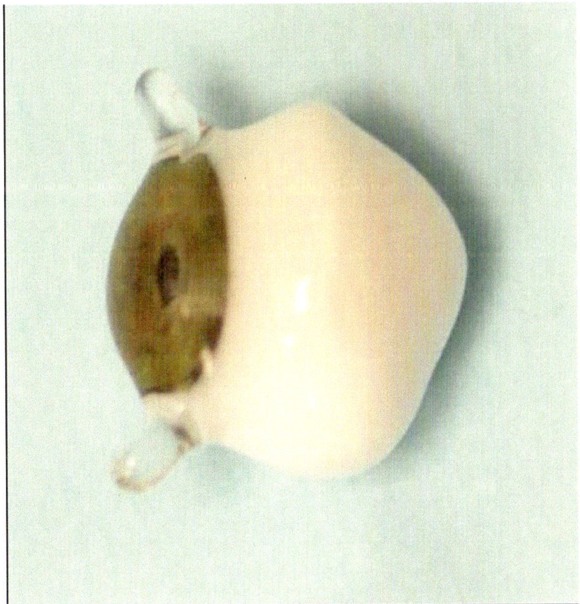

Fig. 19.1 Expansion conformer that respects the posterior pit. Horizontal phalanges assist in expansion of the fissure

entered where maximum expansion has been reached at each stage. The process includes waiting increasingly longer times for rehabilitation and recovery after each expansion, ensuring the socket has sufficient time to heal after each phase.

Following the initial impressions, the conformer shape goes through a "design-to-function expansion", targeting areas that needed to be improved while carefully manipulating the design to precisely maximize the effectiveness of expansion. This part of the process routinely takes place over 1–3-month intervals. The "design-to-function" process must not be too aggressive to allow the tissues of the socket to flourish and function. Timing is important to determine whether the socket is ready for the next stage of expansion. The speed of expansion can proceed quickly or slowly based on the individual response of each patient, and the process goes through alteration processes including vertical changes, horizontal changes, and changes in both thickness and shape. The principal determinant of when and how to make these changes is based on the functionality of the eyelids. It is critical that the eyelids are not overwhelmed to provide normalcy to every patient.

The larger expanders have a projection into the apical pit, which is a key characteristic for successful expansion. After initial expansion, phalanges are placed on the anterior lateral and medial aspects of the expanders to concurrently stretch and gently expand the eyelid tissues (Fig. 19.2). Too aggressive expansion or failure to respect the posterior pit can create a dysfunctional socket with canthal disruption and conjunctival scarring. Once the socket scars, future expansion and prosthetic fitting is a challenge. Socket tissues in children are very pliable when expansion is initiated at an early age [15]. A completely phimotic socket at birth can be successfully expanded to a near-normal configuration using this slowly progressive non-surgical technique (Fig. 19.2).

An ideal expansion conformer accomplishes three goals: expansion of the socket mucous membranes, stimulation of bony growth by orbital volume replacement, and expansion of the lid fissures for promotion of lid growth.

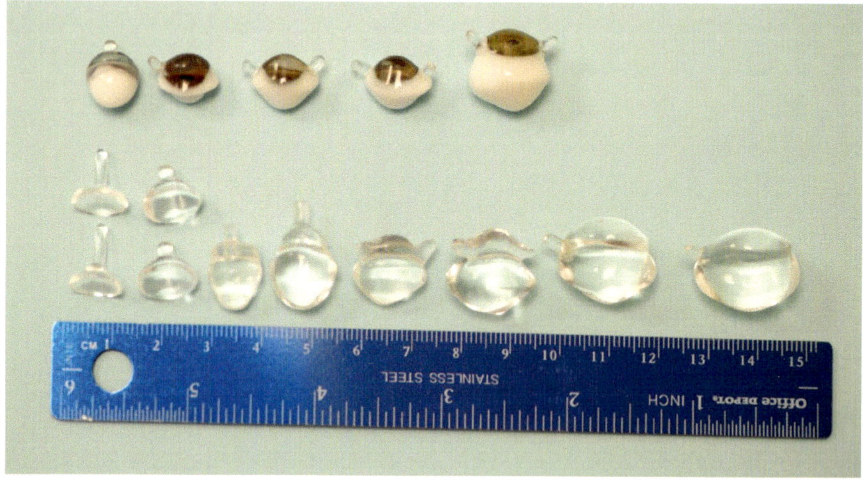

Fig. 19.2 Serial expansion conformers

The parents are counseled on the risk of re-contracture of the tissues should the expander prolapse from the socket. After the ophthalmologist and ocularist agree that the socket has been sufficiently expanded, surgical implantation at around the age of 5 years with a permanent orbital implant is planned. The authors suggest delaying the surgical intervention for at least 3 months after final expansion has been reached to prevent re-contracture. We recommend waiting until the age of 5 years of age for surgical intervention for the following reasons: reduced anesthesia risk, school age that has been reached resulting in increased social pressure, and bony orbital volume that has reached approximately 77% of that of a 15-year-old orbit when the orbit has been expanded correctly. This allows placement of an adult-sized implant [7, 20, 21]. The largest spherical implant that permits closure of Tenon's capsule and conjunctiva without undue tension is placed. If extraocular muscles are found in cases of clinical anophthalmos (true CM), they are sutured to the orbital implant to increase socket and prosthetic motility. Pressure conformers are used after implant placement to allow for additional expansion.

Surgical Intervention

Preoperatively, three pressure conformers are constructed by the ocularist (Fig. 19.3). One of these conformers is placed intra-operatively after implantation to maintain the fornixes and prevent symblepharon formation and contracture during the post-operative period.

Surgical Procedure

General anesthesia is induced, and the patient is prepped and draped in the usual sterile fashion. A lid speculum is placed, and Westcott scissors are used to incise conjunctiva and Tenon's capsule. The orbital contents are carefully inspected for

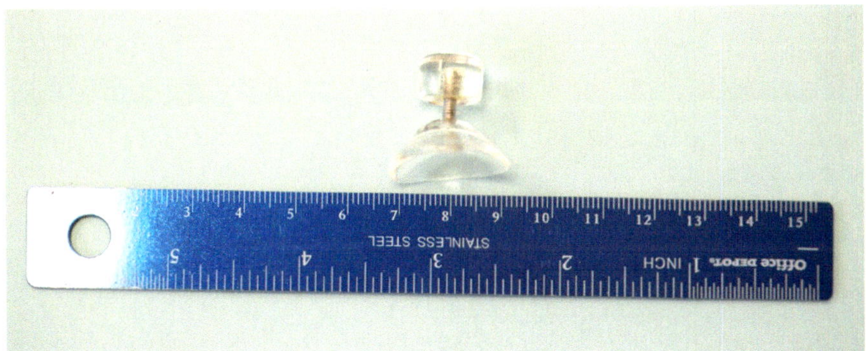

Fig. 19.3 Compression conformer

ocular tissues. If a globe or cyst is identified, the structure is removed in the standard enucleation fashion and sent for histopathologic evaluation (Figs. 19.4 and 19.5). If the extraocular muscles are attached to the identified ocular structure, they are isolated and secured using double-armed 5-0 Vicryl™ suture in standard enucleation fashion. Careful blunt dissection is performed within the orbit to create adequate

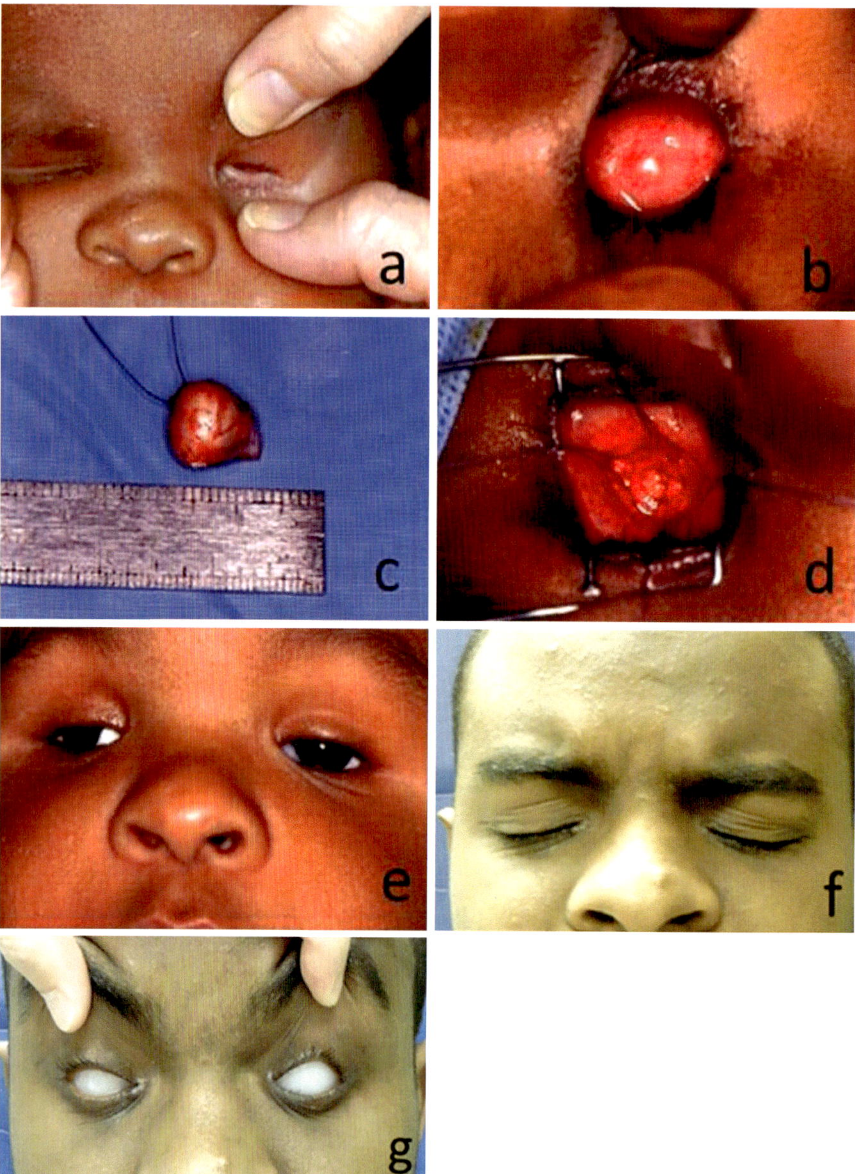

Fig. 19.4 Treatment sequence: socket expansion, enucleation of vestigial ocular remnant, and prosthesis placement. (**a**) Pre-expansion, (**b**) post-expansion, (**c**) ocular remnant removed via enucleation, (**d**) intraoperative orbit after enucleation with Vicryl™ sutures attached to extraocular muscles, (**e**) postorbital rehabilitation child, (**f**) and (**g**) late teenage year with normal bony, soft tissue, and socket anatomy

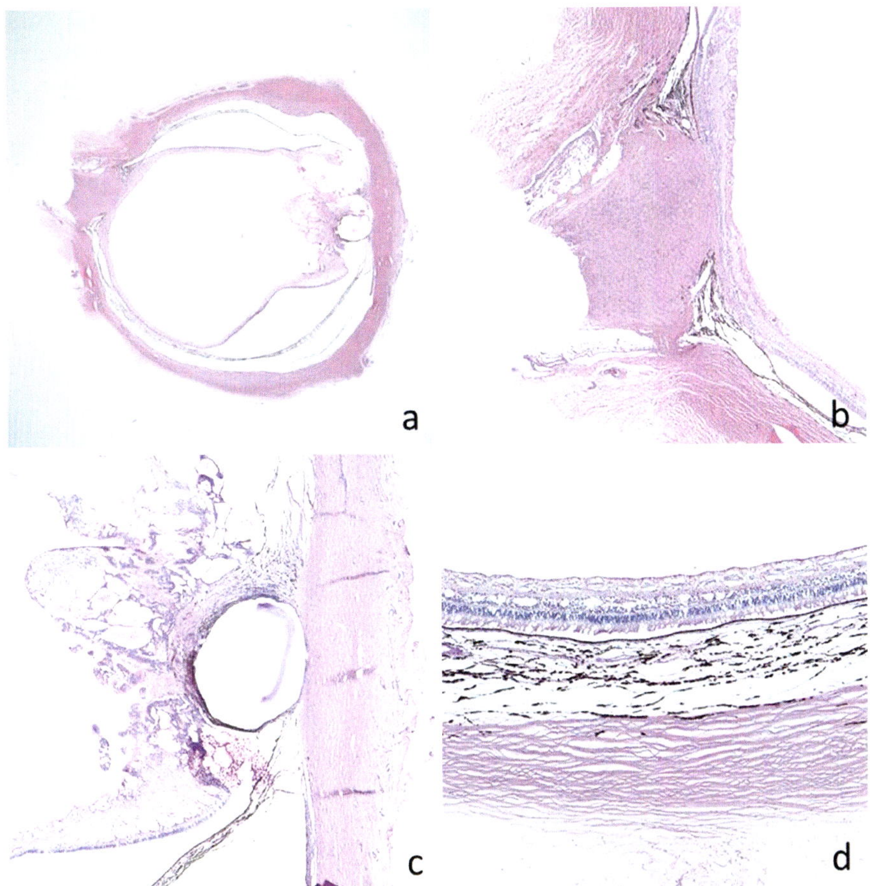

Fig. 19.5 H&E stained vestigial ocular remnant. (**a**) Microphthamic globe. Vitreous filled with dense fibrovascular connective tissue with surrounding disorganized and folded retina. Hematoxylin and eosin, 12.5× magnification. (**b**) Anteriorly pulled optic nerve head with marked optic nerve atrophy. Focal areas of gliosis present in retina. 40× magnification. (**c**) Absence of a clearly defined cornea with dense fibrovascular connective tissue similar to sclera. No distinct lens or anterior chamber is present. Collection of cuboidal cells (ciliary epithelium) is present in the region of lens. 40× magnification. (**d**) Variable loss of photoreceptor cell layer, especially inner and outer segments, and cystic changes within retina. 100× magnification

space for the permanent implant. Generally, the authors prefer to place a 16 mm or 18 mm porous polyethylene scleral-wrapped spherical implant. If the extraocular muscles are identified, four widows are cut in the sclera corresponding to the insertion of each extraocular muscle. The 5-0 Vicryl™ sutures securing the muscles are then passed through the anterior edge of the window to allow the muscle to interface with the implant. If no extraocular muscles are identified, three double-armed 5-0 Vicryl™ sutures are placed from the approximate place of extraocular muscle insertion on the scleral-wrapped implant to the fornixes laterally, medially, and inferiorly and brought out through the conjunctival fornices and tied. This technique improves postoperative motility and stability of the implant. A superior fornix suture is not placed, as this suture can lead to postoperative ptosis. Tenon's capsule and conjunctiva are closed in a layered fashion with 5-0 Vicryl™ and 6-0 plain sutures, respectively. The best-fitting pressure conformer is then placed after antibiotic ophthalmic ointment has been applied. A pressure patch is then placed, and general anesthesia is reversed.

The pressure patch is left in place for 1 week. A pressure conformer remains in place for 5 weeks while the socket is healing. After 5 weeks, a socket impression is taken, and an ocular prosthesis is created by the ocularist.

Discussion

Congenital anophthalmos and microphthalmos comprise significant functional and cosmetic deformities and can be a challenge to treat. In bilateral CA cases, the family must process both the functional blindness and cosmetic disfigurement of the child. In the past, these patients routinely underwent multiple surgical and imaging procedures, increasing the risk of scar formation, receiving unnecessary radiation and anesthesia, and producing psychological trauma to both the patient and the parents [8].

Previous published studies describing the treatment of congenital anophthalmos have several potential pitfalls including multiple surgical interventions, high rates of complications or failures, lack of long-term results, and aggressive surgical approaches leading to the destruction of key orbital anatomy. While there is a large collection of studies on acquired anophthalmos in the literature, far fewer studies address the management of congenital anophthalmos.

Previously described methods risk complications including severely scarred and contracted sockets, disruption of the lateral canthus, serial radiation and anesthesia exposure, failure to complete protocol, and implant migration [13, 16–18]. Therefore, we advocate a conservative expansion technique that preserves the apical pit of the socket and does not surgically disrupt the conjunctival surface or the lateral canthal angle. This expansion is followed by a placement of a large sclera-wrapped orbital implant after maximum expansion has been achieved, usually after 5 years of age.

Respecting the anatomy of the anophthalmic socket plays a crucial role in successful expansion. The shape of the expansion conformers should reflect the shape of the posterior pit of the socket for successful expansion. Additionally, an oval depression in the medial socket is occasionally identified and likely has similar significance in successful expansion. This conservative expansion technique demands patience from all team members, as too aggressive expansion or failure to respect the posterior pit can result in a dysfunctional socket with canthal disruption and conjunctival scarring.

The goals of gradual serial expansion with delayed surgical intervention include successful expansion of the socket mucous membrane, formation of deep conjunctival fornixes, stimulation of bony orbital growth, and promotion of eyelid growth (Figs. 19.6 and 19.7). Failure to respect the posterior pit and medial depression of the socket during expansion prolongs the expansion process and can lead to con-

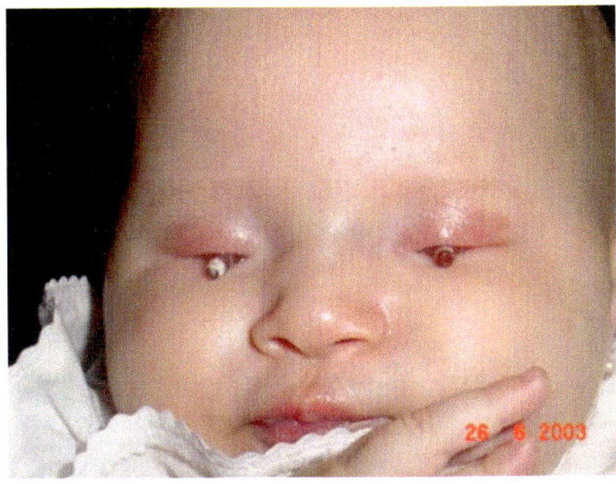

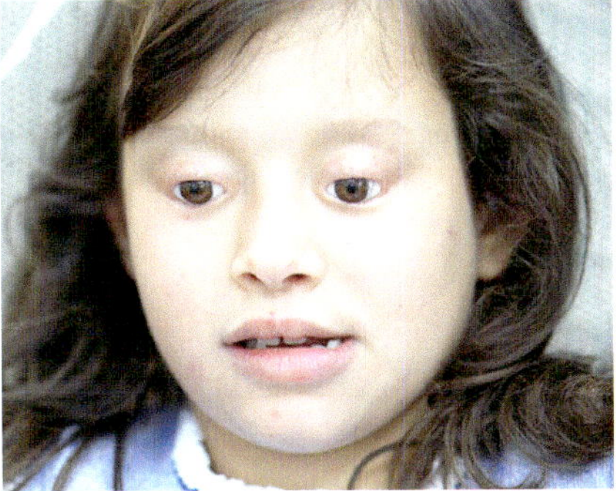

Fig. 19.6 Bony Growth. Improvement in orbital rim prominence, brow to lid margin, and horizontal and vertical fissures from initial conformer to 3 years postoperatively

junctival fibrosis. Preservation and respect for anatomy of the socket and lids, including the lateral canthal angle and conjunctiva, and avoidance of repeated surgeries will prevent progressive irreversible scarring.

The advantages of the described management approach include the elimination of the need for multiple surgeries, radiation exposure, and repeated general anesthesia. Therefore, psychological trauma to the child is decreased by minimizing the number of procedures needed. Surgical intervention is delayed to an age appropriate for non-emergent general anesthesia, reducing the risk of potential future behavioral problems and learning disabilities [20, 21]. Flick et al. illustrated that repeated exposure to anesthesia and surgery before age two is an independent risk factor for the later development of learning disabilities [21]. Instead of repeated CT scans, serial photography and clinical examination are used to measure development of the orbit (Figs. 19.6 and 19.7). By eliminating serial radiographic intervention, the risk for the development of radiation-induced malignancies is reduced, as the use of CTs in children delivers a dose of 60 mGy (2–3 head CTs) and may triple the risk of leukemia and brain cancer [22].

Patients with CA usually have lid abnormalities that may tempt the surgeon to perform a lid lengthening or elevating procedures at a young age. However, surgery to lengthen or raise the eyelid should be delayed until the orbit and lids have been maximally rehabilitated with the appropriate implant and ocular prosthesis [23]. An exception is the correction of lid colobomas that can result in inability to maintain a conformer or prosthesis.

Conclusion

Many paradigms exist for the treatment of congenital anophthalmia, most of which include early aggressive surgical intervention, disruption of crucial anatomical structures, the need for repeated use of general anesthesia, high complication rates,

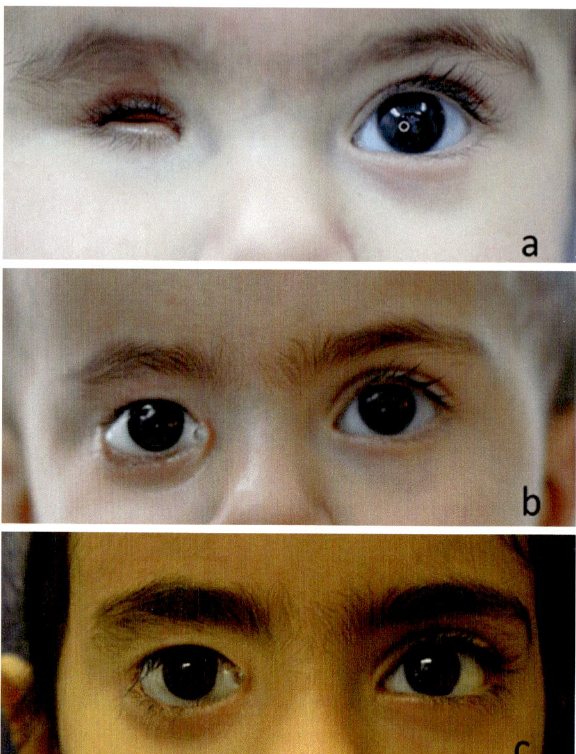

Fig. 19.7 Clinical Series. (**a**) Preoperative (**b**) postsurgical (**c**) rehabilitated orbit with bony symmetry, improved brow to lid margin, and lid fissure dimensions

and lack of long-term results. A conservative management is superior with a low complication rate and one that gives excellent long-term cosmetic and functional results with only a single surgical intervention. The approach also eliminates the need for serial radiographic imaging and multiple surgical interventions, and reduces patient and family psychological trauma.

References

1. Shaw GM, Carmichael SL, Yang W, Harris JA, Finnell RH, Lammer EJ. Epidemiologic characteristics of anophthalmia and bilateral microphthalmia among 2.5 million births in California, 1989–1997. Am J Med Genet A. 2005;137(1):36–40.
2. Kallen B, Tornqvist K. The epidemiology of anophthalmia and microphthalmia in Sweden. Eur J Epidemiol. 2005;20(4):345–50.
3. Morrison D, Fitzpatrick D, Hanson I, Williamson K, van Heyningen V, Fleck B, et al. National study of microphthalmia, anophthalmia and coloboma (MAC) in Scotland; Investigation of genetic aetiology. J Med Genet. 2002;39(1):16–22.
4. Tucker S, Jones B, Collin JRO. Systemic anomalies in 77 patients with congenital anophthalmos or microphthalmos. Eye. 1996;10:310–4.

5. Gregory-Evans CY, Williams MJ, Halford S, Gregory-Evans K. Ocular coloboma: a reassessment in the age of molecular neuroscience. J Med Genet. 2004;41:881–91.
6. Fantes J, Ragge NK, Lynch SA, et al. Mutations in SOX2 cause anophthalmia. Nat Genet. 2003;33:461–3. Gene analysis of some patients with bilateral anophthalmia showed mutation in the SOX2 gene.
7. Farkas LG, Posnick JC, Hreczko TM. Growth patterns in the orbital region: a morphometric study. Cleft Palate Craniofac J. 1992;29:315–8.
8. Drennan M. Balloon expansion therapy of clinical anophthalmos. J Ophthalmic Prosthet. 2000;5(1):9–15.
9. Gossman MD, Mohay JM, Roberts DM. Expansion of the human microphthalmic orbit. Ophthalmology. 1999;106:2005–9.
10. Christiansen SP, Gees AJ, Fletcher GA. A new conformer design to expand the horizontal lid fissure in severely microphthalmic eyes. J AAPOS. 2008;12:212–4.
11. Gundlach KK, Guthoff RF, Hingst VH, Schittkowski MP, Bier UC. Expansion of the socket and orbit for congenital clinical anophthalmia. Plast Reconstr Surg. 2005;166:1214–22.
12. Dunaway DJ, David DJ. Intraorbital tissue expansion in the management of congenital anophthalmos. Br J Plast Surg. 1996;49:529–35.
13. Krastinova D, Kelly MB, Mihaylova M. Surgical management of the anophthalmic orbit, part 1: congenital. Plast Reconstr Surg. 2001;108(4):817–26.
14. Bernardino CR. Congenital anophthalmia: a review dealing with volume. Middle East Afr J Ophthalmol. 2010;17:156–60.
15. Dootz GL. The ocularists' management of congenital microphthalmos and anophthalmos. Adv Ophthalmic Plast Reconstr Surg. 1992;9:41–56.
16. Gundlach KK, Guthoff RF, Hingst VH, et al. Expansion of the socket and orbit for congenital clinical anophthalmia. Plast Reconstr Surg. 2005;116:1214–22.
17. Tao JP, LeBoyer RM, Hetzler K, et al. Inferolateral migration of hydrogel orbital implants in microphthalmia. Ophthal Plast Reconstr Surg. 2010;26:14–7.
18. Tse DT, Abdulhafez M, Orozco MA, et al. Evaluation of an integrated orbital tissue expander in congenital anophthalmos: report of preliminary clinical experience. Am J Ophthalmol. 2011;151(3):470–82.
19. Merritt JH, Trawnik WR. Prosthetic and surgical management of congenital anophthalmia. J Ophthalmic Prosthet. 1997;2:1–14.
20. DiMaggio C, Sun LS, Li G. Early childhood exposure to anesthesia and risk of developmental and behavioral disorders in a sibling birth cohort. Anesth Analg. 2011;113(5):1143–51. Epub 2011 Mar 17.
21. Flick RP, Katusic SK, Colligan RC, Wilder RT, Voigt RG, Olson MD, Sprung J, Weaver AL, Schroeder DR, Warner DO. Cognitive and behavioral outcomes after early exposure to anesthesia and surgery. Pediatrics. 2011;128(5):e1053–61.
22. Peace MS, Salotti JA, Little MP, et al. Radiation exposure from CT scans in childhood and subsequent risk of leukaemia and brain tumours: a retrospective cohort study. Lancet. 2012;380(9840):499–505.
23. O'Keefe M, Webb M, Pashby RC, Wagman RD. Clinical anophthalmos. Br J Ophthalmol. 1987;71:635–8.

Chapter 20
Retinoblastoma and Uveal Melanoma

Brian C. Tse

Retinoblastoma

Retinoblastoma is the most common primary intraocular tumor in the pediatric population, with approximately 250 new cases in the United States each year [1]. Recent advancements in the treatment of retinoblastoma, such as intra-arterial and intravitreal chemotherapy, have increased eye salvage rates in these patients [2]. However, despite these advances, there is still a role for enucleation in the management of retinoblastoma.

Indications

In the International Retinoblastoma Classification grouping system, eyes are grouped according to extent of disease and spread of intraocular tumor. Primary enucleation is generally considered to be the treatment of choice in Group E eyes that have poor visual potential [3]. These eyes can be characterized by diffuse infiltrative tumor, anterior segment seeding, tumor touching the lens capsule or anterior to the vitreous face, neovascular glaucoma, massive intraocular hemorrhage, phthisis bulbi, or massive tumor necrosis. Group D eyes that may have diffuse intraocular tumor dissemination and/or subretinal seeding can also be managed with primary enucleation, although some practitioners seem to be moving toward globe-sparing treatments (intra-arterial, intravitreal, or intravenous chemotherapy) in these eyes [3–7]. Lastly, patients with progressive intraocular disease unresponsive to local and systemic therapy should also be considered for enucleation [3].

B. C. Tse (✉)
Bascom Palmer Eye Institute, University of Miami Miller School of Medicine, Miami, FL, USA
e-mail: b.tse@med.miami.edu

T. E. Johnson (ed.), *Anophthalmia*,
https://doi.org/10.1007/978-3-030-29753-4_20

Laterality of the retinoblastoma also plays a role in deciding whether or not to enucleate. In Group D and E eyes in patients with unilateral retinoblastoma, enucleation can be the definitive treatment [3]. In the absence of high-risk histopathology (anterior chamber, choroidal, optic nerve, or extrascleral extension), the patient may not require any further treatment or systemic chemotherapy following enucleation. In bilateral retinoblastoma, the treatment algorithm is more complex. However, primary enucleation is usually performed on the worse eye if it is classified as Group E, while an attempt will be made to salvage the remaining eye with a combination of focal and systemic therapy [3].

Pre-operative Considerations

Neuroimaging of the orbits and brain should be obtained prior to enucleation to assess for extraocular disease. The optic nerve should be assessed for thickening or enhancement that may indicate optic nerve invasion of the tumor [8]. Magnetic resonance imaging (MRI) is the preferred imaging modality over computed tomography (CT), as it allows for better imaging of the optic nerve, central nervous system, and pineal region (looking for "trilateral retinoblastoma") [9]. Additionally, using MRI as opposed to CT minimizes radiation exposure in these retinoblastoma patients, which can decrease the incidence of secondary malignancies later in life.

Intra-operative Considerations

Eyes with intraocular tumors may not have the external stigmata that one may expect to see in eyes that are being removed for other reasons, such as trauma. Thus, it is important to confirm the correct eye to be removed. The eye to be removed should be pharmacologically dilated in the pre-operative holding area. Indirect ophthalmoscopy should be performed after draping the patient in order to visualize the intraocular tumor and designate the proper eye for removal. The eye that will not be removed should have the eyelids taped shut so as to prevent exposure keratopathy or corneal abrasion. A Fox shield should be placed over this eye as well to protect it intra-operatively.

For the most part, the steps involved in an enucleation of an eye with retinoblastoma are the same as those for an eye without retinoblastoma. Enucleation technique has been described earlier in this book. However, additional precautions should be taken to avoid inadvertent globe puncture during surgery, causing tumor cells to spill into the orbit. Retrobulbar block should not be performed with a needle; rather block may be administered behind the globe on a blunt-tipped irrigating cannula after conjunctival peritomy has been completed. Traction sutures should not be placed through the sclera.

The most common route for extraocular extension of retinoblastoma is through the optic nerve; therefore, another goal of surgery is to remove the globe with as long a segment of optic nerve as possible. In lieu of placing a traction suture, a stump of medial rectus tendon 3–5 mm long should be left at the insertion when removing the medial rectus muscle. Once all the extraocular muscles have been removed, a curved hemostat can be used to grasp the medial rectus stump to abduct the globe. Abduction of the globe serves to move the intraorbital portion of the optic nerve medially so as to aid with obtaining maximal optic nerve segment length. With the globe in abduction, long Metzenbaum scissors are passed in the medial intraconal space between the globe and medial rectus muscle. The orientation of the tips of the scissors should be parallel to the medial wall of the orbit, and the scissors should be closed so as to minimize the risk of inadvertent globe perforation. Once the optic nerve is strummed with the Metzenbaum scissors, the blades are opened to straddle the optic nerve prior to transection. One should aim to obtain an optic nerve segment greater than 10 mm in retinoblastoma patients.

Curved enucleation scissors are generally not the preferred instrument with which to cut the nerve, as their curved nature will shorten the length of optic nerve segment obtained. Additionally, clamping of the optic nerve with a hemostat prior to transection is usually avoided as to prevent crush artifact of the nerve on the pathologic specimen. Finally, after the eye is removed, the gross specimen and socket should be examined for evidence of extraocular extension.

Orbital implant options are discussed elsewhere in this book, with most surgeons tending to place porous implants (polyethylene, hydroxyapatite, or aluminum oxide) [10]. Regardless of the type of implant placed, it is important to adequately replace the orbital soft tissue volume lost after enucleation to avoid cosmetic pitfalls of deep superior sulcus, eyelid ptosis, and enophthalmos. Adequate volume replacement with a large orbital implant can also aid with symmetrical orbital bone growth in this pediatric population.

Once the implant has been placed and the extraocular muscles secured to the implant, meticulous closure of Tenon's capsule is done with interrupted buried 5-0 Vicryl™ sutures. A thorough Tenon's closure can minimize the incidence of postoperative implant exposure. Some practitioners even go so far as to perform a two-layered closure of Tenon's capsule – posterior then anterior. Conjunctiva is closed with either plain gut or Vicryl™ sutures.

Orbital Extension of Retinoblastoma

The management of orbital retinoblastoma is challenging, although luckily rare in developed countries. Patients should be initially screened for distant metastases, which are present in 30–40% of patients with orbital retinoblastoma [9]. Although treatment can differ according to extent of orbital disease, systemic chemotherapy and external beam radiotherapy (45–50 Gy fractionated to the orbit) are mainstays of therapy [9, 11]. These therapies may be combined with local resection of the orbital mass or, in certain cases, orbital exenteration [11–13].

Uveal Melanoma

Uveal melanoma is the most common primary malignant intraocular tumor in adults, with an incidence of 4.3 per million in the United States [9]. The tumor has a predilection for Caucasians that increases with age. Plaque brachytherapy is the most common form of treatment for uveal melanoma. However, enucleation is commonly used in these patients as a primary treatment or secondarily after initial plaque brachytherapy [14].

Indications

The Collaborative Ocular Melanoma Study (COMS) randomized patients with medium-sized choroidal melanomas to receive either enucleation or iodine-125 brachytherapy. Unadjusted 5-year survival rates were comparable in both treatment arms (81% for enucleation and 82% for brachytherapy). Rates of histopathologically confirmed metastases were also similar in both arms (11% for enucleation and 9% for brachytherapy) [15]. The COMS large tumor study randomly assigned patients with choroidal melanoma to either enucleation alone or pre-operative irradiation followed by enucleation. Again, there were similar 5-year survival (43% for enucleation alone; 38% for pre-enucleation radiation) and metastatic rates (40% for enucleation alone; 45% for pre-enucleation radiation) between both treatment arms [16].

Thus, primary enucleation does not appear to be inferior to plaque brachytherapy in terms of overall survival rate in the treatment of uveal melanoma [15]. There is a trend toward eye conservation therapies (usually with plaque brachytherapy) in small- to medium-sized tumors, while primary enucleation may be more favored in eyes where the largest basal diameter of the tumor is greater than 15 mm [9].

Secondary enucleation may also be needed after initial conservative eye therapy for uveal melanoma, with COMS group reporting 12.5% of eyes required enucleation within 5 years [14]. Within the first 3 years after therapy, local tumor recurrence is the most common reason for secondary enucleation after plaque brachytherapy, while ocular pain is the most common reason for secondary enucleation after 3 years. Blind, painful eyes may result from sequelae of plaque brachytherapy such as radiation retinopathy, neovascular glaucoma, scleral melting, choroidal atrophy, and radiation optic neuropathy.

Pre-operative Considerations

Usually a systemic metastatic workup is performed at initial diagnosis, which may consist of liver function tests, chest X-ray, and liver imaging (ultrasound or CT scan). Unless significant orbital extension of the melanoma is suspected, usually no dedicated orbital imaging is needed prior to surgery.

Intra-operative Considerations

Similar precautions as described in the retinoblastoma section should be taken with uveal melanoma patients as well during enucleation.

Orbital Extension of Uveal Melanoma

Extraocular extension of uveal melanoma is seen in 6–14% of enucleated eyes and is a poor prognostic factor [17, 18]. Patients with extraocular extension have a 5-year mortality rate between 45% and 66% [19]. Risk factors for extrascleral extension include increasing tumor height, anterior tumor extension, large basal tumor diameter, diffuse uveal melanoma, high-risk pathology (epithelioid cell type, closed vascular loops, high mitotic rate), and monosomy 3 [9]. There does not appear to be any evidence in the literature regarding gene expression profile classification and risk for extraocular extension, although Class II is associated with higher risk of metastasis [20].

Orbital exenteration should be considered in cases with extensive extraocular extension of uveal melanoma. Shammas and Blodi thought that early exenteration in these patients was beneficial [18]. However, Affeldt and co-authors did not find any prognostic benefit to early exenteration in patients with orbital extension [19]. Additionally, Kersten and colleagues examined 42 patients who had undergone enucleation or early exenteration for uveal melanoma with extrascleral extension and found no difference in survival rates between the two groups [21]. They posited that systemic tumor dissemination had already occurred at the time of surgery. Exenteration in some patients can be palliative in nature in the event that the orbital melanoma is causing massive proptosis (Fig. 20.1) [22].

In more localized (<3 mm) extraocular extension of uveal melanoma, other less invasive options than exenteration can be considered. Plaque brachytherapy can be performed as part of a globe sparing therapy [23]. Enucleation can be performed with localized tenonectomy or orbital fat excision in lieu of exenteration.

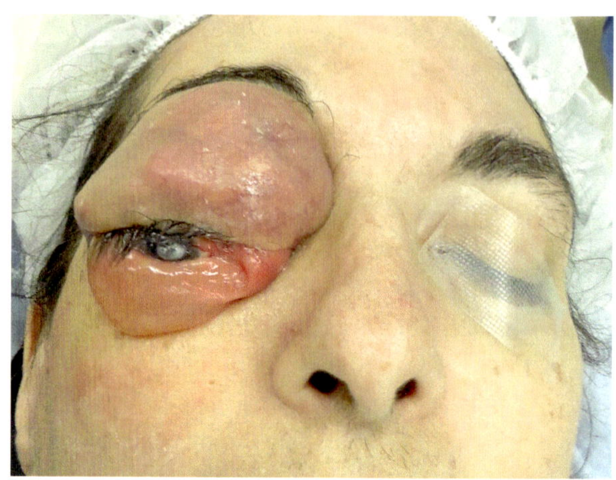

Fig. 20.1 Patient with large secondary orbital melanoma for which palliative exenteration of the orbit was performed

References

1. Ellsworth RM. The practical management of retinoblastoma. Trans Am Ophthalmol Soc. 1969;67:462–534.
2. Abramson DH, Dunkel IJ, Brodie SE, et al. A phase I/II study of direct intraarterial (ophthalmic artery) chemotherapy with melphalan for intraocular retinoblastoma initial results. Ophthalmology. 2008;115:1398–404.
3. Rodriguez-Galindo C, Wilson MW, editors. Retinoblastoma. Boston: Springer; 2010.
4. Schefler AC, Abramson DH. Update on ophthalmic oncology 2012: advances in retinoblastoma and uveal melanoma. Asia Pac J Ophthalmol (Phila). 2013;2(2):119–31.
5. Shields CL, Shields JA. Retinoblastoma management: advances in enucleation, intravenous chemoreduction, and intra-arterial chemotherapy. Curr Opin Ophthalmol. 2010;21:203–12.
6. Abramson DH, Ji X, Francis JH, et al. Intravitreal chemotherapy in retinoblastoma: expanded use beyond intravitreal seeds. Br J Ophthalmol. 2019;103(4):488–93. https://doi.org/10.1136/bjophthalmol-2018-312037.
7. Kiratli H, Koc I, Inam O, et al. Retrospective analysis of primarily treated group D retinoblastoma. Graefes Arch Clin Exp Ophthalmol. 2018;256:2225–31.
8. Razek AA, Elkhamary S. MRI of retinoblastoma. Br J Radiol. 2011;84:775–84.
9. Singh AD, Damato BE, Pe'er J, Perry JD, editors. Clinical ophthalmic oncology. Berlin: Springer; 2015.
10. Wladis EJ, Aakalu VK, Sobel RK, et al. Orbital implants in enucleation surgery. Ophthalmology. 2018;125:311–7.
11. Honavar SG, Singh AD. Management of advanced retinoblastoma. Ophthalmol Clin North Am. 2005;18:65–73.
12. Chatanda G, Fandino A, Casak S, et al. Treatment of overt extraocular retinoblastoma. Med Pediatr Oncol. 2003;40(3):158–61.
13. Doz F, Khelfaoui F, Mosseri V, et al. The role of chemotherapy in orbital involvement of retinoblastoma. The experience of a single institution with 33 patients. Cancer. 1994;74:722–32.
14. Jampol LM, Moy CS, Murray TG, et al. The COMS randomized trial of iodine 125 brachytherapy for choroidal melanoma IV. Local treatment failure and enucleation in the first 5 years after brachytherapy. COMS report no. 19. Ophthalmology. 2002;109:2197–206.
15. Collaborative Ocular Melanoma Study Group. The COMS randomized trial of iodine 125 brachytherapy for choroidal melanoma, III: initial mortality findings. COMS Report No. 18. Arch Ophthalmol. 2001;119:969–82.

16. Collaborative Ocular Melanoma Study Group. The collaborative ocular melanoma study (COMS) randomized trial of pre-enucleation radiation of large choroidal melanoma: IV. Ten-year mortality findings and prognostic factors. COMS report number 24. Am J Ophthalmol. 2004;138:936–51.
17. Coupland SE, Campbell I, Damato B. Routes of extraocular extension of uveal melanoma: risk factors and influence on survival probability. Ophthalmology. 2008;115:1778–85.
18. Shammas HF, Blodi FC. Orbital extension of choroidal and ciliary body melanomas. Arch Ophthalmol. 1977;95:2002–5.
19. Affeldt JC, Minckler DS, Azen SP, et al. Prognosis in uveal melanoma with extrascleral extension. Arch Ophthalmol. 1980;98:1975–9.
20. Harbour JW. A prognostic test to predict the risk of metastasis in uveal melanoma based on a 15-gene expression profile. Methods Mol Biol. 2014;1102:427–40.
21. Kersten RC, Tse DT, Anderson RL, et al. The role of orbital exenteration in choroidal melanoma with extrascleral extension. Ophthalmology. 1985;92(3):436–43.
22. Shields JA, Shields CL. Massive orbital extension of posterior uveal melanomas. Ophthalmic Plast Reconstr Surg. 1991;7(4):238–51.
23. Ganduz K, Shields CL, Shields JL, et al. Plaque radiotherapy for management of ciliary body and choroidal melanoma with extraocular extension. Am J Ophthalmol. 2000;130:97–102.

Chapter 21
Strategies for Orbital Expansion

Benjamin Erickson

Introduction

Both congenital and early acquired pediatric anophthalmia require carefully choreographed and thoughtful management, as orbital volume plays a substantial role in the development of the bony socket and surrounding facial structures. The ability to retain a well-proportioned ocular prosthesis is also instrumental in psychosocial development.

While congenital and acquired anophthalmia share many commonalities, there are certain critical differences, which typically render intrauterine developmental and early postnatal deficits more challenging to manage. Comprehensive systemic evaluation, genetic counseling, and multidisciplinary management are of paramount importance in congenital cases. Additionally, the pediatric facial structure has obtained only 40% of adult size by 3 months of age, but typically reaches 90% of adult size by 5.5 years of age [1]. The paradigm for management of anophthalmia arising after 5–6 years of age is therefore much more closely akin to that for adult-acquired anophthalmia, discussed in detail elsewhere in this text.

Conversely, early defects require distinctive interventions aimed at promoting age-appropriate and symmetrical development of the eyelids, conjunctival fornices, bony orbit, and adjacent midfacial structures. Depending on the extent of the anatomical deficits, this may necessitate a two-tiered strategy: The first aim is the promotion of periocular soft tissue development via staged or progressive tissue expansion with acrylic or hydrogel conformers, supplemented with as needed reconstructive surgery to the eyelids, canthal structures, and fornices. The second aim is the promotion of orbital and midfacial growth with serial implant exchange, tissue expansion with saline or hydrogel implants, or dermis fat grafting.

B. Erickson (✉)
Stanford Byers Eye Institute, Department of Ophthalmology, Palo Alto, CA, USA
e-mail: bericks o@stanford.edu

T. E. Johnson (ed.), *Anophthalmia*,
https://doi.org/10.1007/978-3-030-29753-4_21

Congenital Anophthalmia

Microphthalmia, congenital anophthalmia, and coloboma (MAC) constitute a continuum of developmental disorders that arise from defects in optic vesicle formation [2–4]. 'Clinical anophthalmia' is an entity that encompasses both true anophthalmia and severe microphthalmia without cyst. While rudimentary neuroectodermal tissue may be present in this latter group, the therapeutic challenges are identical due to the absence of a globe or globe-like structure, which is critical to stimulating normal growth of the bony orbit, midface, and periocular soft tissues [4–6].

The reported incidence is between 0.6 and 4.2 per 100,000 live births, although these registry-derived estimates may reflect not only underlying population differences but also inconsistent definitions of anophthalmia [2, 3]. Unsurprisingly given the critical period during which these defects arise, over 50% of cases are associated with significant systemic abnormalities [2]. Postnatally, comprehensive evaluation of the ears, palate, heart, lungs, genitourinary system, esophagus, pituitary axis, and other midline brain structures is therefore indicated [2, 7–9]. Association with other first and second pharyngeal arch developmental anomalies, such as facial clefting and Goldenhar syndrome, may require additional reconstructive interventions [10, 11].

In patients with unilateral anophthalmia, it is important to examine the fellow eye carefully, as more subtle defects such as coloboma, dermoid, sclerocornea, congenital glaucoma, optic nerve hypoplasia, cataract, and retinal dystrophy are present in nearly half of patients [2, 11]. Of note, nearly one-third of those with unilateral anophthalmia are ultimately classified as legally blind, suggesting a need for multifaceted social and occupational support [11]. Overall, only 10% of those affected have isolated anophthalmia with no other ocular or systemic findings [12, 13].

Given advances in the quality of routinely performed fetal ultrasound, in utero detection of anophthalmia is occurring with greater frequency [14]. Postnatally, ultrasound of the orbit is also useful to determine whether an ocular remnant and/or associated cyst is present. It is typically the first-line imaging study, as it does not require sedation or subject the neonate to potentially deleterious radiation. Magnetic resonance imaging (MRI) is the optimal study to evaluate for the presence of intracranial abnormalities, while computed tomography (CT) permits detailed evaluation of the bony orbit, which may be useful in planning for and monitoring the results of orbital expansion [15, 16].

Treatment

As previously emphasized, the first principle of management is to identify and treat any associated complications, which may jeopardize systemic health. In cases of unilateral anophthalmia, the fellow eye should be monitored carefully and treated aggressively for glaucoma, cataract, and amblyopia. Monocular precautions with the use of protective polycarbonate lenses should be instituted to safeguard against trauma to the more developed eye.

Presence of an eye is an important stimulus to growth of the orbit and periocular soft tissues both in utero and throughout the first decade of life [17]. A normally developing globe triples in volume between birth and adolescence, with concomitant expansion of bony orbital confine [4, 18]. The orbit reaches 70% of its adult volume by age 4 and 90% by age 7, with the fastest growth occurring in the first year of life [17, 19].

Accordingly, bony orbital hypoplasia, microblepharon, foreshortened conjunctival fornices, and hemifacial microsomia with secondary hypoplasia of the maxilla and crowding of the brow are all potential functional and cosmetic consequences of anophthalmia [16–18, 20]. Both soft tissue hypoplasia and asymmetric bony growth require early and aggressive management to optimize long-term outcomes [18]. This treatment generally occurs in two stages, beginning with the soft tissues; access to the orbit for volume enhancement and expansion may initially be limited [21].

Palpebral and Conjunctival Management

Starting in the first few weeks to months of life, serial acrylic conformers may be used to enlarge the palpebral fissure and conjunctival fornices (Fig. 21.1). Fitting requires the assistance of an experienced ocularist, as each successive conformer needs to be big enough to promote meaningful tissue expansion without producing significant discomfort or unduly high risk of extrusion [21, 22].

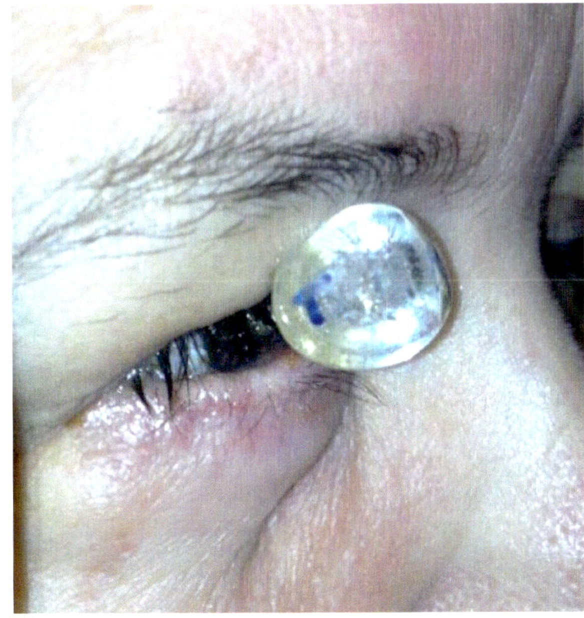

Fig. 21.1 Pressure conformer in place in a right ophthalmic socket. Note that pressure applied to the stem extending externally to the eyelids is transmitted to the conjunctival fornices via the conformer. (Courtesy of Dr. Thomas Johnson)

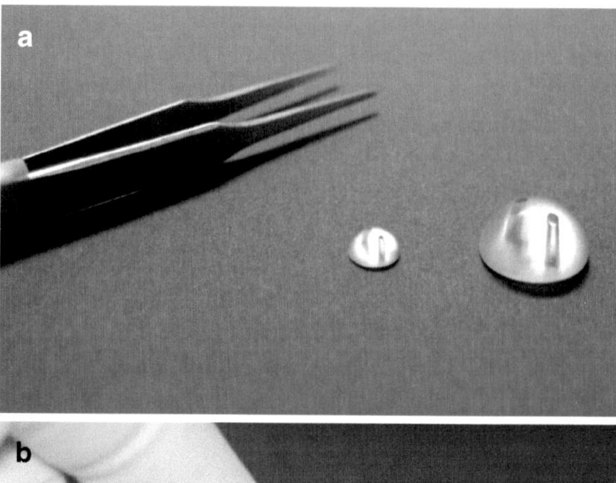

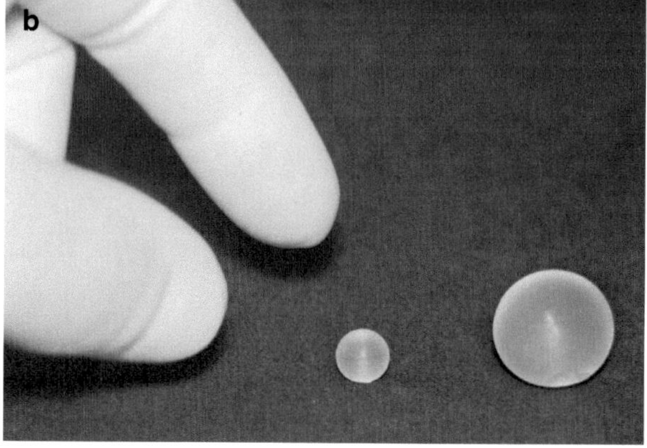

Fig. 21.2 Hydrogel expanders in (**a**) hemispheric configuration for expansion of the conjunctival fornices and (**b**) spherical configuration for progressive expansion of the anophthalmic socket. (OSMED Tissue Expanders, FCI Ophthalmics, Pembroke, MA)

Another option is to position a hemispheric hydrogel conformer in the fornices with subsequent suture or cyanoacrylate glue tarsorrhaphy (Fig. 21.2) [19, 23]. Uptake of tear fluid by the initially anhydrous gel results in progressive osmotic expansion over the course of several weeks. These devices can exert peak hydrostatic pressures of 20–30 millimeters of mercury (mmHg) during early expansion, but tissue adaptation ultimately plateaus when the gel matrix is fully hydrated and the conformer approaches maximum size. Exchange for a larger size must then be performed, but due to dynamic expansion, fewer stages are typically required than when using serial acrylic conformers and the associated pressure spikes associated with initial placement may be lower [21].

This incremental soft tissue expansion helps to symmetrize the palpebral fissures and fornices, and will ultimately permit appropriate surgical access to the orbit for additional expansion with static or dynamic implants. Reconstructive surgery to canthal structures and/or fornices – with oral mucus membrane grafting – is occasionally required early in the course of care but otherwise may be deferred until after definitive orbital expansion [22]. This first stage alone understandably does not have a profound impact on underlying bony hypoplasia or orbital volume deficiency [16, 18, 20].

Orbital Management

Four categories of implants are available for the remediation of congenital orbital volume deficits, and each type can be classified as static or dynamic based on potential for in vivo expansion [15]. Static implants are spheres with fixed dimensions, and may be solid (acrylic, poly[methyl methacrylate]) or porous (porous polyethylene, hydroxyapatite, or aluminum hydroxide). The available dynamic implants are hydrogel spheres, inflatable tissue expanders (with integrated or external ports), and dermis fat grafts [20].

Physiologic orbital pressure in human adults is approximately 3–6 mmHg [24, 25], while the ideal pressure to stimulate growth in a piglet model – resulting in achievement of near-normal orbital volumes – was found to be 20 mmHg [26]. Clinically, no device with the capacity to constantly apply this optimal pressure is available for implantation. Even tissue expanders generate peaks and troughs in orbital pressure, depending on the timing of the most recent injection (if inflatable) or on their state of hydration and remaining capacity to imbibe fluid (if hydrogel). Autologous dermis fat grafts theoretically have the capacity for continuous gradual growth, but don't always enlarge in a predictable linear fashion. The overarching goal is to achieve the most natural and symmetrical growth possible, while minimizing the number of required interventions and degree of cicatricial morbidity to the anophthalmic socket.

Conventional static orbital implants require replacement every year or so in order to encourage ongoing expansion of the bony orbit and midface, with an average of 3–5 total procedures required during childhood. Large incisions are necessary and repetitive trauma to the conjunctiva and orbital fascia can predispose to socket contracture [15, 18, 21]. Unlike their porous counterparts, solid implants do not become tissue integrated, perhaps rendering exchange easier and less traumatic [22].

In order to reduce the total number of socket surgeries, the largest tolerated static implant can be placed during a single stage, but the size will be limited and the resulting pressure spike can increase the risk of extrusion and make it difficult for a prosthesis to be worn comfortably [15]. During the key growth phase, expansion is also proportional to the volume implanted [20]. This strategy is therefore better suited to children 5–6 years of age or older, who have already achieved substantial facial and orbital growth – as opposed to newly identified cases of congenital or early acquired anophthalmia.

Expandable hydrogel spheres confer many theoretical advantages, as the constituent materials employed can absorb up to 2000% of their weight in water, with expansion to 10–30 times their original volume, under laboratory conditions [4, 18, 20, 21]. These parameters can be engineered to influence the rate and degree of implant expansion [21]. As hydrogel implants are inserted in relative dehydrated state, use of smaller lateral incisions can potentially minimizing socket trauma and reduce the risk of extrusion [15, 21].

In practice, there are a number of concerns and limitations. MIRAgel (MIRA, Waltham, MA) – a hydrogel implant previously used for retinal buckling – resulted in a number of well documented delayed onset complications, including excessive swelling, tissue fibrosis, and orbital granuloma formation [27, 28]. While the base compounds and cross-linking characteristics of current commercially available hydrogels are different, some experts still advocate replacement with conventional solid or porous implants once the desired expansion has been achieved [21]. And in spite of the materials engineering promise, staged implant insertions are often still required to promote sustained growth [19]. Removal generally entails aspiration or piecemeal extraction via a conjunctival incision, and can be more challenging than extracting a solid implant [15, 18].

Conventional tissue expanders developed for other indications have demonstrated promise for socket expansion, but present challenges when it comes to maintaining implant fixation, controlling the direction of expansion, and preventing extrusion. Not surprisingly, a poorly anchored expander may have a greater impact on anterior soft tissues than on the bony orbit. Additionally, tunneling the port outside of the orbit entails additional surgical incisions, morbidity, and temporary deformity.

Tse and colleagues developed a purpose-built orbital tissue expander, which consists of an inflatable silicone globe with indwelling port, supported by a titanium T-plate secured to the lateral orbital rim (Fig. 21.3). This bony anchoring serves to control the direction of expansion and reduce rates of extrusion. In an anophthalmic feline model, the expanded orbital volume was only 18% smaller than the normal contralateral side – as opposed to 66% smaller in control animals – after 18 weeks [18]. In nine consecutive pediatric patients with unilateral congenital anophthalmia, the average difference between the volume of the initial implanted and contralateral orbit was $5.68 \pm 2.34\ cm^3$, decreasing to $2.53 \pm 1.80\ cm^3$ after a duration of 18.89 ± 8.80 months [20]. In spite of promising initial results, this implant is not commercially available in the United States at the time of writing.

Dermis fat grafts (DFGs) are a potentially valuable tool in the management of the pediatric anophthalmic socket, but also present significant challenges. As an autologous material, dermis fat avoids many potential issues with biocompatibility, extrusion, and infection. With mucosal epithelialization of the denuded dermal surface, grafts can help to rectify deficits in conjunctival surface area and forniceal depth as well as in orbital volume. Critically – unlike when implanted in the adult orbit – successful grafts tend to expand over time rather than atrophy. However, growth can be unpredictable and is occasionally excessive, requiring surgical debulking [29]. For optimal success, grafts should be harvested and implanted before 3 years of age, after which time they tend to behave more like adult DFGs, with progressive volume loss and atrophy.

In cases of severe under correction or delayed presentation, orbital osteotomy and advancement may be performed by a craniofacial surgeon using techniques introduced by Tessier [15, 19, 21].

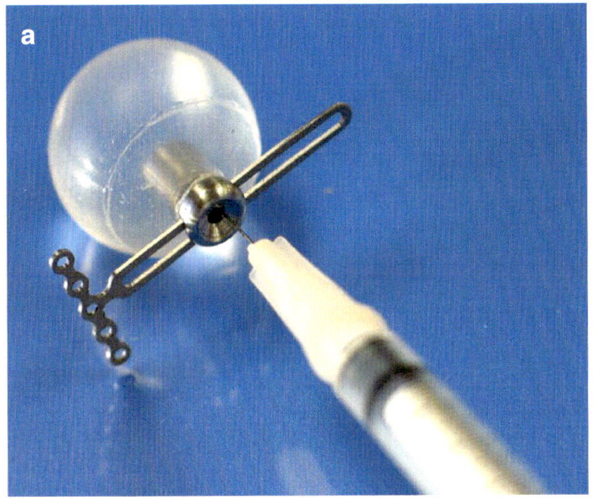

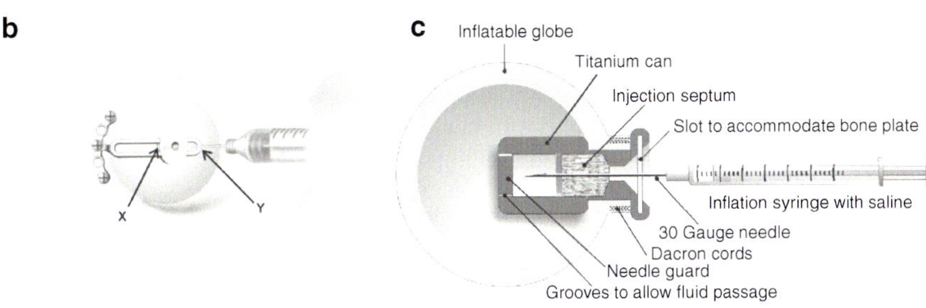

Fig. 21.3 (**a**) Integrated orbital tissue expander with needle in the injection chamber to permit inflation. (**b**) Schematic rendering of the integrated orbital tissue expander in an anophthalmic socket, demonstrating subconjunctival injection port in relation to the titanium T-plate base, which is secured to the lateral orbital rim via screws. (**c**) Cross-sectional structure of the expander demonstrating relationship of the injection chamber to the inflatable silicone balloon. Note that the titanium can and injection guard are designed to prevent inadvertent perforation of the balloon during progressive inflation. (Courtesy of Dr. David Tse)

Additional Management Considerations

It is prudent to evaluate the patient for concurrent nasolacrimal duct obstruction, seen in 10% of cases of congenital anophthalmia. The lacrimal sac may act as a reservoir for bacteria, thereby increasing the risk of infectious complications associated with orbital implants [11, 30].

Conclusion

Management of congenital and early acquired anophthalmia is challenging, requiring systematic evaluation, multidisciplinary management, as well as carefully choreographed and staged intervention in order to maximize orbitofacial development during childhood.

References

1. Farkas LG, Posnick JC, Hreczko TM, Pron GE. Growth patterns in the orbital region: a morphometric study. Cleft Palate Craniofac J. 1992;29(4):315–8.
2. Ragge NK, Subak-Sharpe ID, Collin JR. A practical guide to the management of anophthalmia and microphthalmia. Eye (Lond). 2007;21(10):1290–300.
3. Shah SP, Taylor AE, Sowden JC, Ragge NK, Russell-Eggitt I, Rahi JS, Gilbert CE, Surveillance of Eye Anomalies (SEA-UK) Special Interest Group. Anophthalmos, microphthalmos, and typical coloboma in the United Kingdom: a prospective study of incidence and risk. Invest Ophthalmol Vis Sci. 2011;52(1):558–64.
4. Verma AS, Fitzpatrick DR. Anophthalmia and microphthalmia. Orphanet J Rare Dis. 2007;2:47.
5. Celebi AR, Sasani H. Differentiation of true anophthalmia from clinical anophthalmia using neuroradiological imaging. World J Radiol. 2014;6(7):515–8.
6. Gujar SK, Gandhi D. Congenital malformations of the orbit. Neuroimaging Clin North Am. 2011;21(3):585–602, viii.
7. Macchiaroli A, Kelberman D, Auriemma RS, Drury S, Islam L, Giangiobbe S, Ironi G, Lench N, Sowden JC, Colao A, Pivonello R, Cavallo L, Gasperi M, Faienza MF. A novel heterozygous SOX2 mutation causing congenital bilateral anophthalmia, hypogonadotropic hypogonadism and growth hormone deficiency. Gene. 2014;534(2):282–5.
8. Wang J, Steelman CK, Vincent R, Richburg D, Chang TS, Shehata BM. Two case reports of anophthalmia and congenital heart disease: adding a new dimension to this association. Fetal Pediatr Pathol. 2010;29(5):291–8.
9. White T, Lu T, Metlapally R, Katowitz J, Kherani F, Wang TY, Tran-Viet KN, Young TL. Identification of STRA6 and SKI sequence variants in patients with anophthalmia/microphthalmia. Mol Vis. 2008;14:2458–65.
10. Makhoul IR, Soudack M, Kochavi O, Guilburd JN, Maimon S, Gershoni-Baruch R. Anophthalmia-plus syndrome: a clinical report and review of the literature. Am J Med Genet A. 2007;143A(1):64–8.
11. Schittkowski MP, Guthoff RF. Systemic and ophthalmological anomalies in congenital anophthalmic or microphthalmic patients. Br J Ophthalmol. 2010;94(4):487–93.
12. Lowry RB, Kohut R, Sibbald B, Rouleau J. Anophthalmia and microphthalmia in the Alberta Congenital Anomalies Surveillance System. Can J Ophthalmol. 2005;40(1):38–44.
13. Stoll C, Dott B, Alembik Y, Roth MP. Associated malformations among infants with anophthalmia and microphthalmia. Birth Defects Res A Clin Mol Teratol. 2012;94(3):147–52.
14. Erickson BP, Tse DT. Management of neonatal proptosis: a systematic review. Surv Ophthalmol. 2014;59(4):378–92.
15. Bernardino CR. Congenital anophthalmia: a review of dealing with volume. Middle East Afr J Ophthalmol. 2010;17(2):156–60.
16. Llorente-González S, Peralta-Calvo J, Abelairas-Gómez JM. Congenital anophthalmia and microphthalmia: epidemiology and orbitofacial rehabilitation. Clin Ophthalmol. 2011;5:1759–65.

17. Dunaway DJ, David DJ. Intraorbital tissue expansion in the management of congenital anophthalmos. Br J Plast Surg. 1996;49(8):529–35.
18. Tse DT, Pinchuk L, Davis S, Falcone SF, Lee W, Acosta AC, Hernandez E, Lee E, Parel JM. Evaluation of an integrated orbital tissue expander in an anophthalmic feline model. Am J Ophthalmol. 2007;143(2):317–27.
19. Gundlach KK, Guthoff RF, Hingst VH, Schittkowski MP, Bier UC. Expansion of the socket and orbit for congenital clinical anophthalmia. Plast Reconstr Surg. 2005;116(5):1214–22.
20. Tse DT, Abdulhafez M, Orozco MA, Tse JD, Azab AO, Pinchuk L. Evaluation of an integrated orbital tissue expander in congenital anophthalmos: report of preliminary clinical experience. Am J Ophthalmol. 2011;151(3):470–82.e1.
21. Mazzoli RA, Raymond WR 4th, Ainbinder DJ, Hansen EA. Use of self-expanding, hydrophilic osmotic expanders (hydrogel) in the reconstruction of congenital clinical anophthalmos. Curr Opin Ophthalmol. 2004;15(5):426–31.
22. Chen D, Heher K. Management of the anophthalmic socket in pediatric patients. Curr Opin Ophthalmol. 2004;15(5):449–53.
23. Wiese KG, Vogel M, Guthoff R, Gundlach KK. Treatment of congenital anophthalmos with self-inflating polymer expanders: a new method. J Craniomaxillofac Surg. 1999;27(2):72–6.
24. Kratky V, Hurwitz JJ, Avram DR. Orbital compartment syndrome. Direct measurement of orbital tissue pressure: 1. Technique. Can J Ophthalmol. 1990;25(6):293–7.
25. Riemann CD, Foster JA, Kosmorsky GS. Direct orbital manometry in healthy patients. Ophthalmic Plast Reconstr Surg. 1999;15(2):121–5.
26. Reedy BK, Pan F, Kim WS, Bartlett SP. The direct effect of intraorbital pressure on orbital growth in the anophthalmic piglet. Plast Reconstr Surg. 1999;104(3):713–8.
27. Roh M, Lee NG, Miller JB. Complications associated with MIRAgel for treatment of retinal detachment. Semin Ophthalmol. 2018;33(1):89–94.
28. Thompson JT, Chambers WA. Good ideas gone bad: the MIRAgel saga. Ophthalmology. 2016;123(1):5–6.
29. Heher KL, Katowitz JA, Low JE. Unilateral dermis-fat graft implantation in the pediatric orbit. Ophthalmic Plast Reconstr Surg. 1998;14(2):81–8.
30. Schittkowski MP, Guthoff RF. Results of lacrimal assessment in patients with congenital clinical anophthalmos or blind microphthalmos. Br J Ophthalmol. 2007;91(12):1624–6.

Part V
Prosthetics

Chapter 22
Scleral Shells

Zakeya Mohammed Al-Sadah

A scleral shell is a specific type of craniofacial prosthesis that covers a disfigured or atrophied eye restoring the natural appearance of the eye. There is a greater need for scleral shells nowadays owing to more advanced surgical techniques resulting in more damaged eyes being saved. If corneal sensation is still intact, a conjunctival flap is performed to cover the sensitive cornea. The earliest known evidence of ocular prosthesis was used by Egyptian (Fig. 22.1) and Roman priests as early as the fifth century B.C. The prosthetic eye was worn outside the socket and was constructed from painted clay that was held in place by a piece of cloth [1].

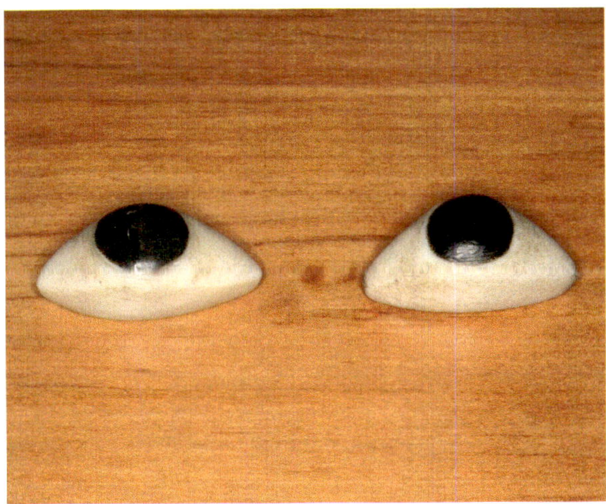

Fig. 22.1 Prosthetic eyes for the dead helped Egyptians "see" when they entered the afterlife (these specimens date from the late Dynastic period, circa 664–332 BCE, or later). (Published with kind permission of Dr. Keith R. Pine. All rights reserved)

Z. M. Al-Sadah (✉)
Ophthalmic Plastic and Reconstructive Surgery, Department of Ophthalmology, Bascom Palmer Eye Institute, University of Miami Miller School of Medicine, Miami, FL, USA

T. E. Johnson (ed.), *Anophthalmia*,
https://doi.org/10.1007/978-3-030-29753-4_22

Two thousand years later, evidence of a different type of ocular prosthesis was found in Persia, where a very light Bitumen paste was used to make a hemisphere. A thin layer of gold was used on the surface of the hemisphere with central circular engraving and sun-ray like lines coming out of it representing the iris [2]. The eye was attached by two golden threads going through two drilled holes on each side of the prosthesis. In addition to this, mention of a prosthetic golden eye worn by a woman was found in early Hebrew texts. In the sixteenth century, glass was used for these prostheses by Venetians instead of gold. This method was only known to Venetians, and the shells were fragile and uncomfortable. The Parisians took over this business two centuries later (Figs. 22.2 and 22.3). Because of their superior glass blowing skills, the center of artificial eye making was then moved to Germany. The United States started making artificial eyes from acrylic polymers after World War II since it was difficult to obtain German products. Reportedly, the first scleral shell was made in 1887 by the Mullers, who were working in the manufacture of prosthetic eyes and within the glass blowing industry. The shell was made for a patient with exposure keratopathy after losing most of his eyelids due to skin cancer. The aim of using that transparent shell was to save vision and provide improved corneal lubrication. After the successful results of that shell, the Mullers started a business of making white shells with transparent centers [3]. Adolf Fick, a German ophthalmologist, was the first person to create a scleral shell for a patient with a blind unsightly eye. He started his trials first on rabbits' eyes where he made mound of their corneas and made glass lenses. Eventually, he continued his studies on

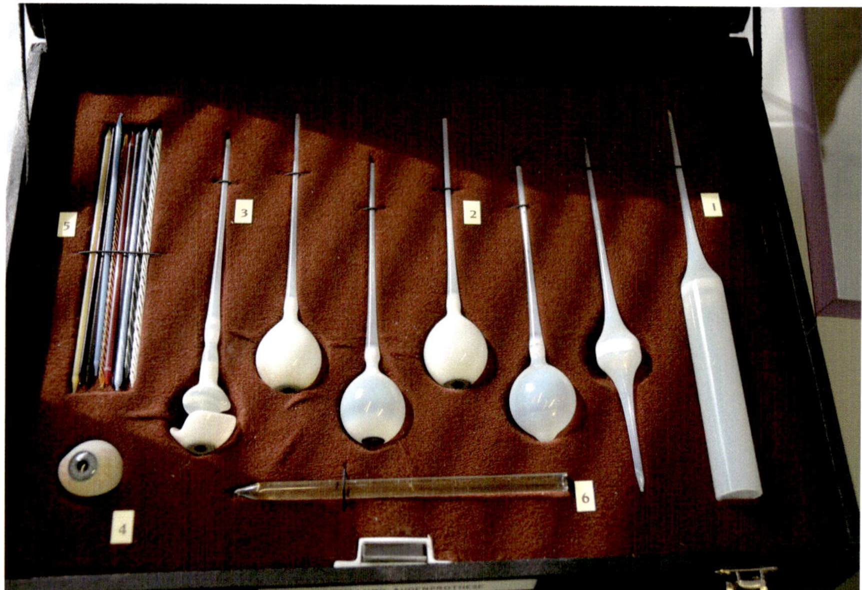

Fig. 22.2 Preformed glass eyes. (Published with kind permission of Dr. Keith R. Pine. All rights reserved)

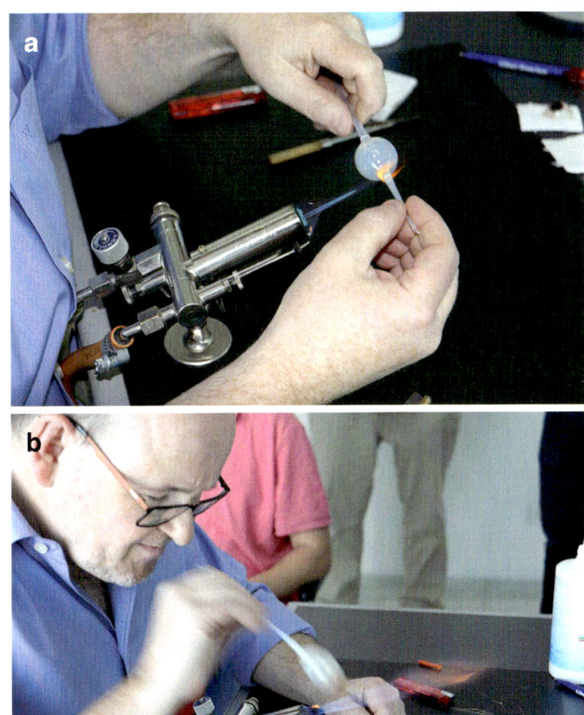

Fig. 22.3 Different steps of the glass eye making: (**a**) The glass eye process begins by softening a pre-tinted hollow glass tube. (**b**) The glass tube is sealed at one end and "blown" to its correct size. (Published with kind permission of Dr. Keith R. Pine.)

human cadavers and tried using glass lenses made at the Zeiss optical center [3]. These days, some European countries are still using glass for ocular prostheses. In North America, most are fabricated using acrylic or PMMA (polymethyl methacrylate). Different methods have been proposed to compensate for the lack of pupillary reaction and subsequent anisocoria of the scleral shell including the use of liquid crystals [4], sources of light [5], photochromics [6], magnetic [7], polarized [8] materials and self-powered, light-sensitive LCD screens [9], but those methods are limited by the size, weight, cost, and the fabrication process, especially when considering production on a large scale.

Excellent motility is usually obtained with a retained eye. Moreover, it also provides a good base for a scleral shell. The fabrication of the scleral shell is technically more difficult than that of a regular prosthetic eye due to its reduced thickness (Fig. 22.4). The thin scleral shells have only a small space for corneal bulge as they are fitted directly onto an underlying, possibly deformed cornea. In contradistinction, the regular ocular prostheses have sufficient thickness to fabricate the shape of a curved cornea with a flat iris behind it (Fig. 22.5) [10].

There are two types of scleral shells, stock and custom shells. Stock shells do not necessarily match the contralateral eye in color or fit perfectly since they are not

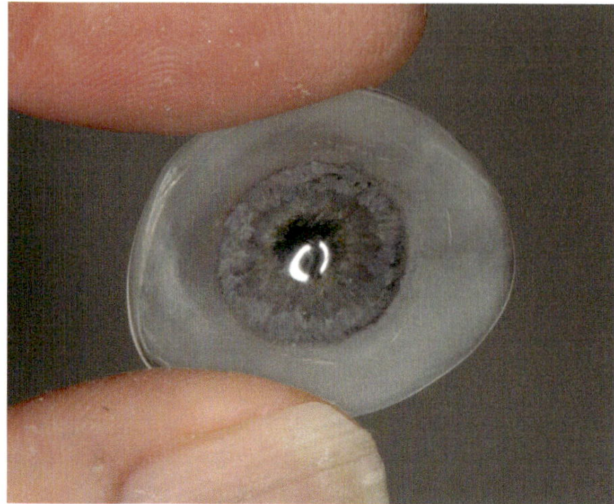

Fig. 22.4 Completed medium-thickness scleral shell prosthesis. (Published with kind permission of Dr. Keith R. Pine. All rights reserved)

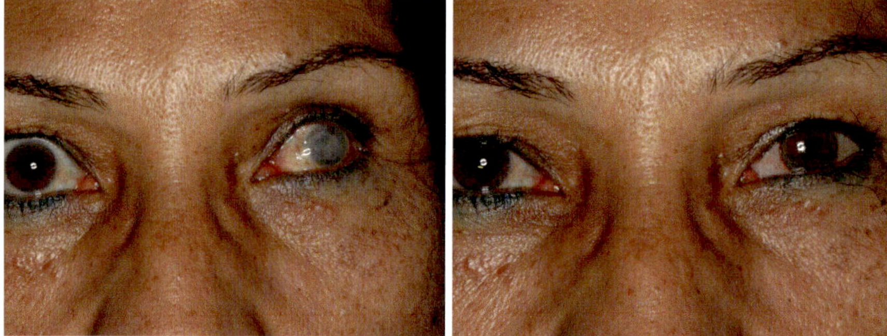

Fig. 22.5 Left strabismic eye with opaque cornea is masked with a scleral shell prosthesis. (Published with kind permission of Dr. Keith R. Pine. All rights reserved)

individually made, and are made with specific parameters by contact lens manufacturers. On the other hand, custom shells are individually and specifically made to match the patient's contralateral eye in all aspects. In addition, custom-made shells will also help promote the development and health of the patient socket. Moreover, they will aid in widening the palpebral fissure of the affected eye by restoring volume, providing eyelid support and preventing ptosis, giving a more natural appearance. Custom-made scleral shells are usually fabricated by board-certified ocularists [1, 10].

Technique [10]

A thickness of 1.5–2.5 mm is used in the manufacture of scleral shells if the palpebral fissure of the affected eye is smaller than the normal eye. The technique used for fabrication is similar to that of a regular prosthetic eye. If the palpebral fissure of the affected eye is the same as the normal eye or just slightly smaller, a thinner shell is usually used and is made in a different technique than the regular one to avoid the discrepancy in the palpebral fissure appearance between both eyes which tends to look larger if a thicker shell was used.

Adequate tear flow is crucial to help eliminate the accumulation of metabolic products that lead to discomfort and burning, limiting the wearing time of the shell. In addition, good tear flow helps prevent corneal edema and neovascularization secondary to corneal endothelial dysfunction.

To maintain proper lid contour and height, the most prominent area of the globe, determined by the corneal position, shape, apex, and contour, has to be determined because this will be the thinnest area of the prosthesis. The thicker areas of the shell will help in the stability, strength, and prevention of irritation and erosion of the sclera. This is aided by making the edges of the shell smoother and rounder.

Scleral shells are more difficult to make than regular ocular prostheses, and require more skill because these shells are too thin to have enough space for a separate iris/corneal segment found in regular prostheses. Therefore, the iris and the cornea are directly painted on the surface of the thin shell. Ideally, about five sessions are needed with an ocularist to fabricate a scleral shell. A trial shell is usually used for proper fitting and adjustments before the final shell is delivered.

First of all, an impression of the eye is taken using ocular trays (Fig. 22.6) after applying topical anesthetic drops, considering the confined space between the globe and the eyelids and the sensitivity of the globe. Using sizers from the ocular tray, the largest one that can be easily inserted into the palpebral fissure is carefully chosen. If the sizer is too small, it will not hold the impression material. If it is too big, it will be difficult to insert the sizer under the eyelids. Polyvinylsiloxane or ophthalmic alginate is used for impression by loading it into a syringe and injecting it into the tray. The lashes are freed from the material once it is set and removed. Next, the impression is cast in a dental stone (Fig. 22.7) to make the trial shell made of clear PMMA. A trial shell is recommended before the final shell is made because the final

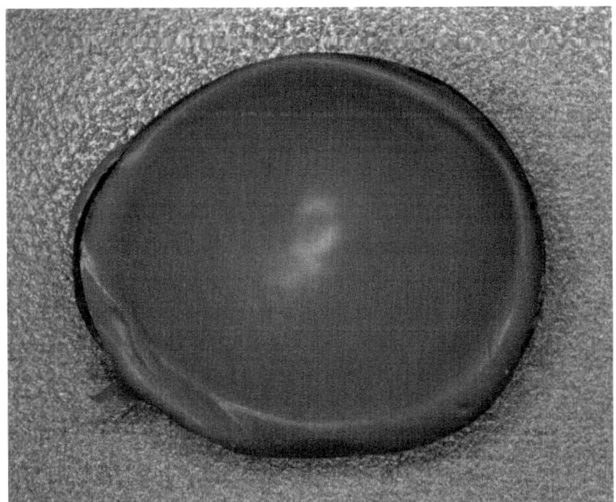

Fig. 22.6 Polyvinylsiloxane impression taken using an ocular impression tray without stem. (Published with kind permission of Dr. Keith R. Pine. All rights reserved)

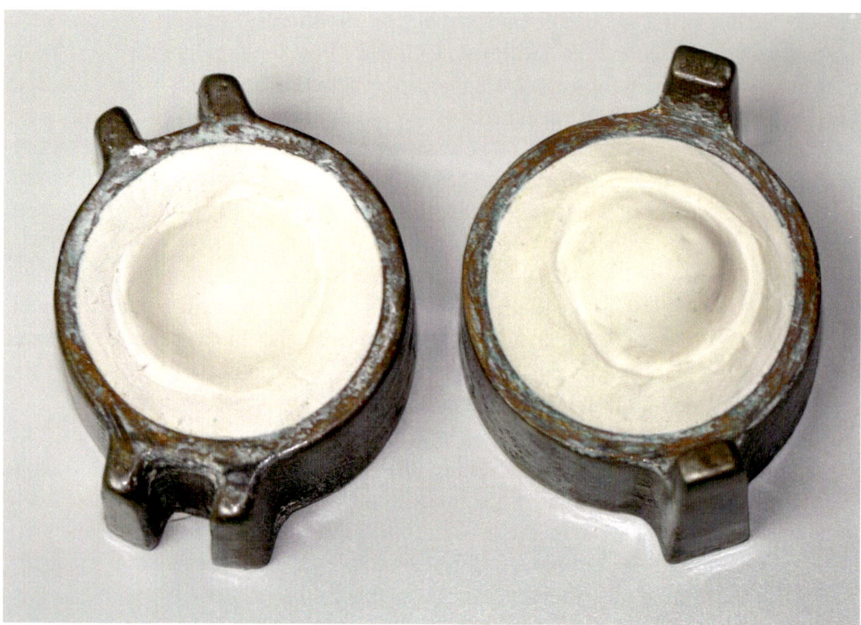

Fig. 22.7 The two-part mold is ready to be packed with clear PMMA dough. (Published with kind permission of Dr. Keith R. Pine.)

shell is so thin that it permits only a limited number of attempts for adjustments to relieve the pressure areas. The trial shell is tested for stability when the patient moves the eye, and adjustments are made accordingly. The fit is checked again using two techniques: by assessing the blanching of the conjunctival and limbal vessels when the shell is inserted, and by checking the fluorescein dye thickness between the trial shell and the cornea. Adjustments are made so that blood vessels are not blanching and a reasonable flow of tears behind the shell is maintained. This is done by polishing and smoothing areas of pressure. The trial shell is then given to the patient to be worn for few days to assess fit and absence of discomfort. Since scleral shells are not oxygen permeable, adequate oxygenation through the flow of tears is crucial to prevent corneal edema secondary to metabolite accumulation which will lead to significant discomfort. Fenestration of the shell has also been used to solve this problem. The fenestrations vary in size, number, and location beginning with a single 1.00 mm diameter fenestration in the temporal area of the scleral shell to multiple 0.5 mm holes around the periphery of the shell [10–12]. The trial scleral shell is used as a mold for the final scleral shell once adjustments are finalized and the patient is comfortable with the fit. The final shell can be transparent, semitransparent, or white depending on the patient's requirement of showing or hiding the structures behind the shell. After trimming, thinning and polishing the

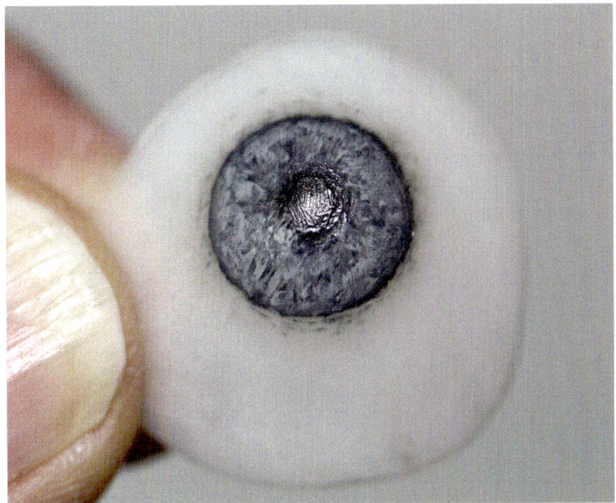

Fig. 22.8 Iris disc painted directly onto the surface of a semitranslucent shell. (Published with kind permission of Dr. Keith R. Pine. All rights reserved)

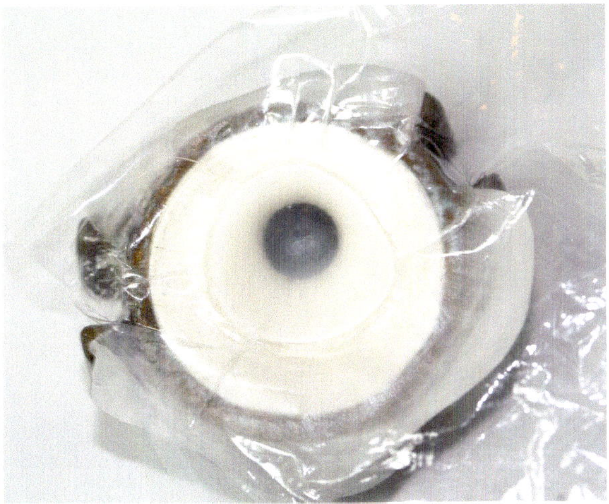

Fig. 22.9 Polyurethane sheet protects the painted surface when a clear PMMA veneer is trial packed. (Published with kind permission of Dr. Keith R. Pine. All rights reserved)

scleral shell into the appropriate size and shape, it is inserted over the patient's eye to mark the pupil position. The iris is painted onto the surface of the shell with a base color, and reinserted again to check for the size and position and adjustments are made accordingly (Fig. 22.8). Once the final shape, size, and position of the iris are reached, the fine details of the iris are painted including the stroma, the pupil, the vessels, the collarette, and scleral details. After the colors are dry, a thin layer of PMMA veneer (Figs. 22.9 and 22.10) is added to preserve the colors, and further polishing is performed. The fenestration holes are drilled after that process, and the shell is fitted again (Figs. 22.11 and 22.12).

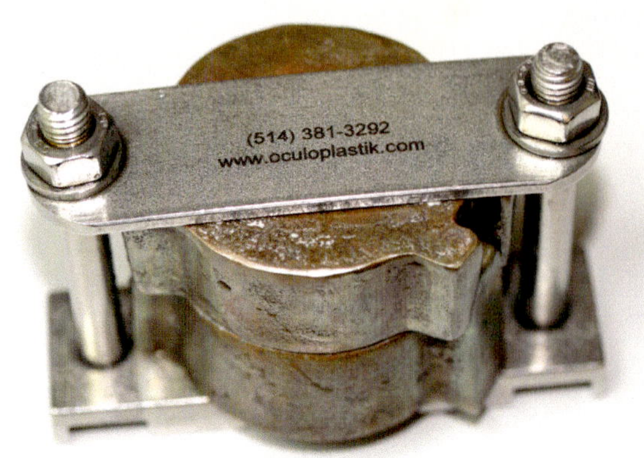

Fig. 22.10 The PMMA veneer is processed according to the manufacturer's instructions. (Published with kind permission of Dr. Keith R. Pine. All rights reserved)

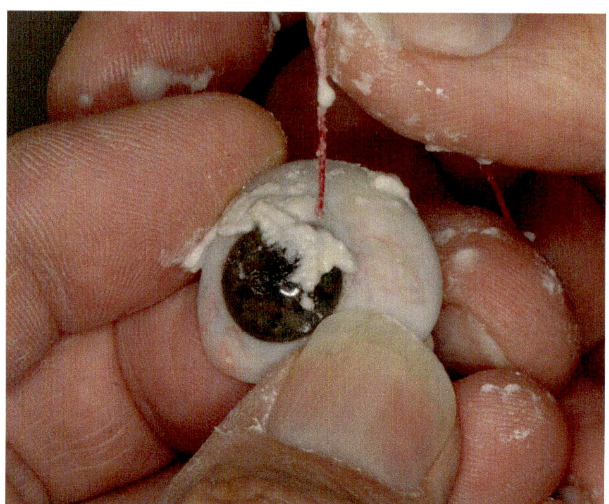

Fig. 22.11 The edges of the hole are smoothed with a cotton thread and pumice. (Published with kind permission of Dr. Keith R. Pine. All rights reserved)

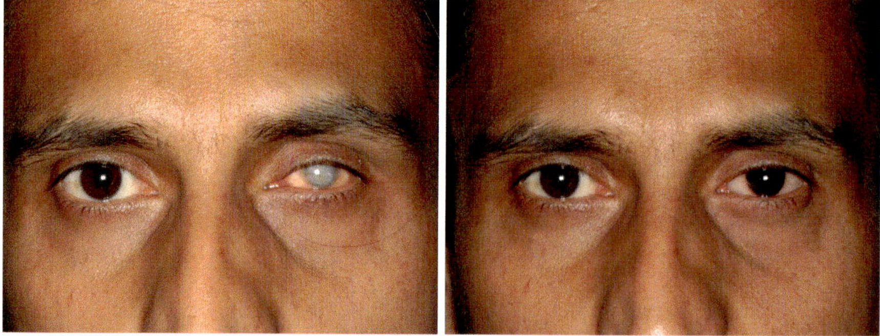

Fig. 22.12 Completed thin scleral shell prosthesis in situ. (Published with kind permission of Dr. Keith R. Pine. All rights reserved)

Pros and Cons of Scleral Shells [1, 10]

Pros:

- Better motility than regular prosthetic eyes where the eye is removed, since the existing eye is used as a base.
- More stable than prosthetic contact lenses because of their larger size, and better cosmetically in lighter colored eyes

Cons:

- Thin scleral shells may require fenestration to help with the tear flow as they fit more tightly than regular post-enucleation ocular prostheses.
- Thicker scleral shells may need to be removed every month to help with the oxygenation of the cornea; thinner ones may need to be removed every night.

Follow-Up and Care

The patient is seen one month after the final prosthesis is inserted to check for fitting and monitor any complications. After that the American Society of Ocularists recommends that infants under 3 years of age be seen every 3 months, under 9 twice yearly and older patients every year by an ocularist and an oculoplastic surgeon [1]. At each visit the surgeon/ocularist examine for proper fitting and possible complications. Polishing of the scleral shell is done every visit to restore the smooth surface of the shell and maintain the health of the tissue around it. It is crucial to stress on the importance of wearing protective polycarbonate glasses ALL THE TIME on each visit which helps protect and possibly improve the vision of the normal eye, and camouflage any cosmetic problems that cannot be fixed with the shell such as motility problems or eyelid retraction/ptosis [1, 10].

The patient is reassured that minimal mucoid discharge is normal, and is managed and minimized by removing and cleaning the shell not less frequently than monthly. A wet paper towel is used to wipe the shell and eliminate the biofilm, deposits, and debris. It is also recommended to avoid hot water and abrasive materials like toothpaste and soap with a fragrance or a moisturizer. When the eye is removed for a longer period of time it should be kept in a dark container with water to avoid the damage to the shell material due to lamination caused by drying [1, 10].

To remove the prosthesis the patient needs to look up and use the forefinger to pull and press down on the lower lid to allow lower edge of prosthesis to slide out (Fig. 22.13). Another way to remove the shell involves using a wet suction cup (Fig. 22.14), pressing it against the shell, and then releasing the squeeze creating a vacuum enabling a grip, then pulling and gently maneuvering the prosthesis out while holding down the lower lid [1, 10].

To insert the prosthesis, the prosthesis is held with the suction cup or between two fingers and orienting the nasal part which is usually sharpest point toward the

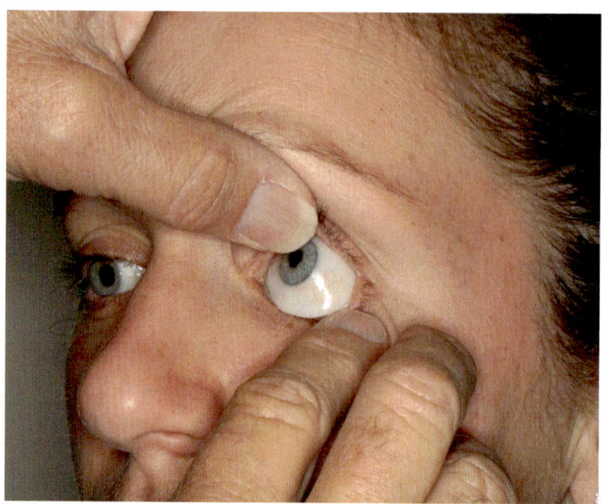

Fig. 22.13 Removing a patient's prosthetic eye. The caregiver's forefinger slides the lower eyelid under the prosthesis while the patient is looking upwards. (Published with kind permission of Dr. Keith R. Pine. All rights reserved)

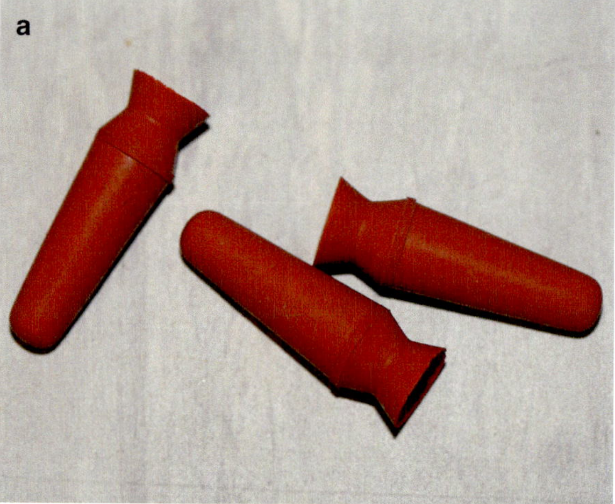

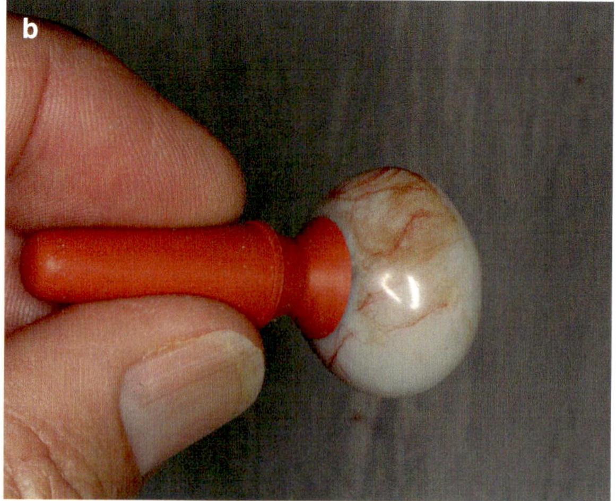

Fig. 22.14 (**a**, **b**) Rubber suction cups make it easier to remove and insert prosthetic eyes. (Published with kind permission of Dr. Keith R. Pine. All rights reserved)

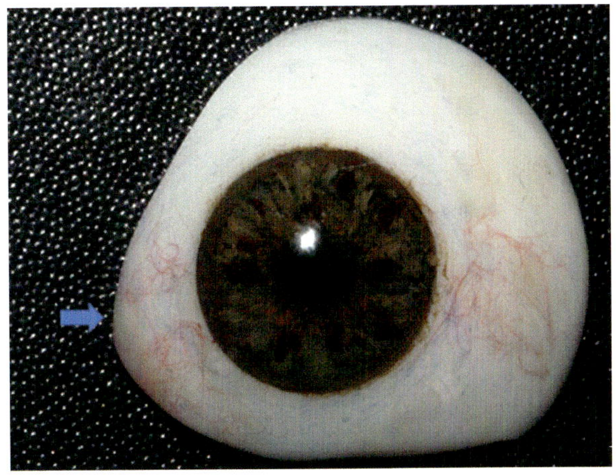

Fig. 22.15 *For orientation*, the sharpest and/or pinkest point (indicated by the *arrow*) is positioned toward the nose. (Published with kind permission of Dr. Keith R. Pine. All rights reserved)

nose (Fig. 22.15). The patient is instructed to look downwards while the other hand lifts up the upper eyelid and sliding the shell under it. While holding the shell in place, the lower eyelid is pulled downwards to push it in place and is then released.

References

1. Ocularist.org.
2. London Times. 5,000-year-old artificial eye found on Iran-Afghan border. 20 Feb 2007.
3. Lamb J, Sabell A. The history of contact lenses. In: Phillips AJ, Speedwell L, editors. Contact lenses. 5th ed. Edinburgh: Butterworth Heinemann Elsevier; 2007.
4. Leuschner FW. Light-controlled pupil size for ocular prosthesis. In: Proceedings of ophthalmic technologies II 1644, 1992. p 320–325.
5. Schleipman F, Schleipman R, Sleet DPV, Duncunson PA. US Patent No. 6,139,577. Washington, DC: U. S. P. a. T. Office Washington; 2000.
6. Friel TP. US Patent No. 5,061,279. Washington, DC: U. S. P. a. T. Office; 1991.
7. LaFuente H. US Patent No. 4,332,039. Washington, DC: U. S. P. a. T. Office; 1982.
8. Young SR. US Patent No. US 7,311 397 B1. Washington, DC: U. S. P. a. T. Office; 2007.
9. Pine KR, Sloan BH, Jacobs RJ. Clinical ocular prosthetics. Cham: Springer International Publishing; 2015.
10. Lapointe J, Harhira A, Durette J-F, Beaulieu S, Shaat A, Boulos PR, Kashyap R. An ocular prosthesis which reacts to light. In: Proc. SPIE 7885, ophthalmic technologies XXI, 788512, 11 Feb 2011. https://doi.org/10.1117/12.874078.
11. Harris MG, Barreto DJ, Matthews MS. The effect of peripherally fenestrated contact lenses on corneal edema. Am J Optom Physiol Optic. 1977;54(1):27–30.
12. Stone J, Phillips AJ. Contact lenses. London: Barrie & Jenkins; 1972.

Chapter 23
Keratopigmentation (Corneal Tattoo) and Prosthetic Contact Lenses

Zakeya Mohammed Al-Sadah

Summary

Prosthetic contact lenses and corneal tattooing have been used for both cosmetic purposes in nonfunctioning disfigured eyes and for therapeutic purposes in functioning eyes. For example, they are used in aniridia to avoid glare and double vision. In blind, disfigured non-painful eyes, these techniques have the advantage of low cost and the avoidance of more invasive procedures such as conjunctival flaps, evisceration, and enucleation. In certain patients with a close to normal-sized globe and minimal disfigurement, contact lenses are preferred for creating the best match to the contralateral eye. The lenses are commercially available in different iris diameters, colors, and base curves. However, if a more precise match is desired, prosthetic contact lenses can be hand painted and customized. On the other hand, when only acceptable cosmesis and lower maintenance are desired, or in patients with intolerance to prosthetic contact lenses, corneal tattooing can be used. Different dye materials, surgical techniques, and results have been described.

The practice of corneal tattooing began over 2000 years ago. It was first described by the Roman physician and philosopher Galen in 150 AD and again by Aetius 300 years later. They used different dyes to stain the scarred cornea of blind eyes after cauterizing them with a heated stylet. Different dye materials were used, including iron, nutgalls, copper sulfate, and pulverized pomegranate bark mixed with copper salts [1, 2]. In 1869, Louis Von Wrecker introduced a new method of tattooing by coating the cornea with Indian ink and using a grooved needle to insert the stain into the cornea stroma obliquely after applying cocaine as a topical anesthetic [2]. To produce a perfectly round pupil and cornea, some physicians used the von Hippel trephine for delineation. Holth and others used a metal cylinder for the

Z. M. Al-Sadah (✉)
Ophthalmic Plastic and Reconstructive Surgery, Department of Ophthalmology, Bascom Palmer Eye Institute, University of Miami Miller School of Medicine, Miami, FL, USA

T. E. Johnson (ed.), *Anophthalmia*,
https://doi.org/10.1007/978-3-030-29753-4_23

same purpose. Armaignac applied china ink in a funnel fixed to the cornea [1]. In order to be more efficient, Taylor used a bundle of needles instead of a single needle. In 1901, an electrical, needle-like fountain pen for tattooing was introduced by Nieden, as he thought it was more practical. Additionally, Morax created a corneal flap and injected the stain underneath it, followed by applying a pressure patch to hold the stain on the eye [2].

Ink Types and Colors

Different types of ink and dyes are described throughout the history of corneal tattooing. The safest and most commonly used are Indian ink and China ink which are believed to impart a long-lasting effect (Fig. 23.1) [3, 4]. Metallic dyes in a powder form (sliver nitrate, platinum, or gold chloride), organic dyes, and uveal pigments from the choroid of animal eyes [5], candle soot [6], and drawing ink [7, 8] have also been tried. Different materials were incorporated to produce colored pigments like gamboge, terra sienna, ultramarine, Prussian blue, and calcium carbonate. However, many of them incited corneal irritation [1]. According to Ziegler, materials used as pigments in corneal tattooing have to be metallic, non-irritant, and

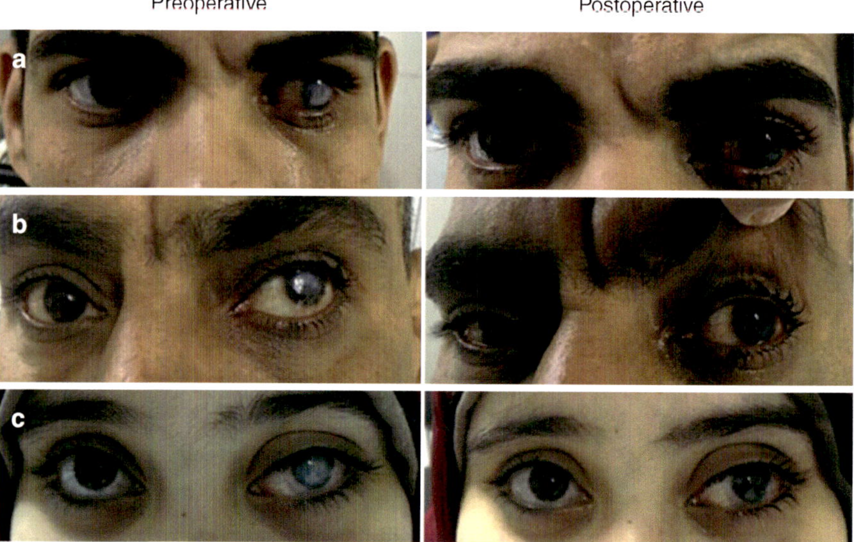

Fig. 23.1 External photos of superficial corneal staining with China painting ink using superficial corneal staining technique via direct superficial intrastromal injection of the pigment material with a 30-gauge needle. (**a**) Pre-tattooing and 3 months post-tattooing of a 32-year-old male. (**b**) Pre-tattooing and 1 month post-tattooing of a 62-year-old male. (**c**) Pre-tattooing and 3 months post-tattooing of an 18-year-old female. (Published with kind permission of Dr. Alahmady H. Alsamman. Hindawi, Egypt.)

miscible in water but not soluble, permanent, opaque, and stabilizable [1]. Histopathologically, it was found that the pigmentary deposits are found as irregular clumps in interfibrillar spaces, keratocytes, and lymphatic and blood vessels where the location and the shape of each deposit are affected by the type of pigment (metallic vs. nonmetallic) [1]. Nonmetallic pigments such as Indian ink were found intracellularly as light and dark granules with sharp edges inside keratocytes due to the process of endocytosis. Metallic pigments such as platinum chloride were found as round, black granules intracellularly in keratocytes and also extracellularly, and induced a foreign body inflammatory reaction secondary to the extracellular component of the pigment [1, 6, 9]. The extracellular material is phagocytosed by corneal fibroblasts. This is thought to be part of the corneal protective mechanism against damage caused by any foreign material and is believed to account for the less stable and the less permanent retention of the metallic dye [6]. Because of that foreign body reaction and irritation, the use of many metallic dyes including chromes, cobalt, cadmium, and gamboge are to be avoided together with their chemical excipients that form irritant chemical compounds such as oxycyanid [1]. In order to decrease the foreign body reaction, reduction of the metal pigment size (e.g., black iron oxide) by a process called micronization was introduced, and this change was found to not induce local toxicity owing to the reduced, ~2.5 micron-size of the micronized pigment particles compared with the larger size of the regular metallic pigments [10]. Using this method, one has a wider range of colors available which in turn provides better cosmetic results by matching the color of the eye [10]. Those small particles are nontoxic, non-irritating, non-soluble and safe, and commonly used in dermatology to treat vitiligo [10] (Figs. 23.2, 23.3, and 23.4).

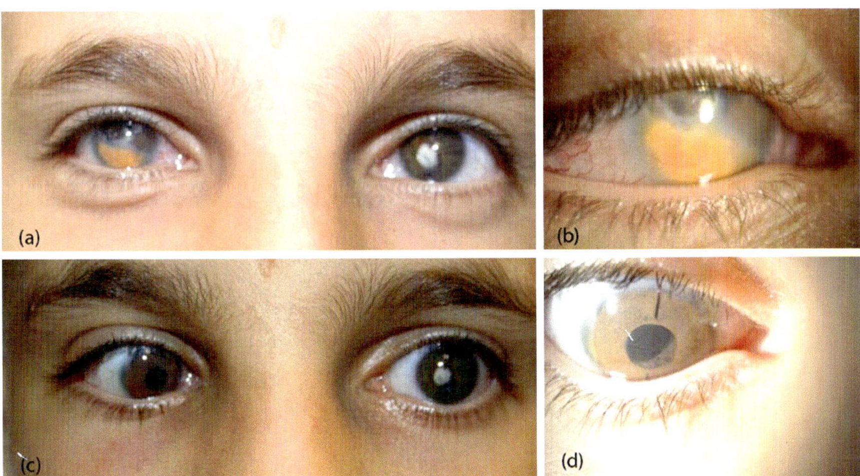

Fig. 23.2 (**a**) and (**b**) Preoperative photos of a case of bilateral retinopathy of prematurity with right eye lipid keratopathy. (**c**) and (**d**) Postoperative photo of right eye intrastromal keratopigmentation with iris and pupil simulation. (Published with kind permission of Dr. Amesty MA and Alio JL. Vissium Spain. All rights reserved)

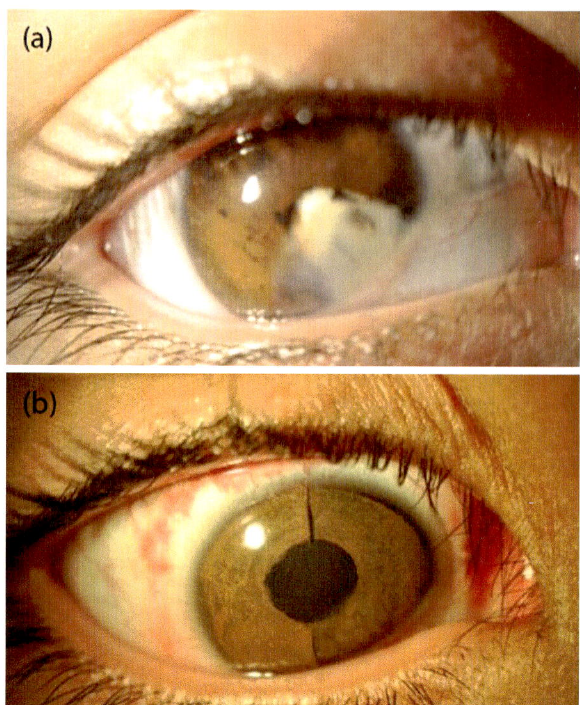

Fig. 23.3 (**a**) Preoperative photos of a case of sectoral corneal opacification secondary to right eye trauma. (**b**) Postoperative photos of sectoral intrastromal keratopigmentation with iris and pupil simulation. (Published with kind permission of Dr. Amesty MA and Alio JL. Vissium Spain.)

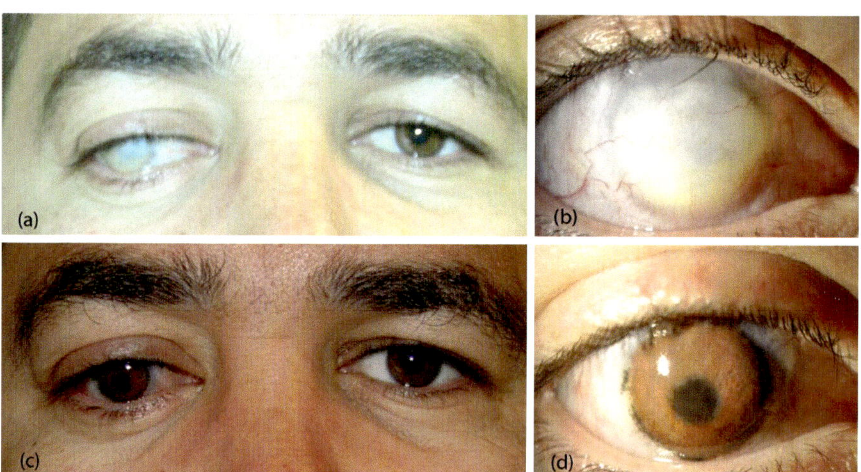

Fig. 23.4 (**a**) and (**b**) Preoperative photos of a case of corneal opacification secondary to right eye trauma. (**c**) and (**d**) Postoperative photos of keratopigmentation with iris and pupil simulation. (Published with kind permission of Dr. Amesty MA and Alio JL. Vissium Spain.)

Keratopigmentation Methods

Two methods are generally used for keratopigmentation: carbon impregnation and dying with platinum and gold chloride. Insoluble pigments like India ink, China ink, lamp black ink and other organic dyes are introduced directly into the corneal stroma in the carbon impregnation method [6]. Conversely, platinum and gold chloride are used in the dying method by inducing a chemical reaction in a de-epithelialized corneal surface which is believed to be easier and quicker, provides a jet-black stain, but fades faster [6]. Several factors play a part in the pigment dispersion including migration and dissolution of the pigment particles and extrusion of the pigment secondary to the inflammatory reaction caused by the chemical irritation to the cornea [1].

Keratopigmentation Surgical Techniques

Cosmetic keratopigmentation can be performed on blind, unsightly eyes that are phthisical, eyes with corneal scars, and leukocoria in blind eyes where surgery is not recommended. However, keratopigmentation can also be used therapeutically in seeing eyes where photophobia is bothersome such as in cases of albinism, iris colobomas, aniridia, and essential iris atrophy (Fig. 23.4). In cases of corneal thinning including descemetoceles and staphylomas, or in cases where there is a risk of corneal ectasia or melt as in autoimmune connective tissue diseases, keratopigmentation is contraindicated. Various methods are described to apply the ink or dye to the cornea. Although difficult in some ink types, sterilization of the ink is important as the presence of bacillus capsule in China ink has been demonstrated [1]. For example, a rod of Indian ink is grated, sterilized and dried at a temperature of 1500° using an electrical sterilizer, and then mixed with water [1]. Alsamman et al. showed that packing China ink in a sterile glass infusion bottle for 20 minutes in a steam autoclave at 121 °C was safe in both rabbit and human eyes [4]. Topical Glycerin can be applied to edematous corneas to help clear them during the procedure. Topical anesthesia is the preferred anesthetic technique. Bandage contact lens and topical antibiotic/steroid +/−cyclopentolate hydrochloride drops are recommended in the first 2 post-operative weeks to help with discomfort, to promote healthy corneal epithelialization, and to stabilize and maintain the pigment and avoid the early fading.

Superficial Corneal Staining

Superficial corneal staining is the most popular technique and is performed by two different methods. The first is a direct superficial intrastromal injection of pigment material using a 30-gauge needle. The second involves placing a drop of ink on the corneal surface after delineation of the area to be stained, followed by multiple, superficial, intrastromal micropunctures with a 30-gauge needle to inoculate the pigment [3, 10] (Figs. 23.5, 23.6, and 23.7). Irrigation is performed intermittently to

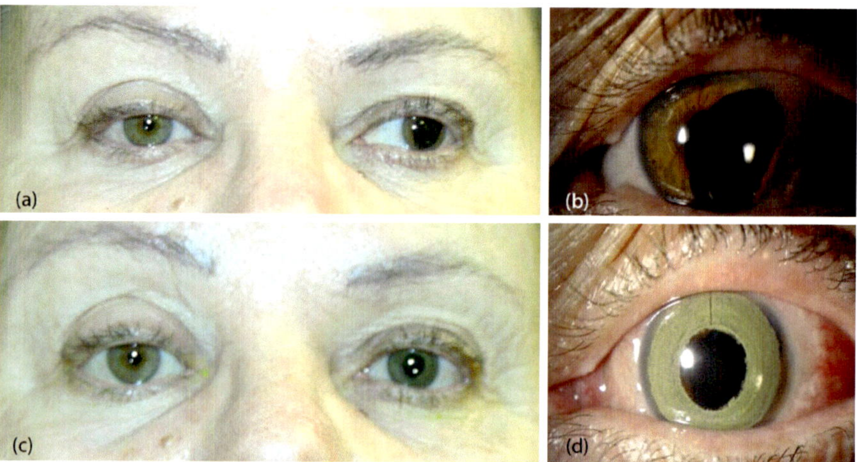

Fig. 23.5 (**a**) and (**b**) Preoperative photos of a case of a left eye traumatic cataract and aniridia. (**c**) and (**d**) Postoperative photos of intrastromal keratopigmentation and strabismus surgery. (Published with kind permission of Dr. Amesty MA and Alio JL. Vissium Spain. All rights reserved)

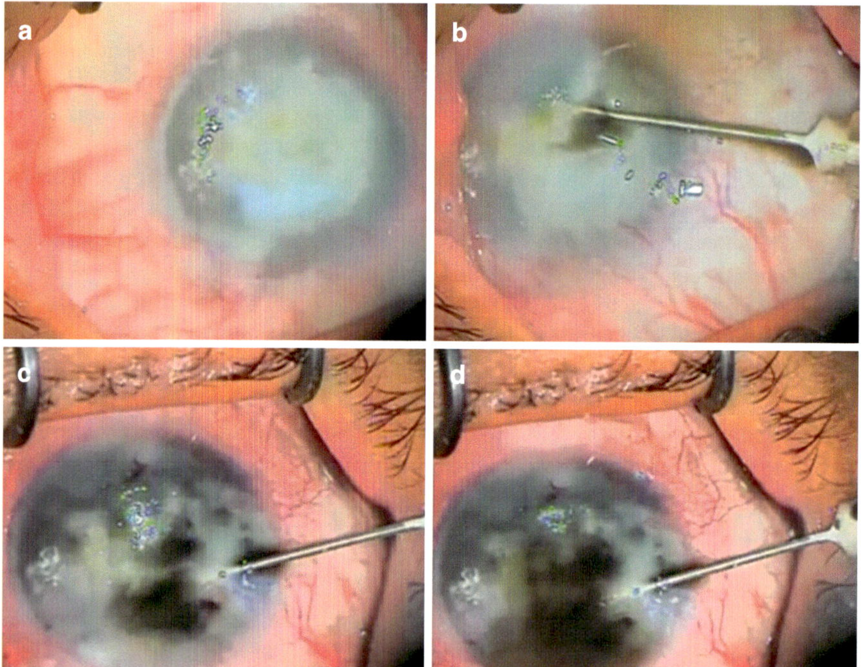

Fig. 23.6 Intraoperative photos of superficial corneal staining with China painting ink using superficial corneal staining technique via direct superficial intrastromal injection of the pigment material with a 30-gauge needle. (**a**) Corneal opacification before tattooing. (**b**) The bevel of the needle was administered intrastromally tangential to the corneal surface, and injection was started. (**c**) Repeated multiple sites injections. (**d**) Full corneal tattooing. (Published with kind permission of Dr. Alahmady H. Alsamman. Hindawi, Egypt. All rights reserved)

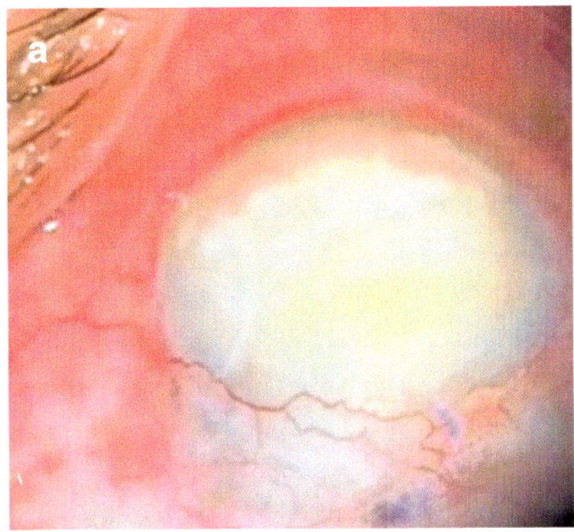

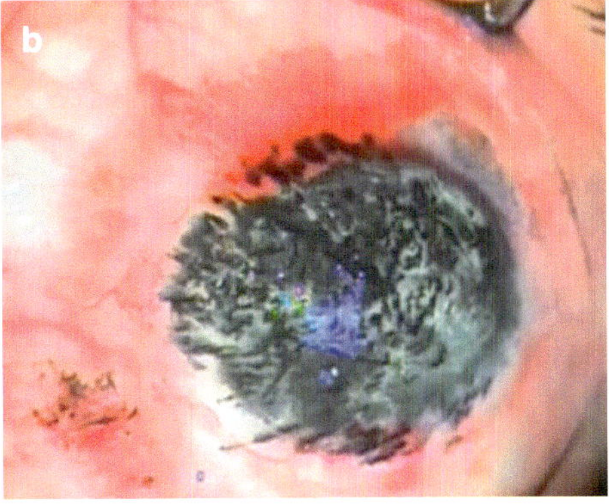

Fig. 23.7 Microscopic photos of superficial corneal staining with China painting ink via direct superficial intrastromal injection of the pigment material with a 30-gauge needle. (**a**) Preoperative photo showing total corneal opacity (**b**) Postoperative photo after corneal tattooing. (Published with kind permission of Dr. Alahmady H. Alsamman. Hindawi, Egypt. All rights reserved)

detect areas that were missed. Also, a three-edged spatula needle can be used in a similar manner [7]. To avoid surgical field obscuration and avoid repetitive irrigation, Theobald injected the eye first and then applied ink with a Daviel curette [11].

Interlamellar Corneal Staining

The low mesopic pupil diameter of the normal eye is measured using infrared pupillometer or a Holladay-Godwin corneal gauge. The center of the cornea is marked, and a radial keratotomy optic zone marker is used to mark the measured pupil diameter. A corneal blade is employed to make 3–4 radial incisions starting from the limbus and extending to the marked pupil. Intrastromal and circumferential dissection up to the nearest incision is performed using a micro crescent blade. Dissection is also performed staring from the limbal border to the marked pupillary area creating a tunnel. Pigment is injected into the tunnel using 30-gauge cannula. Additionally, using a single radial incision, a spiral corneal dissector can be used to create an intrastromal circumferential tunnel by dissecting 180° on each side of the incision [10].

Femtosecond-Assisted Keratopigmentation

One or two intrastromal tunnels are made. The two-tunnel technique is reported to give better cosmesis due to the ability to produce greater resemblance to the normal iris structure. In this technique, a double layer intrastromal tunnel is created, and darker pigment is applied into the deeper tunnel while lighter pigment is applied to the superficial tunnel. Using this technique allows one to more closely match the color of the contralateral normal eye. Appropriate tunnel depth is determined preoperatively with tomography and pachymetry. A superficial incision is made using the femtosecond laser at a depth of 200 microns with an inner diameter of 6 mm and an outer diameter of 9.5 mm and with a vertical incision at 12:00 and an energy setting of 2 mJ. A deeper incision is made at a 400-micron depth with an inner diameter of 6 mm and an outer diameter of 9.5 mm with a vertical incision at 6:00 and an energy level of 2 mJ. The interlamellar tunnels are made using a lamellar corneal dissector. This is followed by using a 30-gauge cannula to inject pigment into the incisions in both layers [10, 12, 13]. Corneal suturing is not required.

Other Techniques

Arif Khan and David Meyer introduced a new method by applying 2% platinum chloride-soaked filter paper on an alcohol de-epithelialized cornea for 2 minutes, followed by placement of a 2% hydrazine-soaked filter paper for 25 seconds [14]. Thomson used a steel pen converted to a cutting edge that provided better visualization of the cornea since there was no need to refill the ink or coat the cornea with ink [15]. Manual lamellar pocket creation followed by injection of dye was described by Chawdhary and coworkers. A trephine was used to create a lamellar 180° hinge, and a filter paper soaked with dye was placed under the pocket for a few minutes [16]. Also, Lee et al. performed corneal tattooing by forming an anterior stromal space using an air bubble infiltration [17].

Advantages and Disadvantages of Corneal Tattooing

Keratopigmentation has a high success rate, low cost, and minimum recovery time. The need for more invasive procedures including penetrating keratoplasty, conjunctival flap, evisceration, and enucleation is eliminated for non-painful blind unsightly eyes when the main indication for the intervention is cosmesis. It is helpful when there is poor tolerance of cosmetic tinted contact lenses and in severe corneal neovascularization where keratoplasty is contraindicated due to the high risk of failure. Tattoo fading after variable amounts of time is encountered after most of techniques, especially the superficial anterior stromal techniques. These patients often need for repeat tattooing (Fig. 23.8) [4, 18]. Also, the fading of the corneal tattooing occurs more rapidly with the use of the chemical dyes [6]. Other disadvantages of keratopigmentation include incomplete coverage of the cornea or insufficient staining (Fig. 23.9) and poor cosmesis due to lack of homogeneity especially in the stromal puncture techniques [4, 18]. Initial discomfort and inflammation are expected on the first few days especially in the superficial techniques secondary to corneal epithelial defects that rarely turn into a persistent epithelial defects or corneal ulcers [10].

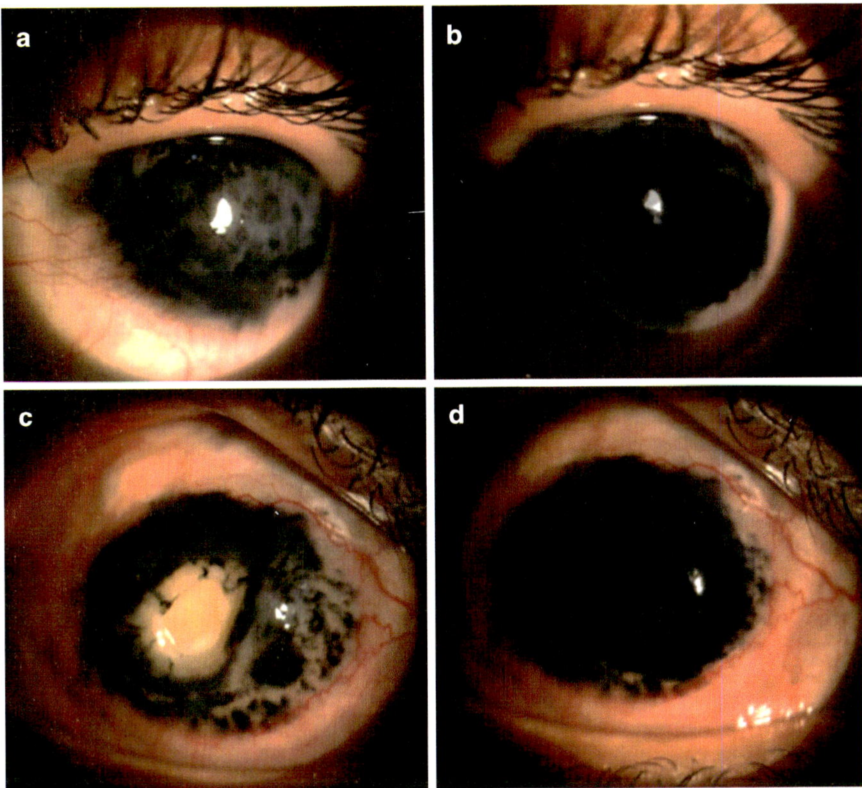

Fig. 23.8 Microscopic photos of superficial corneal staining with China painting ink using superficial corneal staining technique via direct superficial intrastromal injection of the pigment material with a 30-gauge needle. (**a**) and (**c**); fading of tattooing after one month. (**b**) and (**d**) re-tattooing after 3 months which made it homogeneous. (Published with kind permission of Dr. Alahmady H. Alsamman. Hindawi, Egypt. All rights reserved)

Fig. 23.9 Microscopic photos of superficial corneal staining with China painting ink using via direct superficial intrastromal injection of the pigment material with a 30-gauge needle showing insufficient staining. (Published with kind permission of Dr. Alahmady H. Alsamman. Hindawi, Egypt. All rights reserved)

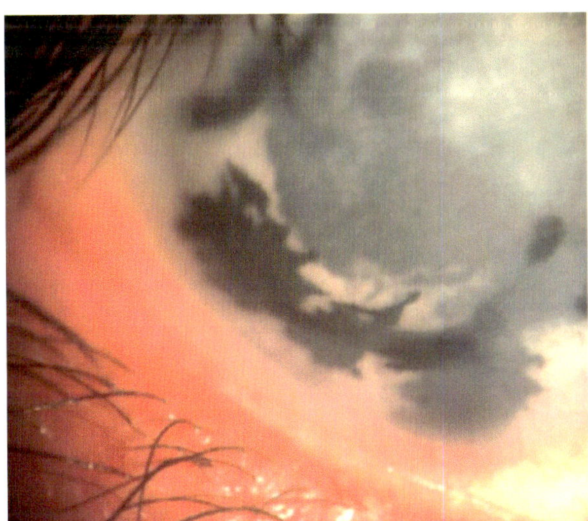

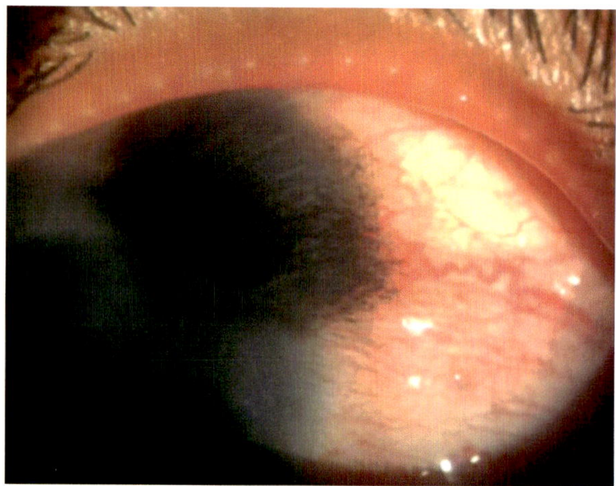

Fig. 23.10 Microscopic photos of superficial corneal staining with China painting ink via direct superficial intrastromal injection of the pigment material with a 30-gauge needle showing dye seepage into the conjunctiva leading to conjunctival space staining. (Published with kind permission of Dr. Alahmady H. Alsamman. Hindawi, Egypt. All rights reserved)

Some studies also describe complications such as hypopigmentation, hyperpigmentation, pigment migration, corneal infections, uveitis, and corneal perforation [19]. Preparation of the micronized mineral pigment by mixing different pigments to produce the desired color provides a wider range of color variety with lower incidence of foreign body reaction, yet can be time consuming [10, 19]. The femtosecond technique and microkeratome dissection methods are expensive, invasive procedures and have the disadvantage of weakening the cornea. Additionally, the flap size limitation might necessitate further dissection to cover the whole cornea. A white epithelial growth masking the tattooed cornea was described by Kim and is treated by simple scraping of the area without the need of repeat tattooing [20]. Kim also described a spread of the pigment into the subconjunctival space with staining through the new vessels of the cornea, and recommended resection of that area in case of inadvertent staining. This problem is best prevented by avoiding injection into new vessels during tattooing (Fig. 23.10) [4, 20].

Prosthetic Contact Lenses [21, 22]

Prosthetic contact lenses are painted or tinted contact lenses designed to mask the flaws and improve the appearance of disfigured corneas, irides, and sclera, as well as defects that occur secondary to congenital anomalies, trauma, and systemic or ocular diseases (Fig. 23.11). Additionally, they are used to reduce photophobia, glare, and double vision and are available in five basic designs, each treating a specific eye condition or deformity (Fig. 23.12). Satisfactory cosmesis is more difficult to achieve in prosthetic contact lens compared with scleral shells because regular corneal shape, good eye alignment, and globe size similar to the contralateral eye are required for the best cosmetic results. In seeing eyes, prosthetic contact lenses

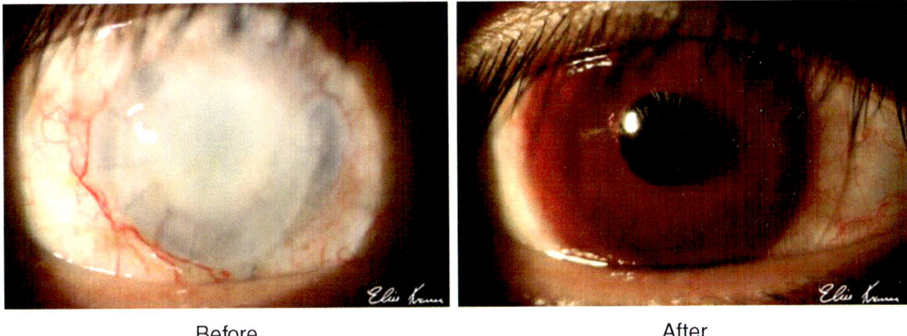

Fig. 23.11 Completely opacified cornea is masked with a prosthetic contact lens. (Published with kind permission of Dr. Elise Kramer, O.D, USA.)

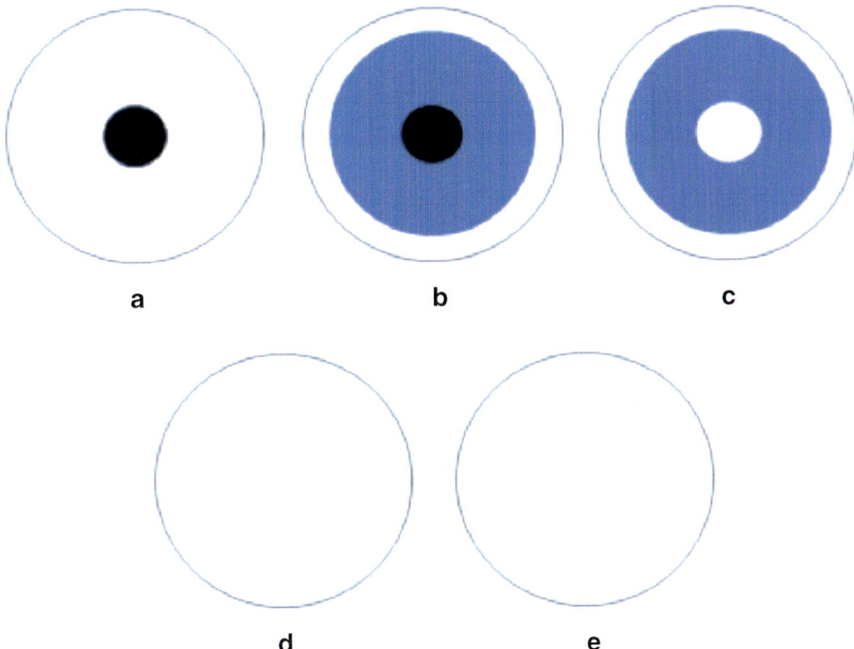

Fig. 23.12 Basic prosthetic contact lens designs. (**a**) Occluding pupil mask with clear iris portion. (**b**) Peripheral mask with opaque black pupil. (**c**) Peripheral mask with clear pupil. (**d**) Translucent tinted lens. (**e**) Translucent tinted peripheral mask with clear pupil. (Published with kind permission of Dr. Keith R Pine, New Zealand.)

come with clear pupils or pupils with a translucent tint. Prosthetic contact lenses also come with opaque, black pupils to improve the appearance of disfigured blind eyes (Figs. 23.13 and 23.14). Different types of lenses are available including poly-

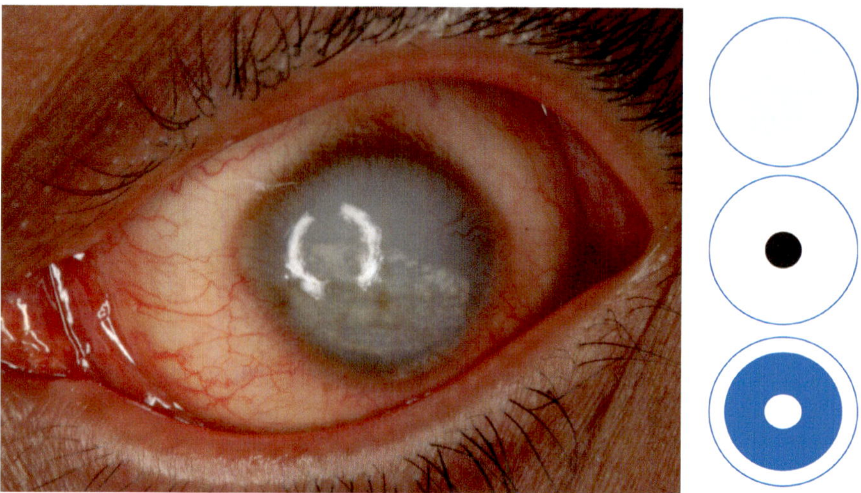

Fig. 23.13 Full-thickness, total corneal opacity. It may be masked with a prosthetic contact lens with an opaque peripheral mask and a black pupil. (Published with kind permission of Dr. Keith R Pine, New Zealand.)

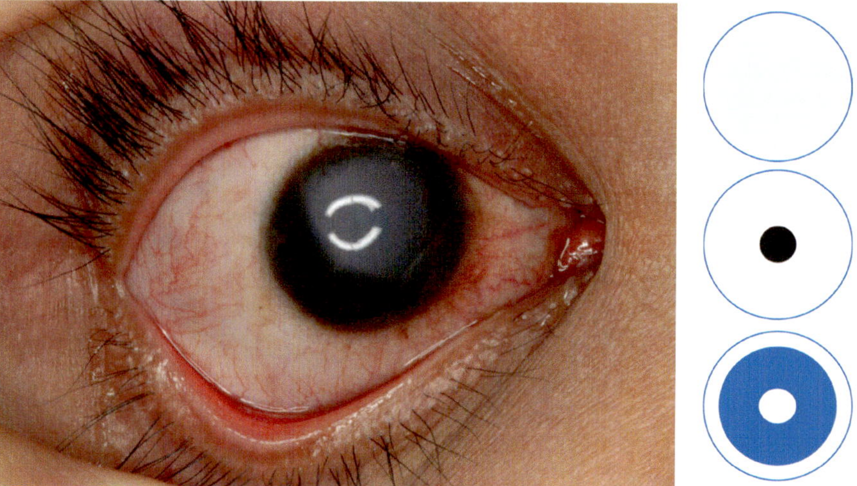

Fig. 23.14 Corneal dystrophy. If the eyes are blind and the pupil is not discernable, clear lenses with black pupils will improve cosmesis. If the pupils are discernable and dark, translucent tinted lenses may mask the grayness of the cornea while not compromising the level of vision. Finally, opaque lenses with clear pupils may be a better option than tinted lenses if a wider range of colors is needed and the optimum level of vision is to be maintained. (Published with kind permission of Dr. Keith R Pine, New Zealand.)

methyl acrylate (PMMA), rigid gas permeable (RGP), scleral contact lenses, and soft contact lenses are available. PMMA and RGP lenses have the advantage of ease of painting to match the contralateral eye. This painting is more difficult to accomplish with soft contact lenses. RGPs and PMMA also improve irregular astigmatism in deformed corneas. For peripheral corneal deformities or larger areas of deformities, soft contact lenses are preferred because of their larger size compared to PMMA or RGP lenses and their mobility over the cornea. In seeing eyes, soft contact lenses are not recommended in patients with irregular astigmatism. Scleral contact lenses are more difficult to design and fit, require a greater level of expertise, and are more expensive. Therefore, they are used as a last resort when all other types have failed, including in patients with difficulty in centration of the corneal contact lens or in those where improvement of the scleral appearance is desired.

Fitting of Prosthetic Contact Lenses [21, 22]

In disfigured corneas, trial lens fitting is performed. Corneal keratometry readings of the disfigured eye and the contralateral eye in case of severe disfigurement are recommended. Generally, PMMA and RGP contact lenses are fitted relatively tight to decrease their movement and made with a larger diameter to cover the cosmetic defect. Trial lenses are used in soft prosthetic lenses to determine the base curve, diameter, thickness, and color (determined by comparing the contralateral eye's color in natural sun light and under artificial light). The flattest soft contact lens is chosen in cases of customized painting because the painting process will cause the contact lens to become tighter. Conversely, scleral prosthetic lenses are fit by taking an impression of the eye and performing trial fitting. The size and the curvature of the sclera are measured followed by measuring the size and curvature of the optical zone.

Inexpensive standard opaque and tinted contact lenses in a wide range of colors and sizes (including curve base, iris diameter, pupil size with clear or black backing) are commercially available. A dark pupil or a peripheral tint can be added to clear contact lenses that are made of soft hydrophilic materials using coloring kits. However, an accurate color match is often difficult to obtain. Therefore, a hand painted prosthetic contact lenses can be ordered and customized (Fig. 23.15) or fabricated by different manufacturers after sending digital photographs of the contralateral normal eye that clearly demonstrates iris color and details. Included in the order are contact lens specifications including base curve and diameter (Fig. 23.16). Only EDTA- free contact lens solution prevents fading of the color of prosthetic contact lenses.

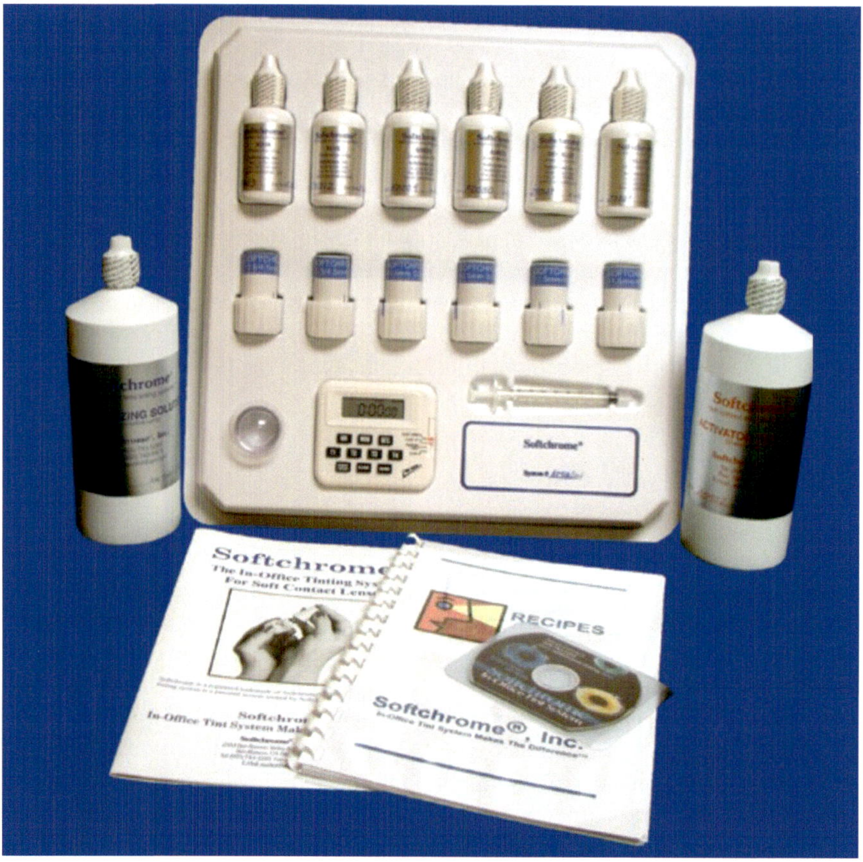

Fig. 23.15 In-house coloring kit for soft contact lenses. (Published with kind permission of Dr. Keith R Pine, New Zealand. All rights reserved)

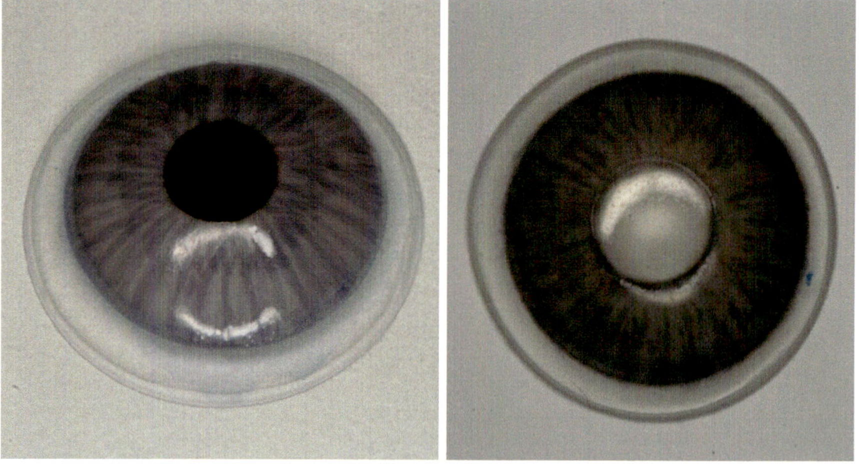

Fig. 23.16 Two examples of soft hand-painted prosthetic contact lenses (Published with kind permission of Dr. Keith R Pine, New Zealand. All rights reserved)

References

1. Ziegler SL. Multicolor tattooing of the cornea. Trans Am Ophthalmol Soc. 1922;20:71.
2. Roy JN. Tattooing of the cornea. Can Med Assoc J. 1938;39:436–8.
3. Vassileva S, Hristakieva E. Medical applications of tattooing. Clin Dermatol. 2007;25:367–74.
4. Alsmman AH, Mostafa EM, Mounir A, Farouk MM, Elghobaier MG, Radwan G. Outcomes of corneal tattooing by rotring painting ink in disfiguring corneal opacities. J Ophthalmol. 2018;2018:6, Article ID 5971290.
5. MJ M, Eghbali K, Schwab IR. Keratopigmentation: a review of corneal tattooing. Cornea. 1999;18:633–7.
6. Remky A, Redbrake C, Wenzel M. Intrastromal corneal tattooing for iris defects. J Cataract Refract Surg. 1998;24:1285–7.
7. Sekundo W, Seifert P, Seitz B, Loeffler KU. Long-term ultrastructural changes in human corneas after tattooing with non metallic substances. Br J Ophthalmol. 1999;83(2):219–24.
8. Pitz S, Jahn R, Frisch L, Duis A, Pfeiffer N. Corneal tattooing: an alternative treatment for disfiguring corneal scars. Br J Ophthalmol. 2002;86(4):397–9.
9. Amesty MA, Rodriguez AE, Hernández E, De Miguel MP, Alio JL. Tolerance of micronized mineral pigments for intrastromal keratopigmentation: a histopathology and immunopathology experimental study. Cornea. 2016;35(9):1199–205.
10. Alio JL, Sirerol B, Walewska-Szafran A. Corneal tattooing (keratopigmentation) to restore cosmetic appearance in severely impaired eyes with new mineral micronized pigments. Br J Ophthalmol. 2010;94:245–9.
11. Jeong J, Lee HJ, Lee SH. Corneal tattooing method using dye injection into the anterior stroma infiltrated with small air bubbles. Acta Ophthalmol. 2013;91(5):e417–8.
12. Kymionis GD, Ide T, Galor A, Yoo SH. Femtosecond-assisted anterior lamellar corneal staining-tattooing in a blind eye with leukocoria. Cornea. 2009;28:211–3.
13. Theobald S. A practical point in the technic of corneal tattooing, the value of which is not commonly recognized. Trans Am Ophthalmol Soc. 1918;16:225–6.
14. Khan AO, Meyer D. Corneal tattooing for the treatment of debilitating glare in a child with traumatic iris loss. Am J Ophthalmol. 2005;139(5):920–1.
15. Thomson W. An instrument for tattooing the cornea. Trans Am Ophthalmol Soc. 1873;2:86.
16. Panda A, Mohan M, Chawdhary S. Corneal tattooing—experiences with "lamellar pocket procedure". Indian J Ophthalmol. 1984;32:408–11.
17. Kim JH, Lee D, Hahn TW, Choi SK. new surgical strategy for corneal tattooing using a femtosecond laser. Cornea. 2009;28(1):80–4.
18. Mannis MJ, Eghbali K, Schwab IR. Keratopigmentation: a review of corneal tattooing. Cornea. 1999;18:633–7.
19. Sirerol B, Walewska-Szafran A, Alió JL, et al. Tolerance and biocompatibility of micronized black pigment for keratopigmentation simulated pupil reconstruction. Cornea. 2011;30:344–50.
20. Kim C, Kim KH, Han YK, et al. Five-year results of corneal tattooing for cosmetic repair in disfigured eyes. Cornea. 2011;30:1135–9.
21. Mannis MJ, Zadnik K, Coral-Ghanem C, Newton K-J. Contact lenses in ophthalmic practice. New York: Springer; 2004.
22. Pine KR, Sloan BH, Jacobs RJ. Clinical ocular prosthetics. Cham: Springer International Publishing Switzerland; 2015.

Chapter 24
Making an Ocular Prosthesis

Yasser Bataineh and Thomas E. Johnson

Introduction

With the development of polymethyl methacrylate (acrylic), the process of fabricating artificial eyes went from an empirical process (as in the case of making stock plastic eyes as well as glass eyes) to the present "state-of-the-art" prosthetic eye-making technique. The progress toward design to function is described in this chapter, as well as the varied steps in artificial eye fabrication.

Eye Socket Impression

Making a negative reproduction of the anophthalmic socket is the first half of the foundation of the "art to function design" process of the making of an ocular prosthesis. Importantly, it is a fact that the posterior aspect of the prosthesis in contact with the anterior socket tissues transfers motility to the artificial eye. Important steps include taking an accurate impression from the socket, initially choosing the correct size, shape, and thickness, and correct dimensions of the tray conformer to ensure a snug fit (without stressing the tissues), and following the contour of the socket. The conformer is perforated in each quadrant by four slits cut parallel to each other, and two small holes are made on each side of a suction cup placed on the anterior-central area to allow excess material to escape. Alginate is mixed with distilled water in accordance with manufacturers' specifications into a smooth consistency. With the patient's head positioned at a 45° angle, the alginate is first placed

Y. Bataineh (✉)
International Ocular Center, Miami, FL, USA

T. E. Johnson
Bascom Palmer Eye Institute, University of Miami Miller School of Medicine, Miami, FL, USA

T. E. Johnson (ed.), *Anophthalmia*,
https://doi.org/10.1007/978-3-030-29753-4_24

superiorly and allowed to flow into the socket using a disposable syringe. The patient is then asked to look down, and when the conformer is filled with alginate, the patient is then asked to gently close their eyes and next open their eyes and look straight ahead. The alginate is left to set 30–60 seconds depending on patient age. Therefore, the impression created is used to produce an accurate reproduction (fingerprint) of the socket anatomy. This process is essential in deciphering and interpreting the anatomy and aiding in determining the exact design needed to correct or minimize the effects of deformities on prosthesis function.

Infants, toddlers, and children are managed slightly differently than adults. After choosing the correct conformer attached to a suction cup, the nasal aspect is marked on the cup. Distilled water warmed to body temperature is used in mixing the impression material and allowed precisely 30 seconds to set. The process is rehearsed with the young patient using a favorite toy and playing music. The alginate is placed with the patient in the supine position using distraction as needed. After the correct time has elapsed, the impression is removed with a rounded extraction tool.

Design

The second half of the foundation is design of the ocular prosthesis. The accurate impression previously described imparts the shape of the posterior aspect of the prosthesis. The next step is to convert the impression from an alginate mass to a wax mass identical to the impression made. The wax mass is pliable and can therefore be manipulated for the art of designing the anterior aspect of the prosthesis. The anterior part of the future prosthesis is systematically transformed by increasing and decreasing the anterior surface area. Each quadrant of the future artificial eye is methodically designed collectively, bringing the design together and aligning and realigning the future iris position by trial and error. This process is continued until the perfect design that fits exactly and delivers correct eyelid position, stimulates eyelid function, and addresses all deformities. This balance act allows wiggle room and allows calculating by design the edging of the artificial eye, allowing flexion and turning of the socket tissues without creating pressure points, strain, or compression of these tissues. Those structures already went through the substantial stress of losing normal orbital structures whether due to acquired or congenital anophthalmias.

In infants, toddlers, and children in general, there is no conversion of the alginate mass to wax. Instead, the impression is converted to a clear conformer and tried in the patients' socket the next day. The design is altered by carving through the finished conformer until the goal is achieved. It may take longer but is less stressful and more accurate. With each alteration one allows 10 minutes of observation accompanied by photographs.

The fabrication process avoids compressing the tissues between the orbital implant and the prosthesis, as both are solid objects. It is necessary to evaluate the socket tissues to ensure there is no evidence that any tissue is under increased stress and there is no breakdown of the tissues. Any breakdown of the anterior tissues of the socket should be promptly evaluated and reported to the ophthalmologist to avoid exposure or extrusion of the orbital implant. Timely communication between the ocularist and ophthalmic surgeon is of utmost importance.

The soft tissues within the orbit are in constantly undergoing anatomical changes. The accumulation of tiny changes over years can create major shifting, especially after surgery, sickness, pregnancy, trauma, or loss or gain of weight. At the same time, the prosthesis still has the same posterior and anterior surfaces, but the prosthesis material has deteriorated over time. Therefore, about every 5 years, a new custom-made prosthesis (CMP) or custom-made scleral shell (CMSS) is made to replace the deteriorated artificial eye and to design a new shape and size to accommodate the anatomical socket changes.

Unique professionals (ocularists) with an emphasis on caring and beauty combine the perfect balance of science, art, imagination, and superior application to create pieces of art that can dramatically improve the quality of their patients' lives.

Patients spend a significant amount of time with the ocularist due to the essential and crucial time requirements for making the prosthesis from the primary evaluation, impression process, design, coloring, fitting, and evaluation after fitting stage. During that time, careful attention is directed to ease the patient's worry and anxiety.

Using compression and molding technique, and after the second half of the mold is completed, it is sealed using at least two layers of liquid separator on the positive side of the mold from both inside and outside. One then waits for the second layer to dry. Next the iris is placed inside the first half mold, mixed with methyl methacrylate to an "early snappy consistency," and packed inside the mold which is then put inside a press, and the pressure is increased slowly every few minutes. The maximum amount of pressure is applied for approximately 15–20 minutes. The next step is curing as described in the Section on Curing. Regular polishing will be alright at this stage as the prosthesis will be placed back in the mold for clear PMMA capping.

Faulty Design of a Prosthesis

Figure 24.1 shows faulty designs of ocular prosthesis with stretching and overwhelming the eyelids and not allowing them to function, leading to deformity.

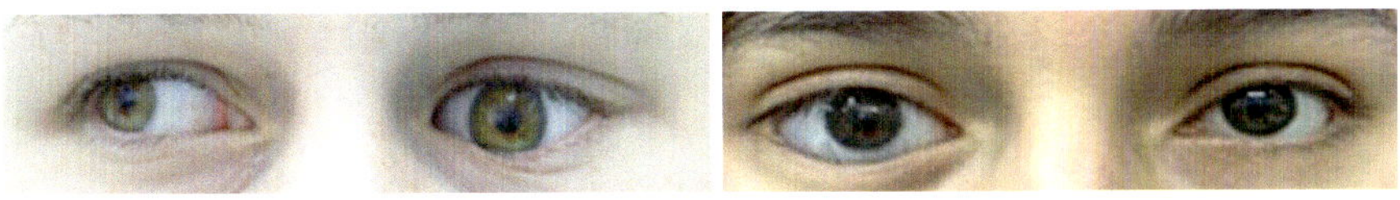

Fig. 24.1 Faulty designs of ocular prosthesis stretching and overwhelming the eyelids and not allowing them to function, leading to deformity

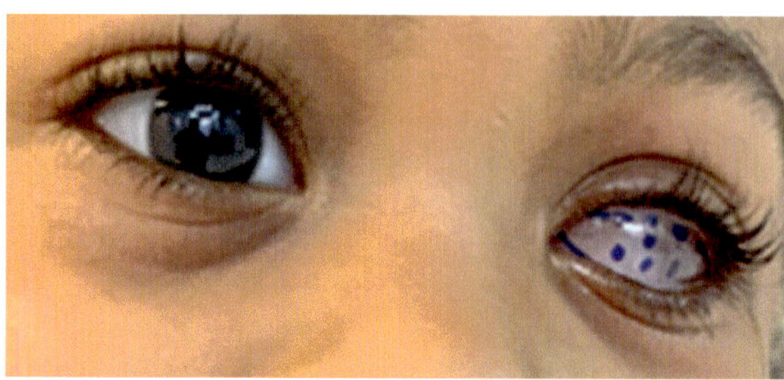

Figs. 24.2 During the design stage

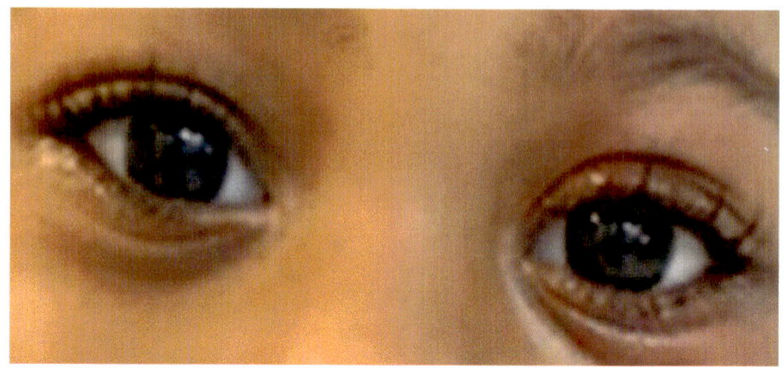

Fig. 24.3 After fitting

Figures 24.2 and 24.3 show ocular prostheses during the design stage and after fitting.

Coloring to Match

After the prosthesis has been cured, the iris is ground down to expose the iris color clear dome. The polished prosthesis with the exposed iris is tried in the patient's socket to check the design and adjust the shape, thickness, and the size of the iris. This is a very important stage that requires the artist to duplicate and simulate the normal eye. Next one adjusts the parameters of the iris 360° and partially tilts the iris upward or downward to achieve symmetry in the curvature and protrusion in comparison to the normal eye. If symmetry can't be achieved, coloring is used to create illusional symmetry, especially in those patients with eyelid deformities.

Coloring is performed while the patient is in the office until a satisfactory result is reached in tone, tent, and texture. In addition, photographs are utilized for studying precise magnified details using a macro lens to capture the iris color in different lighting conditions.

The more layers of color added to the iris, the more lifelike it becomes, adding depth and creating reflection and absorption of light like that seen in natural eyes. A light iris requires between 60 and 100 layers of color using color strokes differing in size and shape, starting from the center of the iris (collarette area) toward the stroma and limbus. Also, it is necessary to add the coloring of the sclera and simulation for veining (using special threads) and tenting.

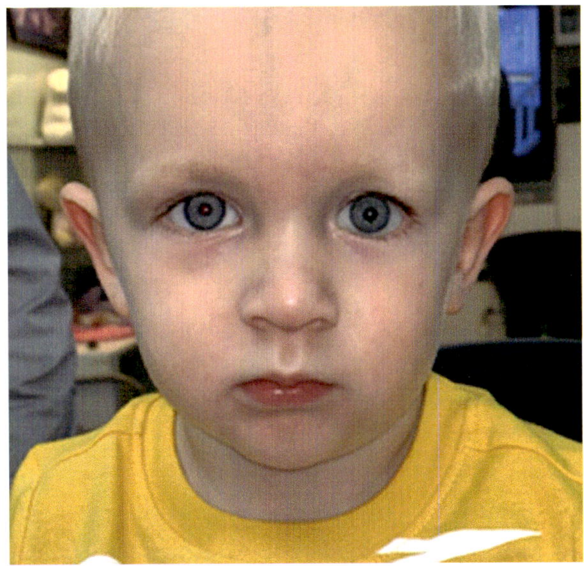

Fig. 24.4 Excellent design, cosmesis, and function of left ocular prosthesis

The mold then is treated with multiple layers of a clear separating agent added to both the front and back. After coloring the artificial eye is completed, the prosthesis can dry using multiple drying techniques. After the drying stage, the prosthesis goes through two different temperature settings to add a crystal-clear layer of methyl methacrylate to protect the color and to create the cornea and conjunctiva of the future prosthesis.

Figure 24.4 shows excellent design, cosmesis, and function.

Curing Method

1. Start with cold water, set to a temperature of 163° F to create a water bath for over night curing, and maximize the pressure before transferring into the next stage.
2. Then place the Press in boiling temperature (water bath) for 1 hour, maximizing the pressure before transferring into the next stage.
3. Immediately after adjusting the pressure to maximum, place the press under low pressure for 20 minutes (pressure cooker).
4. Cool the artificial eye in the cooker until safe to open, and take the Press out to cool at room temperature. No bubbles should be seen within the scleral mass or the clear mass of the prosthesis.
5. Grinding, polishing, fine polishing until optical standard reached, and glazing.

The surface of the prosthesis should be clear of any tool marks, rough edges, and scratches. In short, it is impeccably finished.

Fitting the Prosthesis

The "mission accomplished" stage is reached when the prosthesis is ready to be fitted in the socket, evaluated, adjusted, and readjusted as needed until the best cosmesis is achieved with absolute comfort and balanced function.

This stage is a very methodical stage, and care should be applied to any minor adjustment, followed by evaluation and fine tuning using an extremely high standard of polishing again before delivery. Our "museum" is the beautiful human face, and I feel proud each time I can help relieve a patient's concerns no matter what if possible.

Evaluation after Fitting

Evaluating the fitting after the patient wears the prosthesis for few days to a week gives a critical understanding of the level of patient satisfaction, comfort, cosmesis, and eyelid position and the necessity of any needed adjustments.

To Remove or Not to Remove the Prosthesis

In general, everyone has different needs. If the patient cleans the prosthesis 2–3 times daily with a saline solution by opening the upper eyelid and rinsing, then applying 1–2 drops of lubricant under the upper eyelid (author prefers heavy mineral oil). This should provide enough lubrication to last all day. Removing the prosthesis disturbs the socket tissues and may cause infections. Additionally, pulling on the eyelids frequently is not beneficial, especially if the patient touches and wipes their eyes. At night, a lubricating eye ointment may be helpful to prevent dryness.

Always remind the patient: Lubrication, lubrication, lubrication!

Photography in Evaluation of Treatment in Congenital Anophthalmia and Microphthalmia

Photography is a unique tool to freeze and capture the exact starting point in evaluating, diagnosing, and documenting each patient using a macro lens. Macro lenses are the best option. However, even the new high-resolution smartphone cameras will suffice. Because photography plays an important role, especially in setting a standard for evaluating the protrusion progress in cases of congenital anophthalmia (CA) and congenital microphthalmia (CM) and to differentiate the severity of each case, having a photographic device is critical as the pictures below demonstrate (Figs. 24.5, 24.6, 24.7, and 24.8).

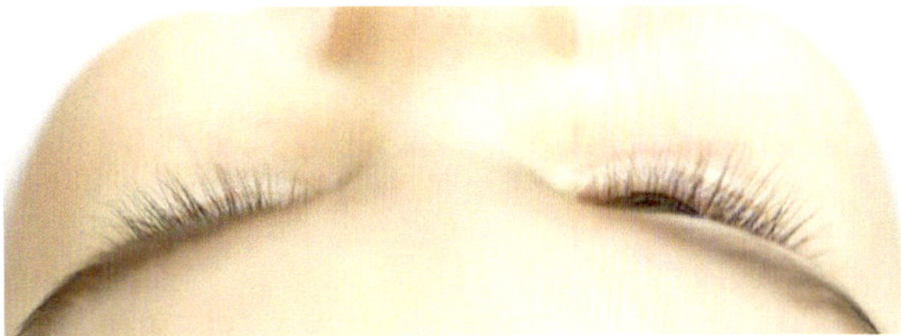

Fig. 24.5 Mild CM, notice depression and difference in protrusion of the left eye versus the normal right eye

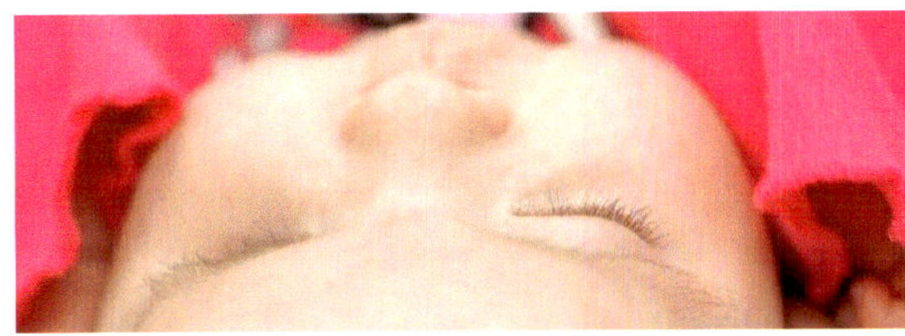

Fig. 24.6 Severe CM left eye with more noticeable difference between the protrusions of the eyes

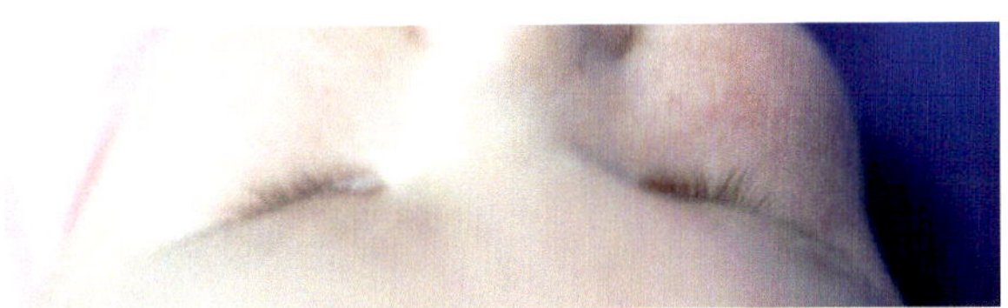

Fig. 24.7 Severe bilateral CA, notice the depressed orbits and the bone hypoplasia, age 3 months

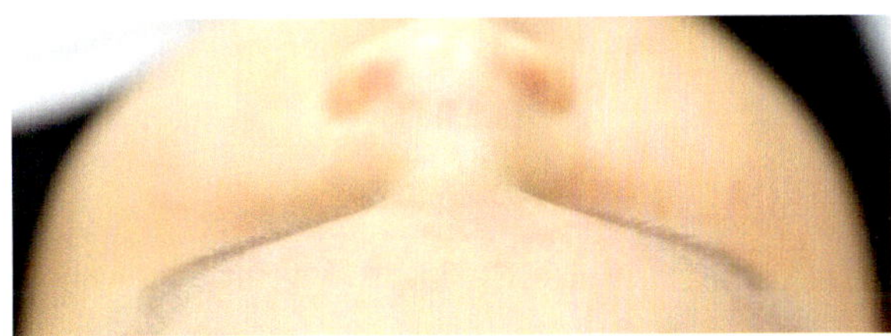

Fig. 24.8 Same patient as Fig. 24.7 but after 18 months with no expansion. Notice the changes including orbits that are more depressed and bony hypoplasia, age 21 months

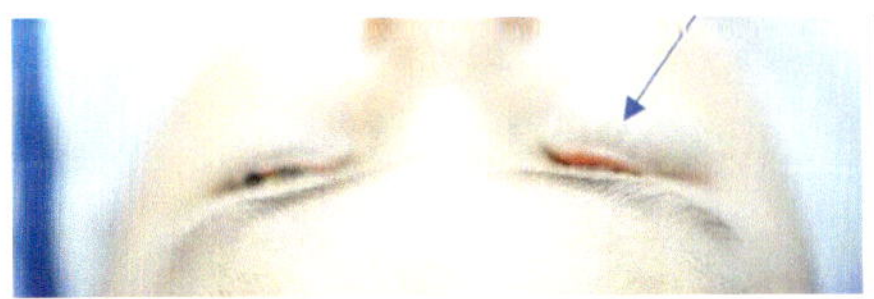

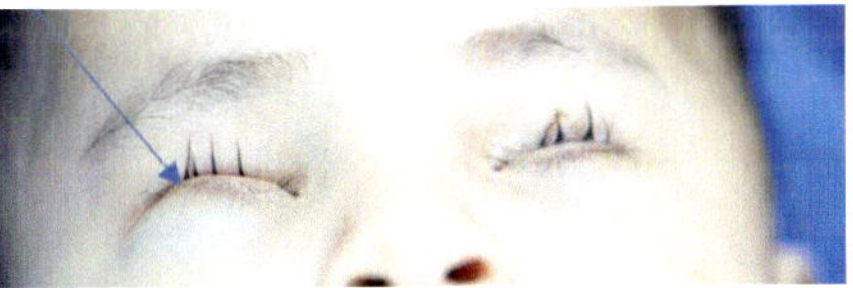

Fig. 24.9 Bilateral CM with cyst OD

In capturing the moment using all angles as a reference, one can appreciate the changes in cases of CA and CM (looking from the top of the head downward toward the bridge of the nose (mid face) that intersects the medial canthus). One can appreciate and compare the protrusion of the eyelids and the development of the face. High-resolution photographs allow one to study the images and compare them during and after the expansion process. The following pictures capture the patient before, during, and after expansion (Figs. 24.9, 24.10, 24.11, 24.12, 24.13, and 24.14).

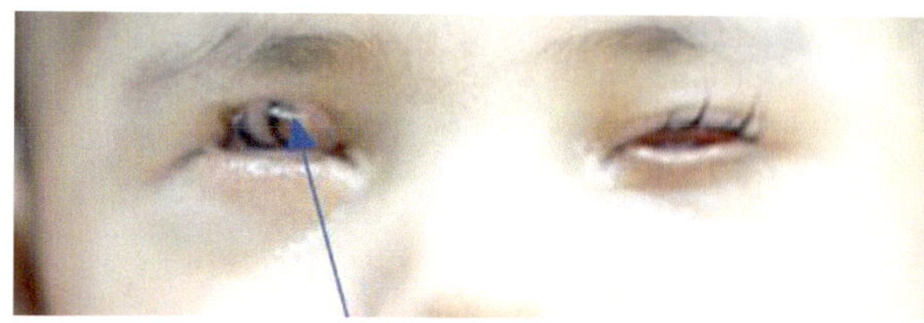

Fig. 24.10 Initial conformer, notice OD conformer tilting upward due to the cyst

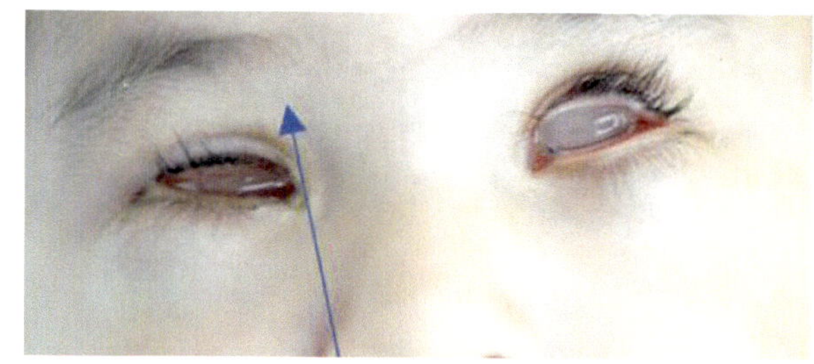

Fig. 24.11 Notice the lid position after a design-to-function conformer is fitted and changed weekly. This result took 2 months to achieve

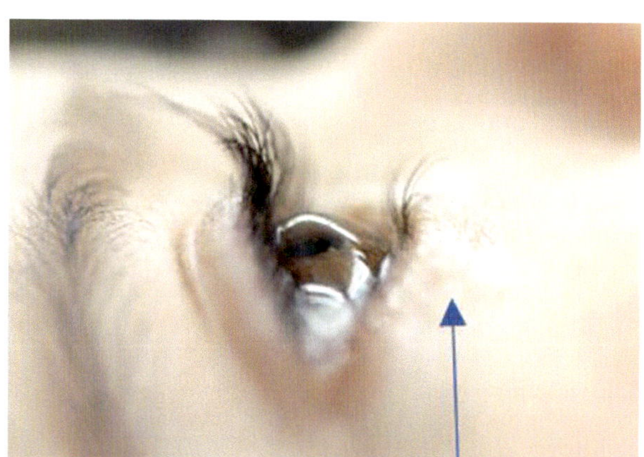

Fig. 24.12 Custom-made scleral shell in place in right socket; notice the disappearance of the cyst

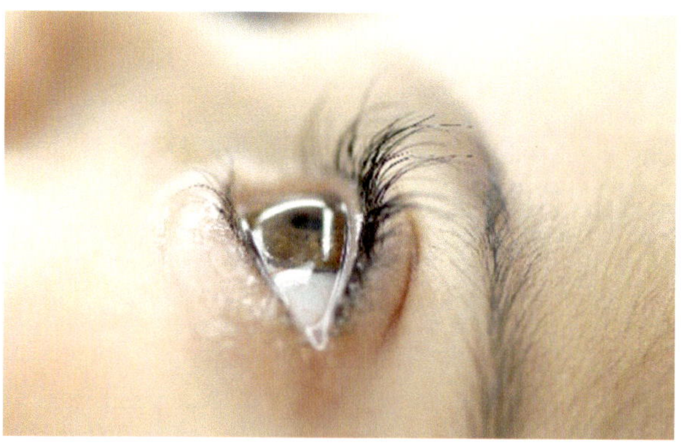

Fig. 24.13 Custom-made scleral shell in place left socket. Notice the eyelid fold. This technique achieved normal functioning of the eyelid

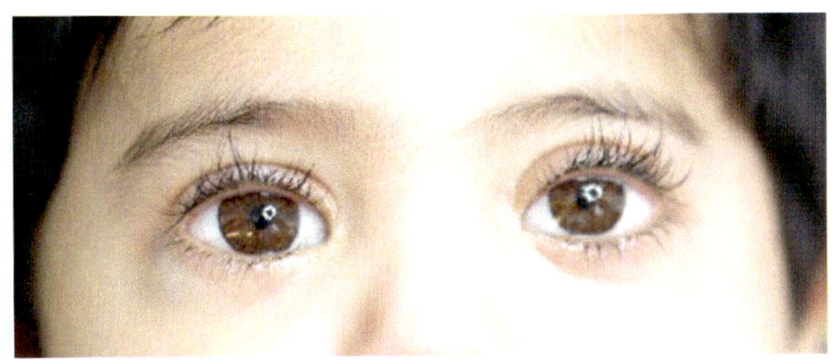

Fig. 24.14 Same patient after fitting custom-made scleral shell

Index

T. E. Johnson (ed.), *Anophthalmia*,
https://doi.org/10.1007/978-3-030-29753-4

P

T

U

V

W

GPSR Compliance

The European Union's (EU) General Product Safety Regulation (GPSR) is a set of rules that requires consumer products to be safe and our obligations to ensure this.

If you have any concerns about our products, you can contact us on ProductSafety@springernature.com

In case Publisher is established outside the EU, the EU authorized representative is:

Springer Nature Customer Service Center GmbH
Europaplatz 3
69115 Heidelberg, Germany

Batch number: 10372213

Printed by Printforce, the Netherlands